THE INTERNET
AND HEALTH CARE

Theory, Research, and Practice

LEA'S COMMUNICATION SERIES
Jennings Bryant/Dolf Zillmann, General Editors

For a complete list of LEA titles, please contact Lawrence Erlbaum Associates, Publishers, at www.erlbaum.com.

THE INTERNET AND HEALTH CARE

Theory, Research, and Practice

Edited by

Monica Murero
Ronald E. Rice

LEA

LAWRENCE ERLBAUM ASSOCIATES, PUBLISHERS

2006   Mahwah, New Jersey   London

Lawrence Erlbaum Associates, Inc., Publishers
10 Industrial Avenue
Mahwah, New Jersey 07430
www.erlbaum.com

Cover design by Tomai Maridou

**CIP information for this book can be obtained by contacting
the Library of Congress**

ISBN 0-8058-5814-8 (cloth : alk. paper)
ISBN 0-8058-5815 6 (pbk. : alk. paper)

Books published by Lawrence Erlbaum Associates are printed on acid-free paper,
and their bindings are chosen for strength and durability.

Printed in the United States of America
10 9 8 7 6 5 4 3 2 1

To Monica's parents—Ezio and Mariú

To Ron's nieces and nephews—Adam, Kendall, Kristen, Matthew, and Zachary

Contents

List of Tables and Figures

LIST OF TABLES

LIST OF FIGURES

Foreword: E-Health Benefits and Risks

Saulo Sirigatti
University of Florence

Health care provision requires rapid and reliable decision-making processes, due to the plethora of responsibilities involved in patient diagnosis, treatment, and eventual follow-up. The decision-making process has a central relevance in daily medical practice. In recent decades, the need to study the processes underneath the formation of medical decision making has become a central issue in health care. Wide variance of medical diagnosis and treatment of the same symptoms or pathology, and the consequent lack of homogeneity in outcomes and costs, are amply reported in literature. Medical doctors often refer to their own experience in the processes of interpreting clinical information, diagnosis, and the choice of treatments. The "traditional" medical approach allows for patients receiving different diagnosis and treatments from doctors who have different etiopathogenetic orientations and different clinical experiences. Conversely, there is a consistent disequilibrium between scarcity of resources and increasing demand and costs of health care in the international context. As a consequence, health care institutions are pressed to develop scientifically based and reproducible strategies ensuring homogeneous level of assistance in medical prevention, diagnosis, therapy, and rehabilitation.

In the last decades, the limits of medical clinical practice based on personal professional experience have facilitated the development of the "evidence-based medicine" approach. According to this praxis, diagnosis and therapeutic decisions are strictly based on the most recent evidence from medical research, with the aim of reducing unjustified variance in diagnosis and treatment. Evidence includes scientific publications, conferences, and continuing medical education.

In this context, medical informatics presents a wide array of resources to health care providers to improve many aspects of their professional activity. Central to this issue, the Internet can be considered as a valuable instrument in supporting evidence-based medicine and improving health care services, by facilitating efficient, rapid, and convenient access to continuing medical education. Moreover, e-health could well become a major element in facilitating the diffusion of scientific knowledge, new methods of assistance and cures, and the promotion of effective policy for the development of sanitary systems in the international context. In this respect, e-health could help reduce the disparities between developed and developing countries in access to health care and medical education.

In developing countries, medical professionals are usually alone in their practice, having to deal with complex clinical conditions and with little or no access to specialist consults. These situations exist not only in developing countries, but also in Western societies, where large discrepancies in health care provision may exist between urban and rural areas, within the same nation.

Medical informatics allows for wider availability of resources and scientific knowledge, and represents a great opportunity for medical education and evidence-based clinical practice, especially for health care providers living in isolated and marginal communities. In addition, e-health can provide new opportunities for fast networking among hospitals and health care institutions within the same nation—or even at the international levels—by offering unprecedented opportunities to harmonize and homogenize diagnostic and therapeutic processes, while promoting citizens' well-being.

In the health care field, the diffusion of electronic services has facilitated access to medical information by "health seekers." The continuous diffusion and availability of the Web represents a huge potential for citizens to participate and collaborate with medical personnel, health institutions, and pharmaceutical companies. Research in this book shows that more and more people, though primarily those who live in Western countries, are not only aware of the potential benefits offered by the Internet, but they actually often use the new sources of information and increase their contact with health care providers.

In the majority of cases, online health information users appear to deal with the need to know more about some aspects of specific pathologies, to look for non-urgent consultations, and gain access to lab test results. The percentage of users who go online to find information not directly related to specific pathologies should not be ignored; in fact, a niche of

Internet users appears to be interested in discovering issues and aspects directly related to the broader field of illness prevention and health promotion. Freedom in accessing unlimited resources, quick retrieval of information, and low cost of the service are all crucial factors in the diffusion of e-health among users.

Although the Internet can offer great opportunities to online users, research (as in this book) has been investigating the risks connected with Internet-based health information. The most evident threats appear to be the lack of control over online content, low reliability, and poor validity of medical information. Freedom of access by users, on the one hand, and free publication of online material, on the other, represent fundamental characteristics of Internet resources, and major strengths in the diffusion of e-health. However, they also hide a possible risk of disseminating and applying inappropriate and erroneous information. To all these risks, we should add the phenomenon of online consultations, including drug prescriptions, without any in-depth patient clinical exam, often at best based purely on online questionnaires.

In recent years the Web can provide patients in-depth information about diseases, and work as a medical consultant offering clinical information; until then, this information was purely the prerogative of the medical doctor. We are witnessing the encounter between medical knowledge—so far subject to the approval of a restricted scientific community—and a new behavior of the patients, who are more aware and informed about their conditions, are acquiring a more central role in the treatment process, and are less likely to play a passive and dependent role in the relationship with their medical practitioner. Both the patient–doctor communication and decision-making processes may be seriously affected. On the basis of superficial, erroneous, or misunderstood information, e-patients may negatively influence the efficacy of therapeutic cure by requesting inappropriate medications or incorrect therapeutic patterns. Sometimes, the medical doctor tries to comply with the patient's requests, knowing that his or her satisfaction may dictate the outcome of treatment and the maintenance of a good professional relationship. In other instances the doctor sees the diffusion of e-patients as a potential erosion of the traditional physician's role, an occasion for possible conflicts, and an increase in workload and time to dedicate to patients that is not always repaid by economic benefits. On the other hand, many foresee in this situation a new type of informed interlocutor who actively contributes to the decision-making process about his or her health care options, evaluates risks and benefits, identifies subjective preferences, overtakes uncertainties, and schedules treatments.

The increasing tendency towards a self-regulated health care from citizens, and the inappropriate publication of information on the Web, suggest the necessity for developing means for "guiding" the user's navigation of the Internet. Unregulated and free publication of online content suggests the necessity to develop new tools to improve users' skills when dealing with large quantities of online information. At the same time, the adoption of standards and ethical codes of conduct for online content providers should allow users to assess the quality of online information.

In 2000 the e-Health Ethics Summit has responded to this major issue by developing and adopting the *eHealth Code of Ethics* whose aim is to offer to the publishers of health care content some criteria for auto-evaluation of Web sites. Among the main principles, we identify candor, honesty, quality, privacy, professionalism, accountability, and responsible partnership. The adoption of the code should guarantee to any online user access to reliable and valuable information and products—in some cases—with full respect of one's privacy and in accordance with commercial and professional best practices.

The most important and contemporary issues, briefly summarized in this foreword, are covered in this book with the competence that distinguishes the authors, following the most updated theoretical and practical perspectives that respect, at the same time, the expectations of the different readers: doctors, patients, web masters, researchers, students, and service providers. The design and development of the various contributions allow the reader to deeply understand and thoroughly evaluate the complexity of contemporary world of e-health, and trace an essential picture about future scenarios, that refer not only to the North American context but also to more widely international settings.

Foreword:
E-Health Research

Lee Rainie

Although it was written about 2,400 years ago, the basic spirit of the Hippocratic Oath still stands as a summary of the attitude of many in the medical establishment about the act of sharing medical information with patients.

> I will pay the same respect to my master in the Science as to my parents and share my life with him and pay all my debts to him. I will regard his sons as my brothers and teach them the Science, if they desire to learn it, without fee or contract. I will hand on precepts, lectures and all other learning to my sons, to those of my master and to those pupils duly apprenticed and sworn, *and to none other*. [emphasis added]

The inference is clear: Well-trained, appropriately pedigreed teachers should be gatekeepers of information that people without proper training could not always be trusted to act on in a fitting way. Doctors know best, in other words.

Although there is much to admire in the ethics embraced by Hippocrates and his successors, their notions about information sharing are not in tune with 21st-century patients. Many have moved dramatically away from the passive posture of their forebears and become emboldened partners in information gathering and decision making when it comes to their care. Rather than being "patients" who submit to the acts deemed suitable by their credentialed caregivers, they are active medical "end users" who crave greater understanding of what is happening to them and an active role in directing what should be done about it. To these *health seekers*—a phrase that this volume helpfully codifies—clinicians can be seen as "tech support" among an array of other health resources they can access via the Internet.

The appeal of this new model of medicine is clear in every imaginable metric. The work of the Pew Internet & American Life Project shows that 79% of American adult Internet users have used the Internet to get medical information (Fox, 2005; Rice, 2006). Here are some of the things they do:

- tentatively diagnose their own diseases
- confirm their doctor's diagnosis and suggested treatments
- check their doctors' and medical facilities' credentials
- research *all* available treatment options—not just those recommended by doctor and often including alternative and experimental treatments
- give themselves a crash course on a specific medical condition when they (or a loved one) is diagnosed
- exchange information and support with other patients with the same disease
- obtain online second opinions
- shop for insurance options and investigate government benefits
- sign up for clinical trials
- seek wellness, fitness, and diet information.

It is indisputable that everything described in this volume will become more prevalent in the future as more people go online and even as current users bring the Internet into the rhythms of their lives. We already see now that new broadband users very quickly change their online behavior as they rely more greatly on the Web to provide the information, products, and services they seek. The Internet-connected computer in their home becomes a privileged information utility that they expect will yield the material they seek (Horrigan & Rainie, 2002).

Yet, for all the change that has already occurred in doctor–patient relations, in patient learning and empowerment, and in the spread of medical innovation, the story of the Internet's role in health is still unfolding. Arguably, we are in the beginning of the second stage of a process that might involve four stages. The first stage could be called the *informational stage*. The Internet is viewed by most e-health users as a vast medical library. They appreciate that they can access the most sophisticated and cutting-edge medical information at any hour of the day. For them, Dr. Google is always in and "he/she" always prints out the information that these patients want to share with their Dr. Fleshandbloods.

The second phase of e-health is the *interactive stage*. This is taking place as people begin to use e-mail to communicate with clinicians, as institutions push towards creation of electronic health records for patients, and as technology allows for greater and quicker data sharing among all the medical stakeholders. So far, only a small portion of the health-seeker population is taking advantage of these Internet-enabled transactions, but, over time, they are likely to become commonplace (Katz, Rice, & Acord, 2004).

The third phase is *instrumental* and it seems to be gaining ground in some of the most advanced medical practices and institutions. Tele-diagnostic tools and instruments are on the drawing board. Some advocates believe that an age of "information therapy" will arrive soon in several senses of the phrase: therapy in the sense that doctors and patients will recognize that the sharing of information is an essential part of their interactions; therapy in the sense that doctors will "prescribe" information as part of their treatment (and be compensated directly for that dimension of their work); and therapy in the sense that people will use home-based devices automatically to pass along important information to their doctors about their conditions such as blood pressure and blood sugar levels without office visits.

The fourth and final step is the *interventional stage*, where actual medical treatment occurs online. Telesurgery and other remote practices would be part of this final stage. It is not hard to imagine psychiatric sessions taking place in immersive virtual environments. Similarly, there will be no technological reason not to have "visits" to a dermatologist or a radiologist in similar environments.

When fourth-stage e-health is commonplace, then Professors Murero and Rice can re-convene this global team of researchers to address the most pressing research question that has yet to be tackled: Does Internet use actually improve health outcomes and a society's overall level of health? We know from several of the authors here that at this early stage of the evolution of e-health, fruitful Internet searches, Internet-based interventions, and physician–patient interactions informed by Internet results, can improve patients' sense of well-being and their sense of control over their lives. That is a good start and, no doubt, the number of scholars preparing to contribute to the second edition of *The Internet and Health Care* is growing all the time.

REFERENCES

Fox, S. (2005). *Health information online*. Pew Internet & American Life Project research. Retrieved May 17, 2005, from http://www.pewinternet.org/PPF/r/156/report_display.asp

Horrigan, J., & Rainie, L. (2002). *The broadband difference*. Pew Internet & American Life Project Research. Retrieved June 23, 2002, from http://www.pewinternet.org/pdfs/PIP_Broadband_Report.pdf

Katz, J. E., Rice, R. E., & Acord, S. (2004). E-health networks and social transformations: Expectations of centralization, experiences of decentralization. In M. Castells (Ed.), *The network society: A cross-cultural perspective* (pp. 293–318). London: Edward Elgar.

Rice, R. E. (2006). Influences, usage, and outcomes of Internet health information searching: Multivariate results from the Pew surveys. *International Journal of Medical Informatics, 75*(1), 8–28.

Acknowledgments

We owe our deep gratitude to all the contributors to this book. They worked diligently with us to produce an integrated publication, were open to all kinds of requests and suggestions, and provided revisions quickly. We thank G. D'Ancona, MD, who read specific chapters and gave us comments and advice; Dr. Vito Cappellini at the Center of Excellence MICC, at the University of Florence, for his collegiality; Linda Bathgate (Senior Editor, Communications) and Karin Wittig Bates (Assistant Editor) of Lawrence Erlbaum Associates for their enthusiastic support for our book proposal; Suzanne Sheppard for the excellent production work; Daisy Lemus, graduate student at the Department of Communication, University of California, Santa Barbara, and Assistant Professor at California State University, Northridge, for reviewing the chapter formats; and Claire Johnson for tolerating Ron's long stints on his computer.

—*Monica Murero, Florence, Italy*
—*Ronald E. Rice, Santa Barbara, California*

About the Contributors

Indrajit Banerjee (MA, Jawaharlal Nehru; PhD, Sorbonne) has been a university teacher and researcher since 1994. He was a postdoctoral research fellow with the GRICIS at the University of Quebec in Montreal, Canada, and has worked at the Ottawa University, Canada, and the University Science Malaysia in Penang, Malaysia. During his stay in Malaysia, he conducted research on the Malaysian Information Infrastructure Initiative, and the Multimedia Super Corridor (MSC). Over the years, he has presented papers at a number of international and regional conferences and seminars. He has also published on various aspects of Asian communications in prestigious journals and books around the world. Dr. Banerjee joined the School in January 2001. Recently he has been awarded two large research grants for conducting media and information technology research. Dr. Banerjee is also currently the Secretary-General of the Asian Media Information and Communication Centre (AMIC), Asia's premier media research, publication, and resource center.

George A. Barnett (BA, MA, University of Illinois; PhD, Michigan State University) is Professor and Chair of the Department of Communication at the State University of New York at Buffalo. He has been editor of *Progress in Communication Sciences* and has written extensively on organizational, mass, international and intercultural, and political communication, as well as the diffusion of innovations. His current research focuses on international information flows in general, and telecommunications flows including the Internet in specific, and their role in social and economic development and globalization.

Suzanne Brunsting is a PhD student at the Amsterdam School of Communications Research ASCoR, Department of Communication, University of Amsterdam. Her project is entitled "Effective Campaign Strategies for Health Education Through Mass Media." Her research concerns developing and testing communication strategies that make the most of the advantages of mass media, to educate people about alcohol use and abuse.

Lorraine Buis (BS, MSI, Michigan State University) is a PhD student at Michigan State University in the Department of Telecommunication, Information Studies, and Media. She is also a research assistant in the MSU Health and Risk Communication Center. Her primary research interests include the study of online health communities and their impact on health outcomes, applications of new technologies in the delivery of health care, and information search and retrieval.

Walter H. Curioso (MD, Universidad Peruana Cayetano Heredia, Lima, Peru; MPH, University of Washington) is a research professor in Epidemiology, STD/HIV, and Health Informatics at the School of Public Health and Administration at Universidad Peruana Cayetano Heredia in Lima, Peru. He's also an affiliate assistant professor in the Division of Biomedical and Health Informatics in the School of Medicine at the University of Washington in Seattle, Washington. Dr. Curioso's research focus is on how to use technology to promote better health in developing countries. His latest projects involve using cell phones to collect and transmit adverse events, and using personal digital assistants to assess sexual risk and antiretroviral medication adherence among HIV patients in Lima. He has written more than 30 articles in health informatics and information technology, evidence-based medicine, public health in developing countries, and clinical medicine. He is an e-health consultant for international and private health organizations, specializing in the design and implementation of information systems and technology.

Mohan J. Dutta-Bergman (PhD, Minnesota) is an Associate Professor of Health Communication in the Department of Communication at Purdue University. He teaches graduate and undergraduate courses in Internet and Health, Social Marketing, Health Campaigns, and Culture and Health. His primary research interest is in the area of health-based new media applications. More specifically, he studies the role of motivations in new media usage, the relationship between new media and traditional media, the different functions of new media, and the uses of the new media in health-related contexts. Professor Dutta-Bergman has published more than 40 articles and delivered more than 50 conference presentations on these areas, receiving awards from the Human Communication and Technology Division of National Communication Association and the Health Communication Division of the Central States Communication Association. His work has appeared in outlets such as *American Behavioral Scientist, Communication Monographs, Health Communication, Health Marketing Quarterly, Journal of Communication, Journal of Consumer Psychology, Journal of Medical Internet Research, New Media and Society, Social Marketing Quarterly*, and so on. Professional experience includes research and strategic work in the advertising, health care, and interactive multimedia industries.

Laura J. Gurak (PhD, Rensselaer Polytechnic Institute) is Professor and department head in the Rhetoric Department at the University of Minnesota, where she also directs the University's Internet Studies Center. She is an internationally recognized researcher with publications including *Persuasion and Privacy in Cyberspace* (1997) and *Cyberliteracy* (2001). She has served as co-principal investigator on two federally funded grants in the University's Medical School, studying the use of the Internet for public health research and intervention.

Lorna Heaton (PhD, University of Montreal) is an Assistant Professor in the Department of Communication, University of Montreal. She is a member of the Interdisciplinary Centre for Emerging Technologies (Centre interdisciplinaire sur les technologies Émergentes CITÉ) and Co-director of the University of Montreal's Laboratory on the Design and Uses of New Technologies (LUDTIC). Her current research centers on the social aspects of the design of computer systems, as well as the integration of technologies in organizations. She has conducted research in the following areas: technology transfer, interface design, crosscultural computing and the evaluation and use of telehealth in various contexts. Other research interests include the adaptability of new media in various work and home contexts.

Brenda Hudson (MS, Boston University) is a PhD student at the University of Minnesota's Department of Rhetoric, where her research interests include the use of the Internet for international HIV/AIDS education and intervention. In addition, she is a science writer for the university's Academic Health Center, covering such topics as stem cell research, cancer, and medical education.

Jennie M. Hwang (MA, Michigan State University) is a PhD student at the Department of Communication, School of Informatics at University at Buffalo (SUNY). Her research interests include media effects, Internet use and information literacy, organizational and international communication.

Ulrika Josefsson (BSc, MSc) is a PhD student in Informatics at the Department of Informatics at Göteborg University in Göteborg, Sweden. Her doctoral research project focuses on how patients use the Internet to cope with illness and how this can contribute to design of emergent forms of Internet use in the relationship between patients and doctors/health care providers.

James E. Katz (PhD, Rutgers University) is Professor of Communication at Rutgers, The State University of New Jersey. Currently he is investigating how personal communication technologies, such as mobile phones and the Internet, affect social relationships and how cultural values influence usage patterns of these technologies. He is also heading a major research project aimed at understanding the normative dimensions of human rights as they influence tobacco control policy. Professor Katz has had a distinguished career researching the relationship among the domains of science and technology, knowledge and information, and social processes and public policy. His books include *Perpetual Contact: Mobile Communication*, *Private Talk and Public Performance* (coedited with Mark Aakhus), *Connections: Social and Cultural Studies of the Telephone in American Life*, *Social Consequences of Internet Use: Access, Involvement, Expression* (co-authored with Ronald E. Rice), and *Internet and Health Communication* (co-edited with Ronald E. Rice).

Gerald Kral (PhD, University of Vienna) has conducted various researches in the areas of clinical psychology, psychotherapy, as well as psychology and clinical implications of Internet use. For his research about online-communities he was awarded the Gesundheitspreis der Stadt Wien in 2002. He is head of the Task Force of the Austrian Psychologists Professional Association in the area of online therapy and is Editor-in-Chief of the journal Psychologie in Österreich.

Helmut Krcmar (PhD, Saarbruecken University) holds the Chair for Information Systems, Technische Universitaet Muenchen, Munich, Germany. Prior to this he worked as Postdoctoral Fellow at the IBM Los Angeles Scientific Center, as Assistant Professor of Information Systems at the Leonard Stern School of Business, NYU, and at Baruch College, CUNY. From 1987 to 2002 he was Chair for Information Systems, Hohenheim University, Stuttgart, Germany. During 2000–2002 he served as Dean, Faculty of Business, Economics and Social Sciences. His research interests include Information and Knowledge Management, and CSCW.

Waipeng Lee (MA, University of Texas; PhD, University of Wisconsin) is an Associate Professor at the School of Communication and Information, Nanyang Technological University. Her research interests include public opinion, persuasion, and the Internet and society. She is a member of the Singapore Internet Project and Singapore Internet Research Centre. She has studied Internet usage patterns, e-health, e-government, and e-religion.

Jan Marco Leimeister (MSc, PhD, Hohenheim University) is a Senior Researcher and Assistant Professor at the Chair for Information Systems, Technische Universitaet Muenchen, Munich, Germany. He manages the research project COSMOS (Community Online Services and Mobile Solutions), funded by the German Ministry for Research and Education. He worked on different occasions for companies such as DaimlerChrysler, IBM, and Siemens Business Services. His teaching and research areas include online communities, ubiquitous and mobile computing, computer-supported collaborative work, and information management.

Cecilia Hsi-Shi Leong (MA, University Science Malaysia) is currently pursuing her PhD at the Nanyang Technological University, Singapore. Her doctoral dissertation is on the role and impact of information communication technology (ICT) on public health care in Singapore. Her other research interests include the impact of ICT on human development, and the role of gender stereotypes in the media. She has 6 years of experience working in the media industry, including 5 years as a current affairs television producer.

Monica Murero (Laurea, cum laude, Iulm University of Milan; University degrees, Iulm, Italy; PhD, State University of New York, Buffalo) is a Professor in Communication and Media Integration at the Center of Excellence for Media Integration and Communication, at the University of Florence in Italy. She is the Director of the E-Life International Institute. Professor Murero consults throughout Europe, including the European Commission. Since 2003, she is appointed in the Board of the International Association of Internet Researchers (www.aoir.org). Professor Murero has received several international awards and grants as outstanding researcher, teacher, and student from European and U.S. universities, where she worked for several years. In 2004, she was awarded the most prestigious prize for academic scientists working abroad, the "Rientro Cervelli" grant (literally: "bring back home the brains"). Since then, she came back to Italy and joined the University of Florence. Professor Murero's research interests revolve around the intersections among new technologies, new media, individual and social change. In particular, she is interested in the interdisciplinary field of Internet research and media integration, the effects of innovation on human behavior, and its steady encroachment into crucial aspects of everyday life, like health care. She has taught courses in new media and multimedia, communication and culture, sociology of consumption, and Internet Research, in the United States and in Europe. Monica Murero has pioneered interdisciplinary studies in collaboration with medical doctors. Her work has appeared in several research funded reports, the *Encyclopedia of Community*, international journals (*Journal of Medical Internet Research*, *Cardiac Surgery Forum*, *Journal of Pediatric Surgery*, etc.), roundtables, and television programs. She coedited the first *International Annual of the Association of Internet Researchers* (2004). In 1998 Monica Murero started building the E-Life International Network of Excellence in Research, a not-for-profit organization whose purpose is to research, support, study, teach, and analyze the diverse and dynamic elements of the mutual impact of Internet and new media on everyday life and social change. Moreover, in 2002 she founded with Susannah Fox (Pew Internet) the International Network of Excellence in E-Health Research (INEHR), while chairing the third worldwide conference of the Association of Internet Researchers in Maastricht (NL).

Bas van den Putte (MS, Communication Science; MS, Political Science; PhD, Psychology, all University of Amsterdam) is Senior Associate Professor at the Amsterdam School of Communications Research ASCoR, Department of Communication, University of Amsterdam. His research interests include the evaluation of mass communicated campaigns and the effects of communication strategies in commercial communication and public health communication.

Ronald E. Rice (PhD, Stanford University) is Arthur N. Rupe Professor of the Social Effects of Mass Communication in the Department of Communication, and Co-Director of the Center for Film, Television, and New Media at University of California, Santa Barbara. He has co-authored or co-edited *Media Ownership: Research and Regulation* (2006); *Social Consequences of Internet Use: Access, Involvement and Interaction* (2002); *The Internet and Health Communication* (2001); *Accessing and Browsing Information and Communication* (2001); *Public Communication Campaigns* (1st ed.: 1981; 2nd ed.: 1989; 3rd ed.: 2001); *Research Methods and the New Media* (1988); *Managing Organizational Innovation* (1987); and *The New Media: Communication, Research and Technology* (1984). He has conducted research and published widely in communication science, public communication campaigns, computer-mediated communication systems, methodology, organizational and management theory, information systems, information science and bibliometrics, social uses and effects of the Internet, and social networks. His publications have won awards as best dissertation from the American Society for Information Science and Technology, best paper from International Communication Association divisions (six awards), and best paper from Academy of Management divisions (two awards). Dr. Rice has been elected divisional officer in both the International Communication Association and the Academy of Management, elected President of the ICA (2006–2007), awarded a Fulbright Award to Finland (2006), and has served as Associate Editor for *Human Communication Research*, and for *MIS Quarterly*. He is on the editorial board of *Communication Monographs*, *Communication Studies Journal*, the *Journal of the American Society for Information Science and Technology*, the online *Journal of Computer-Mediated Communication*, *Communication Theory*, *Human Communication Research*, *New Media and Society*, and *Journal of Management Information Systems*.

Lee Rainie (Graduate, Harvard College; MA, political science from Long Island University) is the Director of the Pew Internet & American Life Project. Since December 1999, the Washington, DC research center has examined how people's Internet use affects their families, communities, health care, education, civic and political life, and workplaces. The Project has issued more than 120 reports based on its surveys that monitor people's online activities and the Internet's role in their lives. All of its reports and datasets are available online for free at http://www.pewinternet .org. Prior to launching the Pew Internet Project, Rainie was managing editor of *U.S. News & World Report*.

Joshua Seidman (BA, Brown University; PhD, MHS, Johns Hopkins School of Public Health) has been on a quest for more than 15 years to improve health care quality—first by influencing health plans and provider behavior, then shifting to a grass-roots approach by activating consumers. In October 2001, Dr. Seidman saw the fusion of these two strategies in information therapy (Ix®)—the prescription of the right information to the right person at the right time to help people make better health decisions. Dr. Seidman is President of the Center for Information Therapy, a not-for-profit organization in Washington, DC, dedicated to advancing Ix practice and science. Before joining the IxCenter, Dr. Seidman served as senior editor and director of quality initiatives for the Advisory Board Company's consumer health initiative. He previously worked there as a researcher and consultant. Dr. Seidman also worked for NCQA as the director of measure development at the American College of Cardiology as assistant director of private sector relations.

Saulo Sirigatti (Graduate, University of Florence; MA, Psychology at Fordham University, PhD in Psychology at the New School for Social Research; honorary Doctorate, State University of Gomel, By) is full professor of Clinical Psychology, Coordinator of the health psychology section, Dean of the Faculty of Psychology of the University of Florence; was President of The XIII Conference of the European Health Psychology Society; is member of the board of the journal *Psicologia della Salute*. Member of some editorial boards: Bollettino di Psicologia Applicata, Scienze dell'interazione, Risorse Uomo, Psicoterapia Cognitiva e Comportamentale, Acta Comportamentalia. Member of several scientific and cultural societies: Accademia dei Fisiocritici, European Health Psychology Society, Associazione Italiana Fulbright, Associazione Italiana di Psicologia, Società Italiana di Terapia Comportamentale e Cognitiva, Ordine Italiano degli Psicologi (elenco Psicoterapeuti), American Psychological Association. Since the 60s he's carried out researches and studies concerning psychosomatics, evaluation of the efficacy and efficiency of socio-medical services, psychological assessment and psychodiagnostics. Later on, he studied stress in adolescents and adults, and burnout in helping professionals, from the point of view of sintomatology and genesis, with regard, also, to coping and prevention. Wrote reviews on psychotherapy efficacy, and studied psychotherapy processes. Recently, other fields of research are represented by quality of life in oncology, and psychological aspects of secondary prevention.

Charles Steinfield (MA, PhD, University of Southern California) is a professor of telecommunication, information studies, and media at Michigan State University, where he is the recipient of MSU's Teacher-Scholar and Distinguished Faculty awards. He conducts research on the applications of emerging communication and information technologies for individuals, groups and organizations. He has received several National Science Foundation research grants, worked in applied research at Bellcore, and was a senior Fulbright Scholar to France. He has been a visiting professor at several European universities and institutes, including the Institut National des Télécommunications and France Telecom Research and Development (formerly CNET), Delft University of Technology and the Telematica Instituut, Helsinki School of Economics and Business Administration, and Roskilde University. He has authored or edited five books, in additional to numerous journal articles and book chapters.

Sarah Stewart is a senior lecturer in midwifery at Otago Polytechnic, Dunedin, New Zealand, and practicing midwife. Sarah is also a PhD student enrolled at the Centre for Online Health, University of Queensland, Brisbane, Australia. Her research is focused on developing and evaluating an online mentoring system for midwives (see her Web site: www .midwife.net.nz).

Evelyn Tang (MA, Nanyang Technological University) is Senior Executive at NetCare Internet Services, a public health organization in Singapore, and works with the information technology division. She is responsible for developing and implementing communications activities of the division. The activities include managing a network-wide web portal that offers e-health services to facilitate physical transactions that patients and staff have with the organization. Evelyn was involved in the revamp of a national Web site that is designed for interaction between the public and government agencies. She also has experience in the print medium, as editor for trade publications and as a freelance writer for lifestyle magazines.

Kier Wallis graduated from the University of California, Santa Barbara, with BAs in Communication and in Law and Society, and a minor in Spanish. Kier is a member of UCSB's College Honors Program, the National Honors Society, and Lambda Pi Eta. Her chapter is part of a Senior Honors Thesis, which allowed her to graduate with distinction in the major. Her research interests include communication and technology, mass communication, and media policy.

Pamela Whitten (MA, University of Kentucky; PhD, University of Kansas) is a professor of communication and a senior research fellow of the Regenstrief Center at Purdue University. Professor Whitten's research focuses on the use of technology in health care with a specific interest in telehealth and its impact on the delivery of health care services and education. She places emphases on social reengineering issues in health organizations deploying communication technologies. Prior research projects range from telepsychiatry to telehospice and telehome care for COPD and CHF patients, as well as the creation of health Web sites for low literate adults. Prior to joining Purdue in 2005, she served on the faculty at Michigan State University for 7 years. She graduated magna cum laude, Beta Gamma Sigma and Alpha Lambda Delta Honor Societies. She serves on the Board of Directors for the American Telemedicine Association.

I

INTRODUCTION

Chapter 1

E-Health Research

Monica Murero
University of Florence, Italy

Ronald E. Rice
University of California, Santa Barbara

MOTIVATIONS FOR THE BOOK

The popularization of the Internet (so far, primarily in developed countries) and its opportunities and challenges have already significantly influenced society. In the health care field, access to online resources and environments is having a major and controversial impact on its stakeholders, users, providers, and institutions. The book presents an in-depth introduction to the field of Internet and health care, from both international and interdisciplinary perspectives. The interdisciplinary and critical perspective combines expertise from social sciences, medicine, policy, and systems analysis. It is the expression of a new generation of e-researchers and practitioners committed to excellence in investigating a new and still little-known phenomenon.

The idea for this book originated in 2002 at the third Association of Internet Researchers (http://www.aoir.org) conference in Maastricht, when Monica Murero and Susannah Fox co-founded the International Network of Excellence in E-Health Research (INEHR). The purpose of the INEHR is to research, study, teach, support, and create diverse and dynamic elements to the impact of the Internet on the health care field. It had become evident that the new field of Internet and health care had grown and matured since the time when people relied only on the words of their family doctor when dealing with a medical threat or deciding to simply keep themselves in good health. Further, much more research and projects have been developed since that time, especially internationally. A search on Amazon.com for books since 2000, using just the two keywords "Internet" and "health," returned 46 books. Some were not relevant, whereas almost all the rest were guides to online resources, manuals on developing health-related Web sites, guides about safe Internet searching, or books for medical specialists or administrators. The two exceptions are the edited books *The Internet and Health Communication: Expectations and Experiences* (Rice & Katz, 2001) and *E-Therapy: Case Studies, Guiding Principles, and the Clinical Potential of the Internet* (Hsiung, 2002).

AUDIENCE

The book is suitable for university educators and students in the social, public health, and medical disciplines, including Internet researchers. Public health and medicine workers will find the book helpful. It is also oriented to professionals in many disciplines who might appreciate an integrative theoretical, empirical, and critical analysis of the subject matter, including developers and providers of online health information. Health care policymakers will be interested in understanding the impact of the recent diffusion of the Internet provided in this book. Methods and data used in the chapters include personal interviews, focus groups, observations, regional and national surveys, online transcript analysis, online controlled experiments, secondary data analysis, case studies, systems analysis, policy analyses, and literature reviews.

RELATED SOURCES

There are several major medical informatics associations and journals, as well as many more associations, conferences, online communities, academic and continuing education organizations, and foundations that emphasize health care, health communication, and the Internet. Examples include:

- The American Medical Informatics Association (http://www.amia.org)
- The Association of Internet Researchers (http://www.aoir.org)
- The Health and Science Communications Association (http://www.hesca.org/index.asp)
- The Health on the Net Foundation (HON) (http://www.hon.ch/HONcode/HON_CCE_en.htm#5)

- The International Communication Association (http://www.icahdq
  .org)
- The International Ehealth Association (http://www.cdh.luth.se/
  cdh/ExternalLinks/ieha/view)
- The International Medical Informatics Association (http://www
  .amia.org)
- The International Network of Excellence in E-Health Research (http://
  www.air-e-health@listserv.aoir.org)
- The Medical Informatics Section (http://www.medinfo.mlanet.org)
  and the Consumer and Patient Health Information Section (http://
  www.caphis.mlanet.org) of the Medical Library Association
- The National Communication Association (http://www.icahdq.org)
- The National Communication Association (http://www.natcom
  .org)
- The Society for the Internet in Medicines (http://www.internet-in-
  medicine.org).

Several international conferences are organized every year, such as MedNet (http://www.mednet2004.com.ar./en/index.php), and hundreds host e-health related panels and roundtables. There are many journals that dedicate articles and special issues to health care, health communication, and the Internet, such as *Academic Emergency Medicine*; *American Journal of Medical Science*; *BMC Medical Informatics Decision Making*; *British Medical Journal*; *Bulletin of the World Health Organisation*; *Computer Methods and Programs in Biomedicine*; *Computers in Nursing*; *Health Care News*; *Health Management Technology*; *International Journal of Medical Informatics*; *InternetHe@lth: Journal of Research, Application, Communication & Ethics*; *Journal of Healthcare Information Management*; *Journal of Medical Internet Research*; *Journal of Online Behavior*; *Journal of Telemedicine & Telecare*; *Journal of the American Medical Association*; *Journal of the American Medical Information Association*; *Journal of the Medical Library Association*; *Social Science & Medicine*; *Student Health Technology and Informatics*; and *Telemedicine Journal and E Health*.

CONTENTS OF THE BOOK

We decided to focus on the relation between the Internet and health care to investigate a very specific but extraordinary innovation, rather than disperse our efforts in the broader field of telemedicine, although other ICTs are considered here in some contexts. The book simultaneously tries to build theoretical perspectives in light of empirical evidence and applications, and to foster integration among researchers, health care providers and health information seekers. The book also highlights some of the challenges that the Internet presents to the health care field, policy-makers, providers and users, in different contexts.

Nonmedical individuals going online to find information and support is a rapidly growing phenomenon in developed countries. The international perspective of the book is crucial: although much of the early work has been done in North America, many exciting developments are happening around the world. In Europe, Asia, Australia, and South America, "online health seekers" are growing rapidly and studies on this new phenomenon are in increasing demand. Thus, we explicitly invited researchers and practitioners from a variety of countries (Canada, Germany, Indonesia, Italy, New Zealand, Peru, Singapore, Sweden, The Netherlands, and the United States). However, although an increasing number of medical and nonmedical public do access the Internet resources, more than one sixth of the world population live in extreme poverty and struggle for survival every day. The book invites policymakers to help remove barriers to the access in developing countries by clarifying problems and opportunities.

The book includes, in addition to Part I which is this introductory chapter, four parts with 17 chapters, subject and author indexes, as well as a chapter entitled "About the Contributors." The next four parts of the volume cover, in sequence: Part II reviews current trends and relevant theory; Part III explores health information seeking and evaluating at the individual level of analysis; Part IV discusses health information at the group or community level of analysis; and Part V implements health information systems at the regional and social level of analysis. Each part of the volume and its chapters are summarized in the following sections.

Part II: E-Health Trends and Theory

Part II provides comprehensive introductions to and reviews of trends in e-health, e-research and e-learning, e-commerce, and health and media use theory relevant to studying and implementing online health care.

Chapter 2: Laura Gurak and Brenda Hudson—"E-Health: Beyond Internet Searches." This chapter examines two key but currently underexamined applications in e-health: clinical service and health care professional education. These applications include electronic medical records and research networks, tele-homecare, and virtual clinics, to name a few. Privacy has significant implications across e-health applications. The chapter review illustrates the powerful ways in which digital technology can enhance human health, but also the problematic issues that are raised, including international and intercultural issues.

Chapter 3: Monica Murero—"E-Research and E-Learning: Could Online Virtual Environments Help Doctors Take Better Care of Patients?" This chapter investigates two contexts: (1) e-learning and e-research virtual environments designed for doctors. It questions two central issues: the validity of e-learning environments to educate and train medical students and practitioners online, by overcoming traditional learning boundaries of space, time and place, and (2) the validity of e-research environments to overcome classic constraints for the production, access and exchange of medical advances within the international scientific community. It also assesses the coverage by 93 medical associations' Web sites. The chapter investigates whether Internet-based learning and research environments have the potential to help doctors take better care of patients. It reflects on the opportunity of introducing attentive policies to help close the digital—and cultural—medical divide, in light of future scenarios that are expected to deeply impact medical research and revolutionize health care in the next few years.

Chapter 4: Pamela Whitten, Charles Steinfield, and Lorraine Buis—"The State of E-Commerce in Health: An Examination, Diagnosis, and Prognosis." This chapter assesses the state of e-health for purposes other than the delivery of health-related information. The examination of commercial e-health activity is directed by two major areas. The first part discusses the current utilization of commercial e-health, both in terms of business-to-consumer (B2C) and business-to-business (B2B) models. The second part presents several barriers and impediments to the growth of online health-related commercial activity and indicate how these barriers have changed over the last 5 years. Overall, a prediction made by Whitten et al. (2001), that "click and mortar" online health enterprises will become more common, is supported. There are many factors that complicate the success of commercial online health services and products. Despite these complicating factors, trends show that B2B commercial activity can be efficient for all involved and B2C commercial activity suggests that more and more Americans expect the presence of online commercial health service and product activity to grow.

Chapter 5: Mohan Dutta-Bergman—"Media Use Theory and Internet Use for Health Care." The use of the Internet for health care has grown dramatically in the last few years. Given the increasing use of the Internet by the health care consumer, it is especially important to examine the theoretical bases of Internet use for health care purposes. This chapter reviews key theories of media use and health behavior in order to provide a theoretical foundation for examining the motivations that drive the uses of the Internet for health care purposes. First, the chapter discusses four key theories of media use: uses and gratifications theory, selective processing theories, elaboration likelihood model, and the theory of channel complementarity. In discussing these, the chapter highlights the functional approach to Internet use for health care, positing the role of consumer motivation in the different uses of the Internet for health purposes and the subsequent information processing outcomes related to these different uses. The functional approach to Internet is further complemented by health behavior theories such as the stages of change model, the extended parallel process model, and the personality-driven health communication model that further articulate the role of audience motivation in health behaviors.

Part III: Searching, Discussing, and Evaluating Online Health Information

Part III considers individuals' use of the Internet to seek online health information, focusing on personal motivations and outcomes, implications for physician–patient interaction, applications in remote locations and nontraditional medical contexts, and quality of online health information.

Chapter 6: Evelyn Tang and Waipeng Lee—"Singapore Internet Users' Health Information Search: Motivation, Perception of Information Sources, and Self-Efficacy." This chapter analyzes and compares e-health seekers' and nonseekers' motivation, perception, and self-efficacy, using the focus group method. Results show that information sources can act as surveillants (to scan the environment), excavators (to acquire specifics), or verifiers (to validate information and treatments). The main reasons for information search are curiosity, personal health management, control, and provision of social support. Overall, participants believe in the Singapore press, are cautious about e-health, and show varying degree of trust toward interpersonal sources. E-health seekers are efficacious in discerning information quality and in handling information overload.

Chapter 7: Ulrika Josefsson—"Patients' Online Information-Seeking Behavior." Patients are increasingly searching the Internet for medical information to cope with illness and a changed life situation. However, few studies have addressed patients themselves and how they find their way through the vast amount of medical information online.

Therefore, with the objective to give voice to the patients, this chapter identifies and analyzes patterns in their online information-seeking behavior. Using a qualitative analysis of 18 in-depth interviews with Swedish patients, the chapter captures important components of the complex picture of patients' information seeking on the Internet. Informed by ideas from information science, the presentation of the empirical data is structured around features in Wilson's (1997) general model of information behavior. Three themes (accessing online information, social support, and information accuracy and applicability) derived from the empirical data serve as the basis for a discussion on the consequences associated with the search behaviors observed in the studies. Balancing factors (coping strategy, resource requirements, and online information-seeking assistance) complement the discussion in order to provide a nuanced picture of the outcomes of the participants' online information seeking.

Chapter 8: Ronald E. Rice and James E. Katz—"Internet Use in Physician Practice and Patient Interaction." The Internet can be part of a technological bridge that can help both patients and physicians better manage health care processes and information because more than half of Internet users in the United States seek health care information online. Although there has been good delineation of the types of activities for which health information seekers and physicians use the Internet, the interface of these two areas—how health information seekers and physicians bring the Internet-assembled information to bear on one another—is less clear. Thus, this chapter looks at these relationships in greater detail. The research review and analyses are organized by use of the Internet by physicians and by patients, and outcomes relevant to physicians and to patients.

Chapter 9: Sarah Stewart—"Delivering the Goods: Midwives' Use of the Internet." Midwives are people who provide maternity care for women and their families. In the New Zealand (NZ) context, a midwife is responsible for the provision of care to a woman from conception until 6 weeks after the baby is born. Midwifery care relies heavily on personal one-to-one communication and physically "being there." Some would argue that e-health is "dangerous nonsense" and there is no place for computers and the Internet in the midwifery practice environment; after all, being a midwife means "being with woman" not "being with computer." However, health consumers are increasingly accessing health information and resources via the Internet, which is bound to have implications with regards to midwifery practice and how midwives utilize the Internet. This chapter discusses the results of a web-based survey that questioned New Zealand midwives about their use of Internet resources. The study sought to find out what resources midwives used and wanted to be developed, and the barriers to use of the Internet. The study also aimed to discover how consumers' use of the Internet affected midwifery practice and how midwives felt about it.

Chapter 10: Joshua Seidman—"The Mysterious Maze of the World Wide Web: How Can We Guide Consumers to High-Quality Health Information on the Internet?" Most existing tools designed to help consumers find credible Internet health information focus almost exclusively on proxy measures of quality, such as the characteristics of the site sponsor and whether the site lists its sources. This analysis of 90 diabetes sites found that these proxy measures do little to explain the comprehensiveness of and accuracy of the information provided. The chapter lays out an alternative strategy for helping consumers find accurate and comprehensive Internet health information.

Part IV: Support Groups and Communities

Part IV analyzes how Internet health information users come together in online support and discussion communities; discusses some of the benefits, dangers, and concerns of this; and how such communities might be intentionally supported through social-science based systems analysis and design.

Chapter 11: Gerald Kral—"Online Communities for Mutual Help: Fears, Fiction, and Facts." The contents and possible effects of virtual self-help or mutual groups are controversial. Moreover, there is little study in German-speaking online environments for self-help. This chapter presents two empirical studies: one study involves an online forum for people suffering from eating disorders and the other, an online forum for people with suicidal thoughts. The study investigated (1) how virtual self-help groups work, and (2) the possible effects for participants. The results indicate that online groups have an important value for mutual emotional support of participants, and there is nearly no evidence for dangerous effects from participating in these online support groups. The two studies are compared and discussed in the light of previous literature.

Chapter 12: George Barnett and Jennie Hwang—"The Use of the Internet for Health Information and Social Support: A Content Analysis of Online Breast Cancer Discussion Groups." This study investigates the content of messages posted by participants of online breast cancer discussion groups. Prior research of online discussion groups primarily focused on the social support provided for breast cancer patients and their families. However, these individuals also tend to have substantial health information needs as they attempt to cope with the disease. This study uses semantic network analysis to evaluate the content of five online discussion groups. The findings suggest that information materials should be constructed to address two major issues: (1) medical treatment (oncology, radiation, mastectomy [surgery] and chemotherapy [the use of tamoxifen]), and (2) social support. These topics should be useful in the production of both print and electronic materials designed to inform individuals about breast cancer.

Chapter 13: Jan Marco Leimeister and Helmut Krcmar—"Designing and Implementing Virtual Patient Support Communities: A German Case Study." Virtual communities can, theoretically, be described as a solution for meeting ubiquitous information and interaction needs. Such needs occur in health care, when, for example, freshly diagnosed cancer patients develop very strong information and interaction needs. But how can such a platform for cancer patients be designed, implemented, and introduced practically? What specifications must a possible technical infrastructure meet? The COSMOS project addresses these topics. Besides these aspects, new technological possibilities like mobile services and mobile devices are influencing virtual communities. Subjects like ubiquitous community access, new possibilities of user identification, and location-related services are of special interest because they might allow real anytime–anyplace access to the community platform. Thus new, value-adding services to community members could be added. But only socially accepted, technically stable, and economically feasible solutions can ensure sustainable success of (mobile) virtual health care communities.

Part V: Practice and Infrastructure

The chapters in Part V provide detailed applications of Internet and related technologies for more regional and societal applications and interventions than individual online health information seeking, or online support communities. Thus issues of infrastructure, designed interventions, and socioeconomic and policy factors are relevant here.

Chapter 14: Kier Wallis and Ronald E. Rice—"Technology and Health Information Privacy: Consumers and the Adoption of Digital Medical Records Technology." New technologies offering improvements to consumers' daily lives are subject to scrutiny regarding the technologies' ability to maintain information security and privacy, important values among today's consumers. Medical information systems that combine digital technology with the highly personal and sensitive information contained in medical records, are increasingly examined as to their ability to achieve their stated medical function, while maintaining a level of privacy consistent with the government's medical privacy legislation. The Santa Barbara County Care Data Exchange (SBCCDE), a major regional health infrastructure project is in the process of implementing digital medical records technology in Santa Barbara County, California, and is subsequently subject to evaluation by its consumers, composed of the general public and medical community. In preparing for the diffusion of digital medical records technology, it is appropriate to investigate those consumer perceptions and concerns that might determine the success or failure of the new system. Therefore, this research investigates—through stakeholder interviews, focus groups, and a survey—consumer concerns, knowledge, and level of awareness regarding several facets of individual medical records technology and privacy.

Chapter 15: Suzanne Brunsting and Bas van den Putte—"Web-Based Computer-Tailored Feedback on Alcohol Use: Motivating Excessive Drinkers to Consider Their Behavior."

This chapter analyzes the effectiveness of computer-tailored interventions targeting excessive alcohol users who are not inclined to seek treatment. The aim of these interventions is to make these people aware of the excessiveness of their drinking and the possible negative consequences. The term *computer tailoring* is explained and illustrated with examples of recently developed interventions, followed by a discussion of the theory underlying computer tailoring. The chapter also contains a description of a small-scale study on the effects of a Dutch computer-tailored intervention. Results of this study are used to raise and discuss several issues, resulting in implications for future research on computer tailoring.

Chapter 16: Lorna Heaton—"Telehealth in Indigenous Communities in the Far North: Challenges for Continued Development."

The chapter begins with a description of the situation in Nunavut, Canada and the challenges of delivering health care across a large number of remote, isolated communities. It draws a portrait of medical practices in this context and describes how telehealth is changing these practices and the relationships between the various parts of the system. The chapter then points to several elements that may be generalizable from this specific case to discuss lessons learned and challenges for continued development. Since telehealth is still in the early stages in Nunavut, this part of the chapter is speculative. Finally, the chapter discusses policy issues and potentials for development, such as the use of the Internet. Insights from telehealth programs in other Northern contexts are introduced in support of the argument.

Chapter 17: Indrajit Banerjee and Cecilia Hsi-Shi Leong—"ICTs in the War Against HIV/AIDS in Asia." In most developing countries in Asia studied in this chapter, universal access is not a certainty due to factors such as the digital divide, economic considerations, or literacy levels. Nevertheless, the Internet does provide an alternative avenue (and in that sense, increases the options) for access to information. More specifically, there are AIDS-related Web sites that are targeted at specific audiences, such as women, adolescents, families affected by AIDS and ethnic minorities. This chapter discusses how ICTs, in particular the Internet, have been used in the battle against HIV/AIDS across South Asia (India, Pakistan, Sri Lanka), South East Asia (Indonesia, Malaysia, Thailand, and Vietnam) and East Asia (China and Mongolia). The chapter reviews the prevalence of HIV/AIDS in these Asian countries, how widespread it has become and also how the Internet is being used by various HIV/AIDS interest groups for support. It also discusses the use of the Internet for HIV/AIDS monitoring, research, and education as well as how networking effects of the Internet have generated synergies between health care providers, researchers, policymakers, and PLWHAs. The chapter reviews what all these mean in terms of implications and challenges for Asia.

Chapter 18: Walter Curioso—"New Technologies and Public Health in Developing Countries: The Cell PREVEN Project." Computers and personal digital assistants (PDAs) are limited in developing countries because of their expense and requirement for additional equipment, such as relatively complex network connections. Cell phones, which are ubiquitous and cheaper than most computers and PDAs, offer a simple solution to a paper-based system. This chapter describes an application of telehealth using cell phones and the Internet to collect, transmit, and monitor data in real-time from female sex workers (FSW) who are part of a 20-city randomized trial in Peru to reduce sexually transmitted diseases (STDs). Early detection and treatment of STDs represents one major strategy for preventing transmission of STDs, including infection with HIV. New technologies and information systems can help public health in terms of prevention, surveillance, and management of public health data. The chapter discusses some barriers, factors, and limitations in collecting data electronically in a developing country. Despite some limitations, cell phones have a valuable role in bridging the digital divide and providing solutions in public health. The chapter also addresses the importance of developing an appropriate technology and collaborating with information technology partners, and provides some lessons learned that can be generalized to other developing and developed countries.

TOPICS ACROSS THE CHAPTERS

In addition to the specific focus, reviews, and results of each chapter, the chapters overall represent a wide array of research, theory, and practice issues relating to Internet and health care. A brief analysis of the 17 chapters reveals 11 general categories of topics: theories and constructs, levels of analysis, methodological approaches, advantages, disadvantages, facilitators, barriers, policy issues, lessons learned, trends, and developments. The following sections provide brief comments about each general category, and a listing of the specific forms of the category across the chapters.

Theories and Constructs

Because of the inherent interdisciplinarity of technology-mediated health care, applicable theories come from a wide variety of domains, such as persuasion, health communication, organizational behavior, psychology, sociology, management, consumer behavior, privacy studies, public health, communication, information systems, and information science (see Table 1.1). Of particular note is the application of theories of human information seeking, community sustainability, system design, and integrated health communication.

Levels of Analysis

In addition to the usual short list of possible levels of analysis—individual, group, organization, community, social, national, cross-cultural— the chapters discuss or imply several other ways to conceptualized levels of analysis (see Table 1.2). One is the important role of professions, which are diverse within health care institutions and cross institutional boundaries. Specific professions have different needs, criteria, and concerns. For example, nurses are concerned both about patient safety and privacy, but also the extent to which technology may interfere with providing personal attention. Another interesting way to conceptualize levels of analysis is that an individual user may have multiple online identities and accounts, whereas multiple users may share the same account. So levels of identity and access become intertwined. A third perspective would consider the intermediary technology users between pa-

TABLE 1.1
Topics Across the Book: Theories and Constructs

- accessibility
- activating mechanisms that generate information seeking
- behavior modeling
- brief/minimal health interventions
- channel complementarity/functional equivalents
- collective knowledge
- community platform engineering process
- comprehensive model of health information seeking
- consumer motivations
- contingencies of practice
- coping strategies (including coping with web-based health information overload)
- critical mass
- diffusion of innovations
- digital divide
- dual (cognitive) processing (elaboration likelihood model, heuristic systematic model)
- economies of scale
- evidence-based practice
- extended parallel process model
- gap between physicians and patients on evaluation and use of Internet health information
- gatekeeping
- health belief model
- health orientation
- health care professionals' practices
- hyperpersonal interaction
- idiocentrism
- information asymmetries
- information behavior model
- information literacy
- information need context
- informed consent
- innovation clusters
- lurking
- media access and control
- media use as functional to different audience segments in different contexts
- message involvement and salience
- need for privacy
- online empathy
- online health business models (click and mortar, online–offline alliance, commission)
- online niche markets
- online self-help groups
- online/virtual community
- prevention versus treatment motivations for health information seeking
- professional identities
- proxy measures of health information quality
- quality of online health information
- quality-of-care measurement
- reinvention
- role model perception

(Continued)

TABLE 1.1
(Continued)

- scalable health community system platforms
- search modes (passive attention, passive search, active search, ongoing search)
- security
- selective processing (exposure, interpretation, retention, recall)
- self-efficacy
- self-monitoring
- self-perceived health risks (such as alcohol consumption)
- sensation seeking
- social influence
- stepwise and emotional model of information seeking
- strength of weak ties
- subjective norms
- supply chain management
- technological fit
- technology acceptance model
- third-party Web site accreditation
- transaction cost theory
- transtheoretical model
- transtheoretical stage transitions
- trust
- ubiquitous health information needs
- uncertainty reduction during threat to quality of life
- uses and gratifications
- web fluency

TABLE 1.2
Topics Across the Book: Levels of Analysis

- accounts may be shared by multiple users
- business-to-businesses
- communicating and collaborating with other professionals in specialty area
- markets and industry, such as B2B and B2C e-commerce
- group/social identity
- individual user may have multiple online identities and accounts
- individuals-to-businesses
- information seekers versus information sources
- intermediary technology users between patients and health care providers
- managers of online support/self-help groups as opposed to individual users of the support group
- online health seekers with same diagnosis
- online support groups allow anywhere from an intimate group of friends to an unknowably large and changing number of people with shared interests to discuss illnesses and treatments, provide behavioral examples and emotional support, and create awareness about otherwise rare conditions
- shift among relationships such as general group support to dyadic chat or offline meeting
- team or sequence of health care providers jointly offering diagnosis and treatment
- transaction chains involving intermediaries

16

tients and health care providers, and managers or moderators of group discussion lists.

Methodological Approaches

The research reported here uses a wide array of methodologies (see Table 1.3). Indeed, studying the complex interactions among stakeholders, users and their family and friends, technology, information, law and regulation, economics, medicine, and social and cultural values requires multiple methodological approaches. Of course, the nature of the Internet provides opportunities for new types and venues for methods and analysis, such as online surveys, Web site features and content analysis, and

TABLE 1.3
Topics Across the Book: Methodological Approaches

- archival/document analysis
- case studies of health organizations
- case study
- content analysis of Web sites
- cost-effectiveness analysis
- developing reliable health Web site evaluation measures
- ethnography
- focus groups
- information systems design requirements and analysis for online health communities
- key stakeholder personal interviews
- literature review
- multidimensional scaling to visually portray relationships among words in online or focus group transcripts
- narrative interviews
- ongoing formative evaluation
- online pre–post field/quasi-experiment
- qualitative interpretation of online discussion group transcripts
- randomized treatment/control field experiment
- recruiting online respondents through snowball sampling
- semantic analysis of online transcripts and focus group discussions
- semi-structured personal or video-based interviews
- survey and focus group pre-testing
- system prototyping
- thematic analysis of focus group discussions
- usage session monitoring forms
- user needs analysis for system design
- using general and medical search engines
- using search engine results as a sampling procedure
- web-based and telephone surveys
- Web site content analysis
- Web site feature analysis

usage monitoring for interface design. The textual and storage nature of online discussions also provide opportunities for analyzing large and over-time transcripts.

Advantages

Potential advantages of Internet and other mediated health information, communication, and service capabilities are familiar and frequently noted, such as reduced cost, increased access, and the ability to overcome time and space (see Table 1.4). Some of these are the flip side of disadvantages, such as benefits to those who are shy or uncertain who are able to "lurk" and learn without posting on discussion groups. Others are more sense-making, whereby discussing one's own experiences and reading others helps develop one's own sense of identity as well as commonality. And others are based on the possibilities for real-time interaction and tailoring of content, and the linking of different media to and from Web sites.

Disadvantages

Additionally, the flip side of some advantages are potential disadvantages, such as anonymous postings fostering deception and lack of accountability (see Table 1.5). Certainly, central concerns involve the fact that as anyone can publish any information on the web (depending on the country of the author), there is little guarantee of the quality, accuracy, and authoritativeness of the information or identity of the author. Another ongoing debate is whether the powerful focus of discussion groups also fosters narrowness and social fragmentation.

Facilitators

Continued diffusion, application, and benefits of Internet health care and communication requires ongoing, and additional, facilitators (see Table 1.6). Obvious ones include broadband infrastructure and funding, but less obvious ones involve patient involvement in their own health care decisions, interconnectivity across systems and media, appropriate regulation and legislation, and support from medical associations and health agencies.

Barriers

As with advantages and disadvantages, the flip side of some facilitators are barriers (see Table 1.7). The fundamental problem of digital divides is that usage of Internet health care information requires technological,

TABLE 1.4
Internet Health Information: Advantages

- access to alternative medicine products and information
- access to emotional and social support from a broad range of others who share same experience and concerns
- adds value
- allows some who are not comfortable posting messages to "lurk"
- anonymity for posting personal health information and problems
- connects those who are geographically or professionally isolated from colleagues
- emotional support
- faster diffusion of medical research
- finding/communicating with/evaluating health providers
- foster development of online communities
- foster development of social and professional health care networks beyond patients/ individuals and beyond system users
- general versus tailored health information
- greater access to diverse sources of health information
- greater provision at lower cost in residential and rural homes
- help patients make sense of their medical experience (such as cancer)
- improve patient empowerment and self-care
- improve processes
- improve self-presentation in discussing medical conditions with others
- increase access
- increased interaction and discussions with physicians (due to e-mail, and bringing in printouts of Internet health information)
- Internet information improves doctor–patient communication and has variety of other positive patient outcomes
- less risk in online self-disclosure
- message tailoring and stages of readiness assessed through interactive choices
- more personalized and customized information and interactions
- not just receive, but also provide social support or the more broad experience of gen- eralized reciprocity and sharing
- online health insurance applications and registration
- physicians interacting with better-informed patients
- provide clinical support to nonphysicians
- provide support for peer counseling
- reduce health care costs
- reduced errors (such as in prescriptions, confusing different patients' medical records)
- reduced social status cues
- reduces face-to-face hierarchical barriers
- reducing errors and delays in obtaining personal medical records
- scheduling flexibility in taking online medical education courses
- switch from telephone calls to online information provision
- therapeutic value of self-disclosure
- wide access to at-risk groups through online health campaigns and interactive inter- ventions

TABLE 1.5
Internet Health Information: Disadvantages

- access to unregulated drugs
- access to unverified alternative medicines and information
- allows some to "lurk" and "free ride"
- benefits require technical expertise and skills and medical knowledge
- bypassing checks for drug interactions
- challenges to physicians by patients with Internet information
- commercial biases in health and prescription sites
- complex and difficult to understand online medical information
- e-mail interaction with patients generates considerable demands on staff and raises liability issues
- inaccuracy of online health information
- inappropriate access by third parties
- may require additional procedures and effort to use a new system
- missing or misleading Web site links
- narrow and self-reinforcing information and interactions
- poor quality information
- pressure on physicians to prescribe Internet-advertised medicines
- reinforcing eating disorders or suicide tendencies
- self-diagnosis and prescribing
- unreliable networks or storage

TABLE 1.6
Internet Health Information: Facilitators

- broadband infrastructure
- collaboratives/cooperatives
- cooperation and coordination among service and infrastructure providers
- government promotion of access and infrastructure and e-health
- HIPAA standards
- interconnectivity across systems and channels
- mobile/wireless devices and interconnections
- more use of general Internet activities
- patients want to be involved in their medical decisions
- physician recommendations of health sites
- positive perceptions of innovation attributes
- reimbursement for online time and services
- support by national medical associations

educational, and economic resources and knowledge. Some aspects may challenge cultural norms and practices. Contention over limited resources and conceptualizations of system purposes by different organizational or political stakeholders can prevent users from benefiting. The same regulations that facilitate and protect the use of health information can also create obstacles, confusion, and complexity. Lack of suffi-

TABLE 1.7
Internet Health Information: Barriers

- access and knowledge
- accountability and responsibility
- computer fears
- computer/ICT skills
- contention for system usage between administrators and health care providers
- cultural divides concerning technology use and social norms toward health behaviors
- differences in data conceptualization by physicians (narratives) and administrators (structured data entry)
- differences in procedures for reimbursement and health coverage across economic sectors and national boundaries
- difficulties in assessing online knowledge acquisition
- digital divide
- high costs of technology overwhelm low cost of access and communication
- HIPAA regulations
- individuals' perceptions of current medical information rights
- insufficient bandwidth
- insufficient control or awareness of third party access to personal medical records
- insufficient health staff
- joint involvement by local service providers/physicians/patients
- jurisdictional conflicts or disagreements
- lack of basic infrastructure
- lack of insurance reimbursement codes for online treatment
- lack of interconnection
- lack of standard evaluation criteria
- lack of support for sustainability of online interventions and health projects
- large gap between those with Internet access and those with many kinds of chronic health problems (such as HIV/AIDS)
- limited vision by government and health care agencies as to potential applications
- majority of health sites in English language
- national and cultural norms and policies
- online privacy concerns
- physician resistance/hesitancy
- poor management of ICT personnel and projects
- standard codes for practices and protocols
- state licensing laws
- sustainability (costs, updating, link stability)
- time required to learn new systems
- usability

cient and trained health care staff is often a more fundamental barrier. Concerns about online privacy and health information quality, resistance by some health professionals to technology mediation of health care, and lack of ongoing support for online projects and interventions are significant barriers.

TABLE 1.8
Policy Issues

- codes of ethics
- cross-state and cross-border drug prescription economics and regulation
- enforcement of online pharmacies
- health insurance portability and accountability act (HIPAA)
- health Web site licensure
- HIPAA
- identity theft
- interstate commerce conditions and criteria
- national/regional/international e-health policies
- privacy (collection, accessibility, security, anonymity, verification)
- telecommunications policy reform in developing countries
- telecommunications tariffs

Policy Issues

Policies—concerning everything from standards for interconnection and health information coding, to privacy, and telecommunications pricing structures—affect the governance and potentiality of all aspects of Internet health care, information, and communication (see Table 1.8). Specific medical associations may establish codes of ethics that health sites have to meet in order to be certified, while national e-health policies direct where funding and system development is targeted. Ineffective or contradictory policies can create both industry and user uncertainty and frustration, and misdirect scarce resources.

Lessons Learned

The traditional focus of many research studies on Internet and health care/communication of course is on factors influencing usage and outcomes, and many of the chapters here provide rich and comprehensive coverage of both the prior research and the reported research. Beyond that familiar sense of lessons learned, the chapters also provide more practical, institutional, and implementation insights (see Table 1.9). For example, assumptions about what users believe about their medical rights, or how search engines actually work, have significant implications for publicity about, and provision of, online health care. Fostering communication among users and stakeholders is as, or more, important, than providing accurate and understandable health information. Long-term planning, realistic expectations, adapting technology to local and cultural contexts, and understanding of how professionals' practice in-

TABLE 1.9
Lessons Learned

- advantages and disadvantages from same kind of use (such as active searching for online health information)
- allow personal recommendations and buddy lists among users
- allow ratings of health sites and content by users
- consumers not well informed (such as about medical rights, implications of privacy statements)
- content analyses of discussion groups sites can help understand users' concerns and interests and guide development of public health messages
- content analysis of discussion groups can lead to better system design and moderator activities
- emphasis on peer-to-peer advice and support than on discussion group moderators
- expectations about and attitudes toward use of a health information technology can influence actual use and outcomes
- few users understand how search engines work
- health care providers (such as midwives) may change/improve their practice due to online professional discussion lists
- health information sources as surveillants/excavators/verifiers
- health institutions and government sites more trusted for credible information
- implement with local partners
- implementation of new health information technologies can change and challenge traditional professional and administrative practice and roles
- information overload a problem but health seekers manage?
- Internet as information source and as communication medium
- Internet health interventions must fit local and cultural conditions and contexts
- lower tech solutions that better match users' contexts and professionals' practices more successful
- manage realistic expectations
- move from information retrieval and transmission to communication and interaction
- need for multiple forms of user involvement in health site design
- need long-term planning
- need to integrate expert judgment with technology
- online discussions may help alleviate some conditions such as suicidal thoughts or eating disorders, but do not seem to motivate users to obtain therapy or treatment
- online health seekers have different general health information source usage patterns
- patients' bringing Internet information to their doctor's appointments affected various outcomes for physicians and patients depending on how the physicians assessed the reliability of the information and their own attitudes toward general popular access to health information
- site map and orientation guides necessary for Web site designs
- social support and interpersonal utility needs
- structural indicators of Web site quality and accreditation seals may not be highly related to accuracy and quality of its medical content
- tendency toward using broad search engine searches instead of specific terms and topic-specific health sites
- understand required human resources
- understand users' needs and perspectives
- use iterative requirements specification in health community design
- use of some media may trigger use of Internet for more information

(Continued)

TABLE 1.9
(Continued)

- use online health information to compare and follow-up interpersonal (include physician) information
- users perceive shortcomings and complexity and credibility problems of Internet, but use it for health information anyway
- users rate online health information quality much higher than do physicians
- visualization of system prototypes helpful for users to understand and comment on design possibilities
- widespread use of Internet by physicians, but much less so for interaction with patients

teracts with new health technologies, are all important lessons learned from some of the studies reported here. Also important is the appreciation that users' beliefs and behaviors may be contradictory (such as about health information accuracy and privacy beliefs compared to evaluations of online searches), and may differ considerably from those of health professionals (such as between physicians and patients).

Trends

The chapters identify and discuss a wide range of general trends in the social, institutional, and professional contexts of Internet health care (see Table 1.10). Many of these are fundamental concerns about health information and communication, whereas some are quite recent entrants to the agenda. Some, for example, represent surprising uses, such as posting or video-streaming online surgeries and births, continuous monitoring of individual health status outside of a medical institution, and physician or hospital web portals. Others are more enduring issues, such as certifying the quality of health information, telehealth, and online publication of medical research.

Developments

There are ongoing developments in technologies and features, and new medical information and practice (see Table 1.11). Many of these are new systems or applications, such as collecting health information locally, transmitting it through text messaging on mobile phones into a web-based database, and tailoring this information for specific groups of users. Online diagnosis tools, miniaturization, voice-response applications, embedded wireless sensors, and high-speed broadband wireless networking are all providing researchers, designers and users new possibilities, as well as new challenges, obstacles, and questions.

TABLE 1.10
Trends

- accuracy and privacy certifications and criteria
- broadcasting baby births through the Internet
- business-related applications
- developing national medical databases such as providing online birth registries
- electronic patient records (digital medical records)
- electronic prescribing services
- electronic publication of medical research
- e-mail between health providers and patients
- health group discussion threads
- hospital and health resource portals
- image-management systems
- increased emphasis on health problems and disparities
- increased system security
- increasing business-to-consumer and business-to-business Internet transactions
- increasing online intermediaries
- massive increase in health care sector investments and expenses
- moderated health discussion sites
- online medical education (physicians, students, patient)
- online medical textbooks and journals
- online test results
- personalized and customized online portals and medical training
- physician referral of patients to health Web sites (including more formally as "information prescriptions")
- physicians turning to the Internet to keep up to date with current research
- point-of-care testing
- real-time and asynchronous monitoring and reporting individual health status as well as disease outbreaks and diffusion
- remote diagnosis
- rise of online transaction processing services
- technology-enhanced clinical applications
- telehealth in remote areas
- traditional print and broadcast media providing links to online health sites
- virtual clinics

CONCLUSION

Clearly the chapters in *The Internet and Health Care: Theory, Research, and Practice* represent a rich and diverse set of contributors, research and usage settings, insights, topics, and theoretical and methodological approaches. These chapters of course represent only a small portion of prior and current research in these areas, and also represent the early stages of a significant and rapidly growing domain of theory, research, and practice. We encourage you to pursue these and related topics in Internet and health care and communication, and to collaborate and communicate

TABLE 1.11
Developments

- context- or location-sensitive services
- disabled patients using embedded sensors to interact with their environment
- electronic learning environments
- electronic research environments
- evaluating e-health behavioral and management interventions
- high-speed broadband wireless Internet
- integration of various treatment and response media (such as online assessment generating advice to contact a telephone hot line or send an e-mail)
- interactive voice-response applications
- miniaturization
- mobile telephone-based or PDS-based health information and communication services
- nanomedicine
- online databases of rare pathologies and cases
- online diagnosis tools
- online health monitoring and personal health management
- online or mobile health monitoring or reminder systems
- online virtual specimen slides
- physically embedded monitoring sensors
- portable digital personal medical records
- regional health information organizations
- use of Internet for medical research networks
- using wireless devices as data entry interface for Internet-accessible databases, digital cameras to capture and transmit medical images
- virtual reality anatomy demonstrations and medical training
- visualization of internal bodily processes
- web-based store-and-forward health information applications (such as for X-rays)

with the current authors and the many others doing work on these topics. Helping to improve the health care and condition of people around the world, through the implementation, application and understanding of the Internet and related information and communication technologies, is one of the most important contributions we, as theorists, researchers, and practitioners, can make. We hope this book aids this effort.

REFERENCES

Hsiung, R. C. (2002). *E-Therapy: Case studies, guiding principles, and the clinical potential of the Internet*. New York: W. W. Norton.

Rice, R. E., & Katz, J. E. (Eds.). (2001). *The Internet and health communication: Expectations and experiences*. Thousand Oaks, CA: Sage.

Whitten, P., Steinfield, C., & Hellmich, S. (2001). EHealth: Market potential and business strategies. *Journal of Computer Mediated Mass Communication*, 6(4). Retrieved March 20, 2005, from http://jcmc.indiana.edu/vol6/issue4/whitten.html

II

E-HEALTH TRENDS
AND THEORY

Chapter 2

E-Health: Beyond Internet Searches

Laura J. Gurak
Brenda L. Hudson
University of Minnesota

Most popular accounts about e-health focus on the use of the web by patients and "health seekers" in Western countries to search for medical information. But as the chapters in this edited volume illustrate, e-health and its implications go well beyond Internet searching to include new ways of delivering health care and influencing public health policy. As readers of this volume know, accessing health-related information has never been easier than in the current "information age," as the Internet's vast content and global reach allows health consumers to quickly connect with the latest information and expertise. In terms of information gathering, the Internet has leveled the playing field—patients and consumers have access to much of the same health information and guidelines as physicians. Beyond this, however, Internet technologies are working their way into the very nature of health care delivery—from medical education to patient–physician communication to technology-enhanced clinical applications. Met with both acceptance and apprehension, the rapidly evolving technological landscape poses interesting implications for health care on a global scale. E-health could play an important role in this century.

E-health, or health-related Internet-based technology, is a broad term, encompassing a wide variety of applications used by consumers, patients, and health care providers. Defined by Wilson (2004) as "[h]ealth-related Internet applications delivering a range of content, connectivity, and clinical care" (p. 241), e-health includes everything from health information Web sites and electronic medical records, to "virtual clinics" used for medical education and teleradiography clinical care—to name just a few. With its promise of cost effectiveness, greater efficiency, and improved patient safety, e-health initiatives are being pursued in various ways and to various degrees across countries and continents. In light of such diverse applications, perhaps e-health is too broad a term to be of much use today. As new applications develop and yet others become more streamlined and specialized, the collective term *e-health* begins to lose its meaning. In fact, we can draw a parallel to the early days of Internet-based business, when the term *e-commerce* was used to reference all aspects of the industry. However, e-commerce has since evolved into many different practices and specializations and, as a result, is now referred to more by its applications than by its generic term. Over time, the term e-commerce, like e-health, seems to have outgrown itself. As a result, we believe an oversimplification of e-health can be limiting when it comes to examining this field. In order to analyze aspects such as cost effectiveness, efficiency, usability, and program quality, it seems necessary to examine them from an application point of view. For instance, in looking at cost savings, electronic prescribing services may have separate considerations from electronic patient records. In this way, it is crucial to approach e-health not as a broad, nonspecific field, but as different applications with differing purposes and uses.

In order to provide a useful overview, this chapter examines two key applications of e-health—clinical and health care professional education—that we have based on categories identified by Richardson (2003; Richardson also includes two other applications: public health information and patient empowerment; and public health policy and prevention, which are beyond our scope here).

Because of space limitations, the following overview provides snapshots of clinical and health care professional education applications, areas that are currently underexamined. We also examine privacy, which we see as having implications across e-health applications. In addition to illustrating the powerful ways in which digital technology can enhance human health, we also examine the problematic issues that are raised. Our analysis will take a particular focus on international and intercultural issues.

AN OVERVIEW OF E-HEALTH

Internet technologies are certainly making an impact in the world of health care, providing patients and consumers with access to information and professional services as well as offering health care providers new ways in managing patient records and clinical techniques. According to Richardson (2003), "The emergence of IT as a way of adding value has been against a background of inexorably rising costs, increased demand for healthcare services, (driven partly by aging populations), and increased patient awareness of healthcare possibilities, ironically, to a large extent, due to health-related websites, some of which are of dubious quality" (p. 151).

Proponents of e-health claim that Internet technologies have the capability to improve patient care, and provide efficiency, ease of access, and savings: "E-health is promoted as a mechanism to bring growth, cost savings, and process improvement to health care" (Wilson, 2004, p. 241). Such benefits, both purported and realized, are driving factors in the implementation of e-health applications. Citing a 2001 survey, Wilson states that "of 440 health care organizations [in the U.S., the survey] found that more than 80% now deliver some form of e-health to their patients, and more than 50% implement advanced e-health applications, including online formularies, prescription refills, test results, and physician-patient communication" (p. 241).

Yet advances in health care technology have not matched recent advances in medicine itself. "The past three decades have seen revolutionary changes in healthcare but only evolutionary changes in healthcare information systems" (Safran, 2003, p. 186). For instance, out of 30 billion annual medical transactions, more than 90% are conducted by phone, fax, or stamped mail; only one third of hospitals have computerized order-entry systems—fewer than 5% require their use; and only 5% of clinicians and 19% of provider organizations use electronic medical records (Novelli, 2004, p. 32).

Nor have advances in health care technology matched that of other industries, such as banking and airlines. *The Wall Street Journal* reports that although "health-care computer spending in the U.S. jumped 9.3% to $23.6 billion [in 2002] . . . much of that went for computer systems that were individually installed at hospitals, clinics and pharmacies" (Naik, 2003, p. B1). Because these systems did not necessarily connect to each other, the "use of computers for improving clinical care remains limited and fragmented."

There are several reasons for the comparative lack of computers in the health care setting, not least reluctance from health care providers themselves, mainly "due to concerns over risk, liability, and initial expense" (Wilson, 2004, p. 241). Other barriers cited include "lack of broadband communication networks, relative unavailability of computing and online connectivity; high costs of hardware and software; lack of political conviction; and lack of a standard code of generally accepted practices and protocols, in particular for information security" (Richardson, 2003, p.

151). To help overcome some of these barriers, various initiatives have been developed over the years. Not surprisingly, these initiatives also portray the scope of e-health applications currently in use. The following is a mere selection.

In Europe, e-health is considered a newly emerging industry in the public health sector with a turnover of 11bn (£7.3bn; $13.1bn) and an estimated spending on e-health by 2010 of "5% of the total of national health budgets—a considerable increase on the 1% recorded four years ago" (Watson, 2004, p. 1155). In 2002, e-health became an "eEurope 2005 policy priority," with targets of an electronic European health insurance card, Health Information Networks to facilitate health information through the health care system, and online health services for health information, electronic health records, teleconsultation and e-reimbursement (Europa, 2005).

In 2000, the United Nations launched the Health InterNetwork initiative to install computers with Internet connectivity at hospitals and other health settings in developing countries (Kuruvilla, Dzenowagis, Pleasant, Dwivedi, Murthy, et al., 2004). A pilot project under this initiative, Health InterNetwork India found that "an important requirement for bridging the digital divide is to ensure that connectivity, content, capacity building, and policy meet real needs" and that Internet technology "will not have a major impact without concerted and coordinated efforts to invest in basic infrastructure, develop human resources, provide relevant content, and implement supportive policies" (Kuruvilla et al., 2004, p. 1196). That is, in order for an integrated Internet communications system to be successful, there must be careful consideration and planning for long-term use, beyond the short-term goal of setting up an information technology infrastructure. Organizations and governments need to work closely with local partners if information technology is to strengthen public health practice.

Electronic medical records (EMR) is another area where organizations and governments need to work with local partners (such as the health care providers themselves) to render digital technology effective in its application (Humber, 2004; see also Wallis & Rice, chap. 14, this volume). In 2004, an executive order from President Bush established the office of the National Coordinator for Health Information Technology. Later that year, the government announced a plan to establish a national electronic medical records system within 10 years, potentially saving $140 billion annually and reducing medical errors (Kalb & Soukop, 2004). Meanwhile in England, the National Health Service (NHS) has embarked on a national Integrated Care Record Service, where it is hoped that "by 2010 every patient in England will have an individual electronic NHS care record" (Coombes, 2004a, p. 1157). The contract to set up and run this service is worth £620 million (932m; $1.1bn) and will connect "more than 30,000 general practitioners and 270 acute community and mental health NHS trusts in a single system" (p. 1157). Also, it is hoped that by the end of 2005, all hospital bookings in England will be done electronically (Coombes, 2004a). In addition to ensuring the technological aspects are sound, collaborators must address concerns of privacy and usability (Humber, 2004).

Other government initiatives aim to incorporate technology and health in a broader sense. In October 2004, the U.S. Department of Health and Human Services announced $139 million in grants and contracts to promote the use of health and information technology (HIT). The awards, administered through the HHS' Agency for Healthcare Research and Quality (AHRQ), will be used to promote access to HIT, to develop statewide and regional networks, and to encourage adoption of HIT by sharing knowledge through the creation of the National Health Information Technology Resource Center (U.S. Department of Health and Human Services, 2004).

In Latin American and the Caribbean, the Presidential Declaration of the 1998 Summit of the Americas articulated that the collective countries of the Americas have a common interest in utilizing information technology for improved health care and as such, identified six areas for government involvement. These areas included information systems and technology promotion; exploring implementation of standards; research and development funding; equitable distribution of resources; protecting rights of privacy, intellectual property, and security; and solving conflicting regulations to ensure cooperation (Rodrigues & Risk, 2003).

In addition to developing new initiatives, however, there is also a push for evaluating the quality and effectiveness of e-health applications. The Robert Wood Johnson Foundation approved a $10.3 million fund for 5 years of research evaluating the effectiveness of e-health applications for health behavior change and chronic disease management (Ahern, Phalen, & Mockenhaupt, 2003). Some projects funded in 2004 include studies that examine: health outcomes of online weight management techniques; the potential of technology to improve chronic disease management and quality of care in diabetics; tailored e-mails to motivate healthy behavior, improve health status and reduce health care costs; and the clinical effectiveness of tele-rehabilitation (Health e-Technologies Initiative, 2005).

Concerns about quality and effectiveness also come from the professions (for instance, Maulden, 2003, regarding neurology; Parekh, Nazarian, & Lim, 2004, regarding residents and orthopedics). From a nursing perspective, Coy Smith made a compelling case that nursing teams "throughout the world are increasingly balancing this equation: What is the value of technology in proportion to its ability to enhance patient safety, retain nurses, provide more direct care time, support the strategic plan, and justify costs?" (Smith, 2004, p. 92). She argued that "[n]urse executives must strategically evaluate the effectiveness of each proposed system or device using a strategic planning process."

Other concerns regarding e-health initiatives include access for disadvantaged or vulnerable populations, ensuring patient safety and privacy, issues of usability, cost-effectiveness, and cultural sensitivity. "[E]valuations need to determine how people use various ehealth features and how such use relates to health outcomes" (Gustafson & Wyatt, 2004, p. 1150). To help ensure quality programs, "ehealth developers must first evaluate users' needs, then the product's risks and benefits, then its feasibility, and then its acceptability to the user" (p. 1150).

Against this backdrop of initiatives, promises, and concerns, in May 2004 the *British Medical Journal* devoted a theme issue to electronic communication and its impact on health care. In an editorial, Richard Smith stated that high-quality information technology will lead to a "radical redesign" in health care; however, he emphasized that the human aspects limit this development more than the technological aspects.

That e-health is here to stay is certain. How best to utilize new technologies to meet the changing needs of the health care field, including how to integrate human considerations to ensure safety, relevance, and acceptance, is an area of debate and concern. We now turn our attention to these aspects by examining two applications of e-health: clinical and health care professional education. We conclude with an examination of privacy and a look to the future of e-health.

CLINICAL APPLICATIONS

The area of clinical applications offers some of the most exciting developments in e-health: interactive telemedicine for remote consultations and diagnoses, managing chronic disorders via the Internet, and tele-home-care, to name just a few.

In his 2004 article, "Medical and Information Technologies Converge," clinical engineer Ted Cohen outlined recent developments in clinical applications of e-health, where information technology has moved from primarily business-related applications (e.g., billing) to systems geared more to clinical applications, such as integrated electronic medical records (EMR) and picture archiving communication systems (PACS). Although there will be a continued need for specialized development of medical devices and software, "once the signal is digitized and external from the body, common computer and communication systems will be used to process, analyze, store, and communicate it to a variety of information systems" (Cohen, 2004, p. 61).

Cohen provided an interesting example of how this may play out in the field:

> For critical patients, point-of-care testing and indwelling sensors will become more commonplace, whereas in the general acute areas of the hospital, more and more laboratory tests will be performed via very automated, robotics-based, off-site laboratories. Nursing unit central stations will become less clinically important as physiological monitor alarms, "nurse-call" requests, and other critical information are communicated directly to the assigned care givers, although the care givers' primary communication tool has not yet been well defined. The acuity level of the inpatient will continue to increase, and more and more technology will be moved to the inpatient's room, rather than moving the patient to the technology. (p. 65)

Telemedicine

Telemedicine, using technology to practice medicine from a distance, encompasses a variety of clinical applications. For instance, it can be used to evaluate patients at remote rural locations and areas without access to particular specialists. Although particularly useful in specialties "where images are crucial to diagnosis, such as dermatology, it is used effectively by many specialties" (Nissen, Abdulla, Khandheira, Kienzle, & Zaher, 2004, p. 259). In fact, one innovative study has Canadian researchers testing telemedicine technology in an underwater laboratory in Florida, using robotic surgery that could be used to delivery emergency diagnostic and surgical care to astronauts in space, as well as to patients in remote areas on Earth (Kilpatrick, 2004, p. 716).

In a clinical setting, consultations between a physician and patient or between physicians can be conducted in a "real-time" transfer so that multiple caregivers and a patient in different locations can simultaneously assess the records. Less technically demanding is store-and-forward, where "clinical images (e.g., information derived from an examination or a procedure) are sent to another site for display, interpretation, and permanent storage," obviating the need for simultaneous consultations (Nissen et al., 2004, p. 259).

New computer technologies are replacing analog technology, traditionally used in video conferencing, making telemedicine applications "easier and less expensive to deploy" (Cohen, 2004, p. 61). These newer technologies include digital cameras, with increased resolution resulting in improved remote diagnosis, and digital communication lines such as ISDN and DSL. However, the newer digital technologies present other challenges, "particularly for real-time applications, in bandwidth, quality of service, security and availability in the rural areas where tele-medicine is most needed" (p. 61).

One study looked at the cost benefit of teleradiography in a rural hos-pital in the Southern United States (Gamble, Savage, & Icenogle, 2004). Typically, teleradiology involves capturing an image on film or electroni-cally that is then transmitted via high-speed data lines to another site in order to be analyzed by a radiologist, who sends a report and communi-cates a treatment plan to the patient's physician. The way in which this process differs from a traditional radiology consult is the use of technol-ogy to transmit the image and report. In a rural area, the radiologist must travel to a rural hospital where the images are held or courier the images from the hospital to his or her office. As Gamble et al. stated: "The radiologist's clinical activities are the same with either model, although use of the radiologist's skills is more efficient with the use of tele-radiography because the need for travel is eliminated" (p. 13). Other po-tential advantages come from improvements in digital imaging, virtual reality, and diagnostic enhancements by means of intelligent computer systems resulting in improved clinical quality and integration with other telemedicine applications.

Of course teleradiology also has potential problems. Computer net-works or servers can crash, which may result in a loss of radiographic images. "The old adage of 'never let the film out of your sight' is not ap-plicable to digital imaging systems where an image could vanish instan-taneously during outages" (Ricci & Borrelli, 2004, p. 67). In addition, whereas historically light is all that is required to view radiographs, com-puter monitors to view digital images are less readily available in com-parison. Despite these issues, the use of telemedicine has very practical and important global implications. For instance, health care services may now become accessible to areas otherwise not served by specialist care, such as geographically remote areas (as in the example just discussed), or less developed countries tapping into medical expertise from another country.

Tele-Homecare

In addition to linking physicians with each other, telemedicine applica-tions work equally well connecting patients in the home with health care providers. Tele-homecare combines telemedicine and home monitoring of physiological variables of patients who are elderly or underserved or homebound with chronic illness. Using PCs, the Internet, and physiologi-cal monitoring devices, these technologies installed in the patient's home facilitate a two-way communication between patient and health care provider. In general, tele-homecare virtual visits might lead to improved home health care quality at reduced cost, greater patient satisfaction with care, increased access to health care providers and fewer patients transferring to higher, more costly levels of care (TeleHomeCare, 2005).

At the University of Minnesota, researchers piloted a tele-homecare program that focused on three health problems that heavily utilize home health care resources: heart failure, chronic obstructive pulmonary disease, and wound care. It involved four clinical partners encompassing both urban and rural Minnesota and found that allowing patients to stay at home while receiving care provided a major positive impact on patient outcomes. Similar technology has since been introduced into nursing homes in rural Minnesota, which allow staff to consult with area hospitals to determine whether a nursing home patient should be transferred to the hospital or receive care while remaining at the home.

Electronic Medical Records (EMR)

Electronic medical records or electronic health records offer the promise of gathering, storing, and using health information more efficiently, and as a result, increase the effectiveness and quality of care and greatly reduce errors and costs (Institute of Medicine, 2001). A 2003 survey found that "87% of EMR users claim enhanced care, 78% claim increased patient satisfaction and 89% claim increased patient adherence to managed care formularies. Also, EMR usage advanced from 22% in 2001 to 30% in 2002, and 34% of the survey respondents said they would implement EMR systems within the next 18 months" (Podichetty & Penn, 2004, quoting Knoop, 2003, p. 94). Yet, according to a 2002 study, 58% of British and 90% of Swedish physicians use EMRs, as opposed to only 17% of U.S. primary care physicians (Podichetty & Penn, 2004, citing Chin, 2002).

We already have mentioned two EMR initiatives, in the United States and England. In England, where the NHS is implementing a national records service, some GPs are concerned that the software system most GPs use has not been chosen as the preferred software system by the local service providers (Coombes, 2004b, p. 1157-a). "We are being asked to change our tried and tested system for one that, in some cases, hasn't even been written yet," one doctor was quoted as saying.

In an effort to address concerns of system integration and national standards, in 2003 the United States' Institute of Medicine issued a report, titled *Key Capabilities of an Electronic Health Record System*, identifying eight core functions that electronic health records should be capable of performing in order to promote greater safety, quality, and efficiency in health care delivery. Specifically, electronic records must protect patient privacy and confidentiality by meeting the standards for security, storage and exchange of data required by the Health Insurance Portability and Accountability Act (HIPAA).

In January 2005, a "road map" for building a national health information network was presented to the government's national health information technology coordinator (Lohr, 2005, p. C1). The report called for an incremental approach with initial government financing and concluded that "patients should control their own records, deciding whether their information can be used in studies for effectiveness of certain treatments and drugs" and that the health network should "operate somewhat like Internet-based email, in which people using different types of computers and software can send and receive messages because the open, standard technology for handling messages is used by everyone" (p. C1).

Another barrier to electronic medical records is the physicians themselves. "Many attempts to get clinicians to use electronic health records have failed, often because of difficulties with data entry" (Walsh, 2004, p. 1184). Clinicians use a narrative-based model for health records, so that most EMR systems, with their requirement of structured data entry, are seen by the physician as too rigid and too much work. For physicians to embrace this technology, developers of electronic records systems should create tools that will support an interactive, social process of record management.

Electronic Research Networks

Leveling patient access to the latest drugs and clinical trials is a goal of the Electronic Primary Care Research Network (ePCRN), a project funded by the National Institutes of Health as part of its "Roadmap" initiative to speed the movement of research from the bench to the bedside. By electronically networking primary care physicians, the ePCRN has potential to tap into a previously underutilized patient base, as primary care providers deliver the majority of patient care in the U.S. (U.S. Department of Health and Human Services, 2001). The network, using Internet2 technology, will give researchers access to potential study subjects throughout the country while establishing a connection that will speed the application of research findings into communities that may not have direct access to research institutions. For instance, the network will alert primary care physicians to patients who might be eligible for a clinical trial. The physician and patient can then discuss treatment options. If the patient decides to participate in the clinical trial, the primary care physician will oversee the protocol locally; meaning, the patient will not have to travel to a research site.

Another benefit to ePCRN is targeted dissemination of information to primary care physicians, through integration with electronic health records. In this way, specific information about potential clinical trials as well as targeted reminders and comparative studies can be communicated to the clinic, helping to keep the practice up to date. It also allows clinics to participate in a national registry in order to track the status of specific conditions or diseases, such as flu or tuberculosis. The program, being led by researchers at the University of Minnesota, includes collaborators at Birmingham University in England (where research networks are already in existence, although on a lesser scale) and the University of California, San Francisco.

E-Prescribing

E-prescribing, included in the United States Medicare law, also is predicted to provide enormous savings. According to a 2004 editorial in the journal *Modern Healthcare*, e-prescribing could mean "a reduction of administrative costs of about $4 per prescription for an estimated total savings of $13 billion annually; a reduction estimated at $10 per prescription for mail-order drugs, worth about $11 billion annually; savings on formulary or generic drugs, estimated to be as much as $36 billion annually; savings because of a reduction in prescription errors, a possible $36 billion; and untold billions of dollars saved in the decline of prescription fraud and abuse" (Novelli, 2004, p. 32). Other estimates are more conservative. The *British Medical Journal* cites a savings in the United States of at least $29 billion: $27 billion from fewer prescription duplications, automatic suggestions of cheaper generic drugs, and warning of potential problems with drug interactions and incorrect dosages, and another $2 billion from "fewer prescribing errors resulting in doctors' visits or stays in hospitals" (Hopkins Tanne, 2004, p. 1155).

In addition to physician e-prescribing, patients are able to directly access online pharmacies. A recent article examining the controversies and legal issues of using the Internet for filling prescriptions (Fung, Woo, & Asch, 2004) states that online pharmacies fall into three major categories: "independent Internet-only sites, online branches of 'brick-and-mortar' pharmacies, and sites representing partnership among neighborhood pharmacies" (p. 188). Online pharmacies offer potential benefits of "increased access, lower transaction and product costs, and greater anonymity." However, concerns around online pharmacies include "the use of 'cyberdoctors,' dispensing drugs without prescriptions from other sites, and importation of prescription medications." For instance, patients using "cyberdoctors" by completing online questionnaires with selections that help obtain the medication in question, may not disclose symptoms to their local provider or may even avoid consulting their local physician altogether. A danger of dispensing drugs without prescriptions was highlighted following the anthrax cases in 2001, when it became clear that ciprofloxacin had been obtained without a prescription. In addition, patient safety may be compromised when obtained in this way, possibly exposing themselves to dangerous drug interactions and/or adverse effects. Finally, Fung et al. (2004) noted there is continued concern over the importation of foreign drugs via the Internet. Although the "importation of unapproved, misbranded, or adulterated drugs is unlawful" and in the United States "[f]oreign-made versions of U.S.-approved medications are also generally not permitted," it is possible that some sites may " 'dispense expired, subpotent, contaminated or counterfeit product[s]' " (p. 191).

In a somewhat different vein, in Canada there is concern that online sales of drugs to the United States, estimated at C$1 billion a year, "could threaten the domestic supply and Canada's low prices" (Westell, 2005, p. 10). As a result, the Canadian government is examining proposals to protect the Canadian system, such as requiring Canadian doctors to see a U.S. patient prior to approving a prescription. In response, a consortium of Canada's online pharmacies says they "are prepared to move to Britain if the federal government follows through on proposals that would in effect put them out of business" (Westell, 2005, p. 10). It's clear that the issue is complicated, with implications of safety, access, regulation, and commerce all playing a part in the debate.

E-Mail Communication

Another major area with great potential for increased efficiency and access, yet with concerns, is the use of e-mail for patient communication (see Rice & Katz, chap. 8, this volume). Enhanced patient and clinician communication was identified by the Institute of Medicine (2001) as one of the five key areas in which information technology could contribute to improved health care; specifically that " 'the health care system should be responsive at all times . . . and that access to care should be provided over the Internet, by phone . . . in addition to face-to-face visits' and that 'a 2-minute email communication could meet many patients' needs more responsively and at a lower cost' " (Patt, Houston, Jenckes, Sands, & Ford, 2003, quoting IOM, 2001, p. e9). Not surprisingly, more and more physicians are increasingly using e-mail to communicate with their patients. Among physicians who use e-mail with patients, Patt et al.'s (2003) study found that e-mail communication enhanced chronic-disease management. "Physicians reported better and more consistent communication with patients who have chronic diseases and require frequent, small changes in management" (p. e9). In addition, physicians noted other benefits, including "continuity of communication with patients (particularly patients who travel), ability to respond to nonurgent issues on their own time, avoidance of phone tag with patients" (p. e9), as well as tending to drug refill requests and sending out educational information, such as links to reliable Internet sources. Barriers to use of e-mail included potential overuse of e-mail by patients, inappropriate or urgent e-mail content, confidentiality issues, and lack of reimbursement for this service.

Some of these perceived barriers are being addressed by the American Medical Association and the American College of Physicians. For instance, these organizations have urged insurers and health plans to explore ways to compensate doctors for using e-mail, either per message or the episode of illness or through a set per-patient or global practice fee (Delbanco & Sands, 2004). Despite suggestions that e-mail may recover costs of telephone calls, missed or unnecessary appointments, medication errors, prescription requests, many physicians are not convinced of e-mail's potential cost savings. "Two thirds of doctors say that they would use e-mail, but only if they were paid for the time involved" (p. 1706).

HEALTH CARE PROFESSIONAL EDUCATION

Although Richardson (2003) identified this category as continuing education for health care professionals, we have broadened it to encompass all health care professional education—from first-year health care students to practicing physicians, nurses, allied health care professionals, health care administrators, and medical technicians.

It is interesting to note that some of the same technologies being used in clinical applications are also being used for educational purposes. For instance, lectures are transmitted to remote or satellite locations, similar to telemedicine. Likewise, surgical techniques are shown via the Internet technologies as distance learning. A particularly interesting example of online learning is called "Supercourse," a free online library of about 1,700 public health lectures, funded by the National Library of Medicine and the National Institutes of Health (Yamey, 2004). Led by Ron LaPorte, professor of epidemiology at the University of Pennsylvania–Pittsburgh, the PowerPoint-compatible lectures are aimed at "teaching the teachers" of public health, particularly to help "information deficiencies" in developing countries (Yamey, 2004, p. 1158). Because many developing countries have a problem with bandwidth capacity, LaPorte solved the problem by copying the Supercourse into local servers. Says LaPorte: " 'While a journal article is linear, we can be multidimensional.' And while it takes years for researchers to share their findings via medical journals, they can share them immediately by posting a lecture on the Supercourse" (p. 1158). To ensure quality control, lectures are reviewed before posting and updating content is encouraged by posting several different lectures on each topic and providing a function for adding comments or updates. The Supercourse series receives an estimated 75 million hits a year.

In addition to increased access to information, Internet technologies allow medical students to encounter their curriculum in new ways. At the University of Minnesota's Medical School, students practice clinical care at a "virtual clinic." The Minnesota Virtual Clinic (MVC) is a web-based virtual clinic supported by a simulated electronic medical records system. Students "visit" the clinic on a weekly basis to learn new information about their patients and are exposed to a number of the realities of medical practice, such as missed appointments and financial constraints. Students follow their patients and families throughout the first 2 years of the medical school curriculum. Patients represent a range of situations, from unusual diseases to pregnancy. Progression occurs in real time; that is, in the MVC a pregnancy typically lasts 9 months. Patient conditions have been carefully designed to match concepts taught in the courses during the medical students' first 2 years.

Internet technologies also can change the way a specific course or field is taught—such as anatomy. New "virtual" methods of teaching anatomy are being explored as "developments in computer capabilities and data processing offer the potential for more realistic and educationally valuable experiences than ever before" (Shaffer, 2004, p. 1280). Although virtual dissection may address some problems surrounding traditional methods, such as storage of cadavers, being time-consuming, and expensive, it is also much more complex, "requiring three dimensions and ideally including tactile information" (p. 1280).

Internet technologies also allow sharing of information that otherwise would be inaccessible. At the University of Minnesota, researchers have developed a way to show how an actual human heart beats—from the inside. The method, developed at the University in conjunction with Medtronic, a medical device company, uses an isolated heart apparatus to artificially stimulate a donor heart to beat outside of the body. A special videoscope is then inserted into the heart's interior, and because a clear fluid is used instead of blood, the inner workings of the heart—the valve action, the contractions of atria and ventricles, and the heart's architecture—can be seen as the heart beats. This visualization is a benefit to students studying cardiac anatomy, as well as to those in the medical device industry interested in developing cardiac instruments, such as pacemakers and valves. Equally important, these images are being made available on the Internet for students throughout the world to access.

Yet, it is important to remember that newer technologies in and of themselves do not result in better education. Information is one thing;

the ability to apply it in clinical settings is another. In other words: "The strength of e-learning is also its weakness. . . . The information revolution is just another, albeit amazingly effective, way to deliver information, but it only makes the challenge of selection more stark. [T]he real challenge to e-learning enthusiasts is to enhance the judgment of practitioners, to find ways to ensure that that 'expert judgment' can be transferred to doctors in the field" (Klass, 2004, p. 1148).

PRIVACY

Privacy is a top concern among users and consumers of e-health, with implications across e-health applications. Indeed, entire books, collections, and special issues of journals have addressed the broad and varied concerns of privacy in an e-health setting, including right of access and intended use of personal data. For our purposes, we provide an overview of privacy, followed by specific examples illustrating the unique implications in this field (see also Wallis & Rice, chap. 14, this volume).

Kelly and McKenzie (2002) identified the main features of online privacy to include: individuals' right to determine what information is collected and how it is used; ability to access personal information held and know that it is accurate and safe; anonymity in web-usage (not being tracked); and, ability to send and receive e-mail messages or other data "without being intercepted or read by persons other than the intended recipient(s)" (p. e12). To help maintain privacy, the authors suggest using firewalls, message and browser encryption, and digital signatures. However, ensuring privacy in e-health applications requires more specific and complex safety measures, beyond mere technology to include human judgment; for instance, deciding when electronic communication is appropriate (Bodenheimer & Grumbach, 2003).

In the United States, the federal government mandated privacy standards for patient health information in the form of the Health Insurance Portability and Accountability Act (HIPAA) of 1996, which took effect April 2003. HIPAA establishes minimum standards for protecting the privacy of individually identifiable health information, including information that is transmitted electronically (U.S. Department of Health and Human Services, 2005).

Of course, the technology itself must be able to accommodate privacy compliance standards. Ricci and Borrelli (2004) discussed HIPAA regulations in terms of teleradiology, warning that lower cost systems may not be HIPAA-compliant in preserving patient privacy. Systems must be able to provide secure data transmission with encryption and password protection and sometimes older or lower cost equipment cannot meet these requirements.

Cohen (2004) offered some specific measures to ensure information system security. Although too detailed for our purposes here, we mention a few: systems that force regular password changes; passwords of eight or more digits including letters, numbers, and special characters; automatic logouts; controlled access to data closets and server rooms; virus scanners that do not interfere with medical applications; logging server administrator access, failed login attempts, and auditing the logs.

More broadly, various initiatives cover ethics beyond privacy. One such initiative, the Internet Healthcare Coalition developed an "e-Health Code of Ethics," which examines the following areas: candor and honesty, quality, informed consent, privacy and data security, professionalism in online health care, responsible partnering, and accountability (Crigger, 2002). Although not legally binding, unlike HIPAA, these codes and others like them are voluntary standards that outline expectations for how participants will behave. In addition, codes of ethics let participants and the public know what's at stake in regards to e-health practices and applications, as well as identifying best practices. Issues of patient and medical privacy will only increase in importance, especially since privacy and related laws are culture and context-specific.

E-HEALTH: THE FUTURE

In a recent article, U.S. Senate Majority Leader, William Frist, MD, speculates what e-health will be like in the year 2015 with a fictionalized account of patient Rodney Rogers.

> Because of the widespread availability and use of reliable information, which has generated increased provider-level competition, the cost of health care has stabilized and in some cases has actually fallen, whereas quality and efficiency have risen. Rodney periodically accesses his multidisciplinary primary medical team using e-mail, video conferencing, and home blood monitoring. He owns his privacy–protected, electronic medical record. He also chose to have a tiny, radio-frequency computer chip implanted in his abdomen that monitors his blood chemistries and blood pressure. . . . Unfortunately, chest pain develops one day while Rodney is on a weekend trip several hundred miles from home. The emergency room physician quickly accesses all of Rodney's up-to-date medical information. Thanks to interoperability standards adopted by the federal government in 2008, nearly every emergency room in the United States can access Rodney's health history, with his permission . . . [and then the] hospital transmits the computerized information about Rodney's treat-

ment seamlessly and paperlessly, to Rodney's insurer for billing and payment. (Frist, 2005, p. 267)

Frist (2005) goes on to articulate what is required to make this scenario viable, where the "inefficient health care sectors of 2005" are transformed into a "retooled, dynamic, streamlined health care system for 2015" (p. 268). By introducing policies for a "patient-centered, consumer-driven, and provider-friendly health care system," he envisions a system supporting "not only the finest technology and research but also the most efficient, the lowest-cost, and the highest-quality clinical care in the world" (p. 268). But what does Frist's scenario mean, in practical terms? In reviewing the literature surrounding e-health, what we see here is a call for both quality and cooperation: quality in available information and secure systems, for instance, and cooperation between providers, disciplines, and countries. Yet, although e-health applications are poised to expand and take advantage of the reach, speed, and other powerful features of the Internet, the medical community views this trend with guarded optimism and sometimes with very practical concerns, noting, for example that "[t]he benefit to physicians of using e-health systems is evident through improved quality of patient care, improved patient–physician communication, reduction of abundant paper records, and gaining a more knowledgeable patient population. However, e-health meets with resistance because of the time investment required to learn computer skills, questionable Internet resources, computer phobia, and a fear of decline in patient–physician relationship" (Podichetty & Penn, 2004, p. 94). Yet it is clear to many that:

> [t]he health system cannot remain oblivious to our rapidly changing technological landscape and mindset. Perhaps for the first time in history, we have the tools to create flexible services that meet the needs of the population and health professionals alike, regardless of who or where they are. The Institute of Medicine, in its 2001 report *Crossing the quality chasm: A new health system for the 21st century*, makes the following statement about health care in the U.S.: "Between the health care we have and the care we could have lies not just a gap, but a chasm." (p. 1)

This statement is all the more accurate with regard to health care on a global scale. The gap or chasm between what most people of the world have for health care and what they might have is enormous. The World Health Organization, for example, notes that "[m]ore than one billion people—*one sixth of the world's population*—live in extreme poverty, lacking the safe water, proper nutrition, basic health care and social services needed to survive" (World Health Organization, 2005a, emphasis added).

What role is the Internet currently playing, what future roles might the Internet play? Can Internet technologies help bridge these gaps in health care access, education, and interventions across the world? "Realising the potential of the revolution in electronic communications will require a major shift from our ethic of competition and narrow self interest, focused on gadgets—to one of generosity and collaboration, centred on people" (Jadad & Delamothe, 2004, p. 1144).

Perhaps one of the most potentially wide-ranging initiatives covering these areas is the World Health Organization's eHealth for Health Care Delivery (eHCD) program. This program is designed to support digital health applications in the following areas: prevention, patient diagnosis and patient management and care (World Health Organization, 2005b). The program's overview sounds like the perfect prescription for taking e-health to the next level on a global scale:

> Through these applications, it is possible to take specialized care to primary health-care centers in remote areas and thereby broaden and improve the quality of the services they offer. By connecting primary health workers to primary health-care centres and connecting these centres electronically to departments and referral centres in hospitals for the exchange of data a significant improvement in access and cost-effectiveness may be effected. Primary health care is thus the main target of the eHCD programme. (p. 4)

It will be exciting to be part of this new century of developments in e-health. Success will require a global approach and strong use of interdisciplinary teams. If ever the time was right to explore the power of the Internet for human health, it is now.

REFERENCES

Ahern, D. K., Phalen, J. M., & Mockenhaupt, R. E. (2003). Science and the advancement of eHealth: A call to action. *American Journal of Preventive Medicine, 24*(1), 108–109.

Bodenheimer, T., & Grumbach, K. (2003). Electronic technology: A spark to revitalize primary care? *Journal of the American Medical Association, 290*(2), 259–264.

Chin, T. (2002, September 2). Americans trail much of Europe in adopting EMRs. *American Medical News*, p. 34.

Cohen, T. (2004). Medical and information technologies converge. *Engineering in Medicine and Biology*, 59–65.

Coombes, R. (2004a). All hospital bookings to be done electronically by end of 2005. *BMJ, 328*, 1157.

Coombes, R. (2004b). GPs worried about having to change to new untested software systems. *BMJ, 328*, 1157-a.

Crigger, B. (2002). Foundations of the eHealth code of ethics. *Internet Healthcare Coalition.* Retrieved March 10, 2005, from http://www.ihealthcoalition.org/ethics/code-foundations.html

Delbanco, T., & Sands, D. Z. (2004). Electrons in flight—email between doctors and pa-tients. *New England Journal of Medicine, 350*(17), 1705–1707.

Europa: Europe's Information Society Thematic Portal. (2005). *Information can save your life.* Retrieved February 12, 2005, from http://www.europa.eu.int/information_soci-ety/qualif/health/index_en.htm

Frist, W. H. (2005). Health care in the 21st century. *The New England Journal of Medicine, 352,* 267–272.

Fung, C. F., Woo, H. E., & Asch, S. M. (2004). Controversies and legal issues of prescribing and dispensing medication using the Internet. *Mayo Clinic Proceedings, 79,* 188–194.

Gamble, J. E., Savage, G. T., & Icenogle, M. L. (2004). Value-chain analysis of a rural health program: Toward understanding the most benefit of telemedicine applications. *Hospital Topics, 82*(1), 10–17.

Gustafson, D. H., & Wyatt, J. C. (2004). Evaluation of ehealth systems and services. *BMJ, 328,* 1150.

Health e-Technologies Initiative. (2005). *Web portal awards.* Retrieved March 10, 2005, from http://www.hetinitiative.org/sub-call_for_proposals/cfp-grantee_info.html

Hopkins Tanne, J. (2004). Electronic prescribing could save at least $29bn. *BMJ, 328,* 1155.

Humber, M. (2004). National programme for information technology. *BMJ, 328,* 1145–1146.

Institute of Medicine, Committee on Quality of Health Care in America. (2001). *Crossing the quality chasm: A new health system for the 21st century.* Washington, DC: National Acad-emies Press.

Institute of Medicine, Committee on Data Standards for Patient Safety. (2003). *Key capabili-ties of an electronic health record system: A letter report.* Washington, DC: National Acad-emies Press.

Jadad, A. R., & Delamothe, T. (2004). What next for electronic communication and health care? *BMJ, 328,* 1143–1144.

Kalb, C., & Soukop, E. (2004, August 9). Get ready for e-medicine. *Newsweek, 144*(6), 53.

Kelly, G., & McKenzie, B. (2002). Security, privacy, and confidentiality issues on the Internet. *Journal of Medical Internet Research, 4*(2), e12.

Kilpatrick, K. (2004). Telemedicine: On, under and out of this world. *Canadian Medical Asso-ciation Journal, 171*(7), 716.

Klass, D. J. (2004). Will e-learning improve clinical judgment? *BMJ, 328,* 1147–1148.

Knoop, C. A., Lovich, D., Silverstein, M. B., et al. (2003). *Vital signs: e-health in the United States.* Boston, MA: The Boston Consulting Group.

Kuruvilla, S., Dzenowagis, J., Pleasant, A., Dwivedi, R., Murthy, N., Samuel, R., & Scholtz, M. (2004). Digital bridges need concrete foundations: Lessons from the Health Inter-Network India. *BMJ, 328,* 1193–1196.

Lohr, S. (2005, January 19). Road map to a digital system of health records. *The New York Times,* p. C1.

Maulden, S. A. (2003). Information technology, the Internet, and the future of neurology. *The Neurologist, 9,* 149–159.

Naik, G. (2003, December 3). England plans major revamp of health care. *The Wall Street Journal,* p. B1.

Nissen, S. E., Abdulla, A. M., Khandheira, B. K., Kienzle, M. G., & Zaher, C. A. (2004). Working Group 6: The role of technology to enhance clinical and educational efficiency. *Journal of the American College of Cardiology, 44*(2), 256–260.

Novelli, B. (2004). The promise and the reality. *Modern Healthcare, 34*(33), 32.

Parekh, S. G., Nazarian, D. G., & Lim, C. K. (2004). Adoption of information technology by resident physicians. *Clinical Orthopaedics and Related Research, 421,* 107–111.

Patt, M. R., Houston, T. K., Jenckes, M. W., Sands, D. Z., & Ford, D. E. (2003). Doctors who are using e-mail with their patients: A qualitative exploration. *Journal of Medical Internet Research, 5*(2), e9.

Podichetty, V., & Penn, D. (2004). The progressive roles of electronic medicine: Benefits, concerns, and costs. *American Journal of Medical Science, 328*(2), 94–99.

Ricci, W. M., & Borrelli, J. (2004). Teleradiology in orthopaedics. *Clinical Orthopaedics and Related Research, 421,* 64–69.

Richardson, R. (2003). eHealth for Europe. In B. Blobel & P. Pharow (Eds.), *Advanced health telematics and telemedicine* (pp. 151–156). Amsterdam: IOS Press.

Rodrigues, R. J. (2000). Ethical and legal issues in interactive health communications: A call for international cooperation. *Journal of Medical Internet Research, 2*(1), e8.

Rodrigues, R. J., & Risk, A. (2003). eHealth in Latin America and the Caribbean: Development and policy issues. *Journal of Medical Internet Research, 5*(1), e4.

Safran, C. (2003). The collaborative edge: Patient empowerment for vulnerable populations. *International Journal for Medical Informatics, 69,* 185–190.

Shaffer, K. (2004). Teaching anatomy in the digital world. *The New England Journal of Medicine, 351*(13), 1279–1281.

Smith, C. (2004). New technology continues to invade healthcare. *Nursing Administration Quarterly, 28*(2), 92–98.

Smith, R. (2004). Can IT lead to radical redesign of health care? *BMJ, 328*(7449).

TeleHomeCare. (2005). *About TeleHomeCare.* Retrieved January 27, 2005, from http://www.telehomecare.umn.edu/about.html

U.S. Department of Health and Human Services (HHS). (2001). Public Health Service, Centers for Disease Control and Prevention. National Center for Health Statistics. Data unpublished.

U.S. Department of Health and Human Services (HHS). (2004). *HHS awards $139 million to drive adoption of health information technology.* Retrieved February 12, 2005, from http://www.hhs.gov/news/press/2004pres/20041013.html

U.S. Department of Health and Human Services (HHS). (2005). *HIPAA privacy rule.* Retrieved February 12, 2005, from http://privacyruleandresearch.nih.gov/pr_04.asp

Walsh, S. (2004). The clinician's perspective on electronic health records and how they can affect patient care. *BMJ, 328,* 1184–1187.

Watson, R. (2004). EU wants every member to develop a 'roadmap' for e-health. *BMJ, 328,* 1155.

Westell, D. (2005, January 10). Canada's online drug dispensaries mull UK shift. *Financial Times,* p. 10.

Wilson, E. V., & Lankton, N. K. (2004). Modeling patients' acceptance of provider-delivered e-health. *Journal of the American Medical Informatics Association, 11*(4), 241–248.

World Health Organization (WHO). (2005a). *WHO highlights health in the 2015 development blueprint.* Retrieved February 12, 2005, from http://www.who.int/mediacentre/news/releases/2005/pr06/en/index.html

World Health Organization (WHO). (2005b). *Strategy 2004–2007: eHealth for Health-care Delivery.* Retrieved February 12, 2005, from http://www.who.int/eht/en/eHealth_HCD.pdf

Yamey, G. (2004). The professor of "telepreventive medicine". *BMJ, 328,* 1158.

Chapter 3

E-Research and E-Learning: Could Online Virtual Environments Help Doctors Take Better Care of Patients?

Monica Murero
University of Florence-MICC, Italy

NEW E-RESEARCH
AND E-LEARNING ENVIRONMENTS

In the last century, medical advances have been perhaps humanity's greatest achievement (Epstein, 2004). More and more sophisticated computer-based systems have contributed to medical accomplishments and education in every discipline, from radiology to genetic engineering and cloning.

At the same time, medical educators are under considerable pressure to enhance the quality and safety of medical care (Ruderich, Bauch, Haag, Heid, Leven, et al., 2004). International patient safety movements and policymakers demand that simulation-based medical education becomes an ethical imperative to Hippocrates's maxim "first do no harm" (Gallagher & Cates, 2004). Education preparation is a key factor in patient care, as it has a direct impact on morbidity and mortality rate. In 2000 Starfield reported that in U.S. hospitals there are more than 100,000 deaths per year due to various errors. Another study found a strong correlation between the educational level of nurses working in hospital and patients' mortality after common surgeries (Aiken, Clarke, Cheung, Sloane, & Silber, 2003).

Nowadays, medical training on "real" patients is no longer acceptable (Gallagher & Cates, 2004). There is an increasing demand for simulation-based medical training and patients' security. The recent diffusion of the

Internet is facilitating the creation and development of "new" learning and research environments for physicians, promising to push the medical armamentarium and patients' care further ahead. For example, continuing advances in Virtual Reality (VR) technology, now available through the Internet at increasingly low cost and at the convenience of multi-synchronous and remote access, have the potential to open new frontiers—but also new barriers—in medical education and practice all over the world (Murero, 2006). Moreover, new Internet-mediated research environments for physicians facilitating unprecedented access, production, and exchange of crucial medical discoveries, have the potential to accelerate new achievements for the study and cure of severe diseases that are affecting humanity, such as cancer and HIV/AIDS, because more and more physicians are using e-research and e-learning environments (Harris Interactive, 2003; Rice & Katz, chap. 8, this volume).

Yet, the validity of "new" virtual learning and research environments is still controversial, and needs to be further investigated (Murero, 2006). This chapter contributes to that goal by analyzing an extensive interdisciplinary literature and numerous examples. Moreover, the chapter investigates two contexts in particular: e-learning and e-research virtual environments designed for doctors. We question two central aspects: (1) the validity of e-learning environments (E-LEs; Murero, 2006) to educate and train medical students and practitioners online, by overcoming traditional boundaries—space, time and place—characterizing the traditional learning experience, and (2) the validity of e-research environments (E-REs) to overcome classic constraints for the production, access, and exchange of medical advances within the international scientific community.

The chapter also (3) assesses 93 medical associations' Web sites' coverage of the topics doctors declared to use the most when online—e-research and e-learning—in highly trusted and influential medical virtual environments.

Finally, (4) the chapter questions whether Internet-based learning and research environments have the potential to help doctors take better care of patients. It reflects on the opportunity of introducing attentive policies to help close the digital—and cultural—medical divide, in light of future scenarios that are expected to deeply impact medical research and revolutionize health care in the next few years.

WHAT ARE LEARNING ENVIRONMENTS?

Wilson (1995) defined a "learning environment" as an instructional metaphor—a classroom, a museum, or an operating room may become a learning environment. Following a constructivism theoretical approach,

Wilson defined VLEs as computer-based or virtual learning environments. Computer-based programs simulating the human anatomy are an example of VLEs.

With the diffusion of the Internet, deep differences emerge between "online" and "offline" virtual learning environments. When computer-based simulations of medical procedures became available on the Internet, multispace and polysynchronous accessibility can be granted to multiple users beyond geographical constraints. Learners interact with other networked participants, and with distributed information tools allowing for increased consulting, training and telementoring (Edelson, Pea, & Gomez, 1996). Telementoring is the use at a distance of audio, video and other ICTs, including the Internet, to exchange medical information, guidance, or instructions for the diagnosis or treatment of a medical condition between more experienced medical personnel (mentors) and trainees or less experienced health care providers.

Recently, Murero has defined *online virtual environments for learning* (E-LEs) as Internet-mediated or -located learning environments, which can overcome traditional boundaries of space, time, and place, and are accessible via the Internet and new information and communication technologies (see Weiss, Nolan, Hunsinger, & Trifonas, 2006). E-LEs present several advantages compared to traditional offline VLEs (Hiltz & Goldman, 2004; Winn & Jackson, 1999), but they also represent design challenges and concerns (Wilson, 1995).

E-LEARNING AND MEDICAL EDUCATION

Medical Simulations and VR Before the Internet

Before the diffusion of the Internet, computer-based patient simulations (CBPS) and virtual reality (VR) technology offered—and continue to offer today—very important educational advantages. Since the 1960s, medical trainees have acquired "risk-free" medical skills by practicing on virtual subjects, rather than real patients. Several authors have validated the usefulness of VR in medical training (Torkington, Smith, Rees, & Darzi, 2001). Recently Grantcharov and colleagues (2004) showed that in the surgical field, VR training significantly reduces students' errors in keyhole gallbladder surgery and, therefore, should be implemented in surgical training programs, confirming previous results (Ali, Mowery, Kaplan, & DeMaria, 2002; Seymour, Gallagher, Roman, O'Brien, Bansal, et al., 2002).

Virtual reality simulations now available in E-LE, virtual hospitals, and virtual patients, offer increased benefits for learners, such as risk-free practice (avoiding hurting real patients), low-cost and convenient multi-synchronous and remote access, case reproducibility, and flexibility for improved skills acquisition that may help shorten the learning curve of diagnostic and treatment procedures (Ahlberg, Heikkinen, Iselius, Leijon-marck, Rutqvist, et al., 2002; Gallagher & Cates, 2004; Gerson & Van Dam, 2003; Grantcharov et al., 2004; Murero, 2006; Ogan, Jacomides, Shulman, Roehrborn, Cadeddu, et al., 2004; Riva, Bacchetta, Cesa, Conti, & Molinari, 2002; Rizzo, Strickland, & Bouchard, 2004; Seymour et al., 2002; Torkington et al., 2001; Winn & Jackson, 1999). E-LEs are helping doctors take better care of patients in areas such as cardiology, radiology, and pathology (Gomez-Arbones, Ferreira, Pique, Roca, Tomas, et al., 2004; Grunewald, Gebhard, Jakob, Wagner, Hothorn, et al., 2004; Marchevsky, Relan, & Baillie, 2003).

Gerson and Van Dam (2003) suggested that medical educators should always associate innovative VR-based endoscopy simulation with traditional—for example, real patients—teaching protocols. VR systems are enormously beneficial for medical training, but still operate within the constraints of the "traditional boundaries" of the learning experience.

Web-Based Medical Courses

The recent development of online learning environments is promising to push medical education and patients' treatment further ahead. Web-based university courses have recently appeared in several countries where the courses were previously inaccessible to students and trainees were unable to attend courses on schedule. In France, for example, WeBS-Surg offers online virtual reality-based applications to train medical students living in remote areas (Grunewald et al., 2004; Marescaux, Soler, Mutter, Leroy, Vix, et al., 2000). At the University of Minnesota, the medical school provides training to young students through a web-based medical virtual clinic (MVC), which gives access to the records of virtual patients. In a 2-year period, students practice their newly acquired skills as patients virtually get older, pregnant, have financial constraints and suffer all sort of new medical problems over time (Speedie & Niewoehner, 2003; see also Gurak & Hudson, chap. 2, this volume). Another interesting example is provided by MIT, which allows free access to hundreds of online courses materials in several disciplines, including health care and technology, to anyone who has Internet access (see http://www.ocw.mit.edu/OcwWeb/Health-Sciences-and-Technology/index.htm). Courses vary from Acoustics of Speech to Genomics and Computational Biology. More than 20,000 professors and researchers (including six Nobel Prize winners) in 151 countries, have shared their medical lectures and built the Supercourse, a multiple-language *Library of Lectures* and courses that aims to train teachers from a distance, and smooth the progress of medical education, particularly in developing countries.

The diffusion of E-LEs stimulates new ways to teach a course as well. In Australia, Kumar and colleagues (2004) described the successful implementation of teaching microscopic pathology with online virtual slides, to closely simulate examination of glass slides with a real microscope. The online system enhanced the effectiveness of teaching histology and histopathology to trainees in remote and asynchronous environments. Moreover, E-LEs can help personalize the learning experience on the basis of individual needs. For example, CAMPUS (http://www .medicase.de) helps German-speaking practitioners examine medical cases online, and acquire advanced skills for patients' diagnosis as the system personalizes the training on the basis of users' characteristics and expertise (Ruderich et al., 2004).

E-LEs for Continuing Medical Education

In New York, a physician sits at home at her laptop computer and follows a "virtual classroom" alongside a slide presentation on emerging treatments for osteoporosis delivered by a specialist at the Mayo Clinic. She sends an e-mail question and receives an answer from the instructor. Finally she takes an online exam, and a few days later, receives a CME certificate in the mail granting her credit. For some physicians the days of travels to conferences and workshops to obtain CME credits are simply history (Gabriel, 2000). Thanks to E-LE, physicians can keep their license and learn about medical science any place, any time, without having to travel. The University of Iowa's *Virtual Hospital* offers free access to a digital health library that contains medical resources for students, teachers, and practitioners, but is also accessible to anyone online. The Web site provides hundreds of free online continuing medical education (CME) courses and books, where practitioners can also access virtual patients' records, including lab exams, ECG, and x-rays online at their convenience—overcoming limits of space, time, and place. In many countries, medical practitioners are required by law to attend continuing medical education courses in order to keep their license valid over time. Users can learn online about previous diagnosis and treatments of real cases, from several medical specialties (see http://www.hv.org). This new phenomenon is still limited to a privileged minority at the present (late 2005).

In sum, e-learning environments, including virtual reality online simulations, virtual courses, hospitals and training on virtual patients can help educate doctors and students by overcoming traditional boundaries, with virtually no risk to real patients.

Barriers still limit the diffusion of e-learning environments. VR systems of e-learning are still very scarce and very expensive to create and maintain over time. Demanding tasks are required to organizations and professional designers of medical education systems to maintain the efficiency of online learning environment over time; that could impede the diffusion of these important training systems. For example, the development of sophisticated E-LEs like CAMPUS often means hundreds of hours of preparatory work for web designers, who need to stimulate and integrate users' feedback into practice to improve current systems for personalized online medical training (Ruderich et al., 2004). In the future, more efficient design tools and new technologies should increase VR systems management.

E-RESEARCH ENVIRONMENTS

A Theoretical Approach

This section analyzes the second major context of our investigation. In our view, *online virtual environments for research* (E-REs) are Internet-mediated or -located research environments, which can overcome classic barriers connected with the research experience—space, time, and place—and are accessible via the Internet and new ICTs. As with E-LEs, E-REs also present several advantages compared to traditional offline computer-based environments (Winn & Jackson, 1999), but barriers as well.

E-Research in Context: Sharing Medical Knowledge

Advances in medical research are crucial means to foster progress in the study and cure of diseases such as cancer, heart, and brain impairments, or chronic conditions. However, when new medical discoveries are not effectively communicated within the international scientific community, there is a concrete risk that crucial information and knowledge is lost or duplicated, with the result that the cure of life-threatening diseases could be delayed. The creation of web-accessible databases organized by medical disciplines and updated by the international medico-scientific community is a growing reality that could well be extended to several medical research programs in the coming years. For example, use of the Internet can prevent loss of precious information by providing new environments for collecting knowledge about rare pathologies with a difficult nosographic classification that could lead to a patient's death without a certain diagnosis. At the present, these cases are rarely published or can be retrieved only with great difficulty. The Online Database of Unknown

Clinical Cases (ODUCC) provides an example of a novel Internet-based project that intends to fulfill this gap in medical research (Masoni, Guelfi, Conti, Conti, & Gensini, 2004).

Not only databases, but also virtual institutes of research are now created on interactive Web sites, to effectively foster exchange of medical findings within a scientific community. The Epigone Virtual Institute integrates online 63 leading European medical research teams from 10 countries to produce joint research programs and exchange knowledge in an interactive Web site, about epigenetic mechanisms (inheritable changes in the genome function, but without a change in the DNA sequence).

Similarly, in 2004, the British National Cancer Research Institute (NCRI) launched an important initiative to bring together international scientists in a virtual community to access and share findings to fight cancer disease, from genomics to clinical trials, in a common format across disciplines (Pincock, 2004). Moreover, the European Association for Palliative Care has created an online research network to share and promote existing knowledge among the members of 30 National Associations in 20 European countries, representing a movement of some 50,000 health care workers and volunteers. Palliative care is the active, total care of the patients whose disease is not responsive to curative treatment (see http://www.eapcnet.org/about/about.html).

The Internet also fosters many ways to improve communication among physicians. Online *mailing lists* and *forums* offer the opportunity to discuss emerging scientific issues and trends with peers in "real time," a growing phenomenon in major medical associations in several countries. The value of and access to online forums is particularly evident when compared to offline environments, like those hosted by periodicals—letters to the editor or to an author—and in workshops or conferences.

Transcending Distance, Place, and Time

Although barriers could limit access to e-research designed for doctors, particularly in developing countries, E-REs are facilitating information exchange and knowledge among the medical international community, by overcoming traditional boundaries (Masoni et al., 2004; Pincock, 2004). However, a limiting factor to consider is the sustainability over time of E-REs, mainly due to costs of maintenance. CliniWeb was one of the first e-research environments for doctors provided by the University of Oregon (USA) and described in the scientific literature in 1996. However, in 2003, it was removed from the World Wide Web because of the impossibility of providing up-to-date medical and biomedical information.

Public organizations and policymakers should develop and support E-REs over time. For example, the U.S.-based National Center for Biotechnology Information (NCBI) has become one of the most popular sites among physicians all over the world—but available for free to anyone online, as for the majority of the examples illustrated in this chapter. Furthermore, every month, 60 million searches are performed using PubMed (http://www.ncbi.nlm.nih.gov/entrez/query.fcgi), a major medical database available on the NCBI Web site, to retrieve thousands of abstract articles, online books, clinical research findings in many disciplines and even the whole Genome sequence. The significance of E-REs is particularly evident when compared with traditional library-based ways of doing medical research.

ARE E-REs AND E-LEs GROWING
PHENOMENA IN MEDICINE?

An Empirical Analysis

A 2002 study from Harris Interactive (2003) revealed that increasing numbers of physicians—90% compared to only 19% in 2001—reported using the Internet to research clinical information, 74% to search for medical journal articles, 63% to communicate with colleagues and (25%) with patients, whereas 58% of the sample use it for continuing medical education (CME), and 30% to access electronic medical records. Interestingly, e-research (clinical information, medical journals) appears as the most popular activity doctors do online, followed by communication and e-learning (CME).

However, there are few studies that clarify whether highly trusted and popular sources of information and communication for doctors (i.e., national and international medical associations and transnational medical organizations) are contributing to the growth and diffusion of e-learning and e-research in different contexts and countries. Medical associations are highly trusted and prestigious sources of information, communication and direction for peer physicians. In order to investigate more the growing interest for e-research and e-learning among doctors, we analyzed 93 Web sites of official medical associations in June 2005.

The phrase "medical associations" was entered in Google, which indicated there were 11,200,000 Web sites. We evaluated the first 50 results and selected the second Web site listed in those results, as it listed 93 links to medical associations' Web sites provided by Yahoo. Fourteen of the 93 were dropped because they were not valid for the analysis (i.e., not relevant, language barrier, or absence of valid links). In total, we selected 79 valid cases for our analysis in six areas of the world (Australia, Asia, Europe, Caribbean, North America, and South Africa). Fifty-eight Web sites were American and 21 were non-American, including three international associations.

In each Web site we first searched for the site map. This allowed us to identify the main content titles, as well as areas restricted to the members. Alternatively we used site-specific search engines when available. We content-analyzed all the Web sites to verify whether each one of them offered virtual e-resources to physicians in 4 major areas: (1) medical science; (2) communication—that is, virtual forums or mailing lists; (3) e-learning and CME; and (4) research or job opportunities. Of all the Web sites, 42% (33/79) offered job and research opportunities to young and senior doctors, a very valuable source of information. A large majority of medical associations' Web sites (61/79, or 77%) offered medical science resources, and 67% offered or provided links to educational courses, including CME and e-learning (though e-learning is offered only on the U.S. sites). This can be explained, in part, by the fact that CME courses are mandatory in several countries, including the United States. Approximately one third of the Web sites provide online forum or mailing lists for exchange of information, and discussion of medical issues among peers (23/79). Overall, in a few cases Web sites did not provide any of the four main features, or showed only one out of four. Those sites tended, instead, to provide legal and "people"-related information, such as members of the board, or the association's president.

Interestingly, online virtual environments for medical research and education are largely present in *official* medical association Web sites for physicians, in several countries and disciplines. When we analyze American associations in the light of previous studies on physicians using the Internet in the American context (Harris Interactive, 2003), it is interesting to note a very strong coincidence between the activities doctors declare to do the most, and the activities available in the Web sites, such as e-research and e-learning. This could be explained in part by the fact that medical associations are influenced by empirical research conducted on their members, that those studies are highly valid in representing doctors' needs and behavior, and that medical association Web sites are providing a good service to their members, in line with physicians' needs.

Further research should clarify the validity of e-research and e-learning resources provided to doctors in official and trusted peer-based organizations by including more countries in the analysis to provide a transnational and transcultural perspective. We are continuing our investigation by analyzing a very large database with associations from many countries and all continents.

COULD ONLINE VIRTUAL ENVIRONMENTS HELP DOCTORS TAKE BETTER CARE OF PATIENTS?

In sum, improved medical knowledge acquired online through E-LEs and E-REs that build "collective knowledge" (Levy, 1997) could well help doctors provide better diagnoses, tests and treatments, and patient care.

Future research should further clarify if online training based on VR systems has proved successful, as offline versions did, in reducing patients' morbidity and death rates in several different medical disciplines. According to the results of this chapter, E-LE-based VR simulations should confirm their validity. In surgical disciplines, an interesting future study could compare patients' postsurgery outcomes—error rates—in light of the previous training received by the operator, over time (i.e., VR systems offline and online versus traditional training).

The effects of using E-REs to help doctors provide better quality of patient care seem less evident than for E-LEs. Perhaps this is because e-research knowledge acquisition is a more abstract entity, more indirect, less explicit and more complex to measure; it cannot be easily summarized by improved patient care. The impact of E-LEs on surgical training, as in our example, can be more directly measured through changes in patients' health status after treatments, than other typologies of e-learning (CME) and e-research can; but that does not mean that the phenomenon is not occurring. Thus studies of the effectiveness of E-REs need different process as well as outcome measures.

Other variables might intervene in the relation between use of E-REs for medical scientific purposes and improved patients' care and should be further identified and tested in future studies, which would require longitudinal and before/after research designs. However, we think that using E-REs and E-LEs is not *per se* a sufficient condition to improve patients' care, but a very crucial one. For example, patients need high-quality diagnostic instruments, good facilities, professional nonmedical staff, good disinfection systems, as well as new scientific discoveries and a highly trained and knowledgeable doctor. Future research should provide scientific support to policymakers in safeguarding physicians' practice and patients' care, and clarify the nature and impact of online virtual environments over time.

E-LE AND E-RE: LIMITATIONS

A Techno-Educational Divide?

Cultural, technological, and financial barriers could invalidate the e-learning and e-research potential for health care provision. For example, in spite of the tremendous impact that offline and online virtual reality systems are having on the health care field, clinicians and surgeons remain unaware or skeptical of their actual potentiality in medical training and practice, and their possible future applications (D'Ancona, Murero, Bergsland, & Karamanoukian, 2001; Grantcharov et al., 2004). We agree with Gallagher and Cates (2004) who observed that further empirical evidence is required to persuade conservative members of the medical community to use advanced tools for virtual reality simulations in their teaching methods. Further studies should clarify why medical instructors are not using highly sophisticated simulation-based learning environments. Are these systems not available? If they are, what cultural, technical and financial components might impede their adoption? What effects on patients' care do health providers perceive? Does this phenomenon have the potential to create an "educational divide" in doctors' knowledge and care? Could the lack of supporting agents be an impeding factor towards the adoption of online virtual environments? Results of such studies should be taken into consideration in peer debates within medical associations about the impact of VR in accelerating skill acquisition, and by Web site designers for the development of future "user friendly" online environments.

Are Doctors Too Old to Learn New Tricks?

Doctors' resistance towards the use of e-learning environments could be explained, in part, by a lack of proficiency in using computer-based systems like VR (LaRose, Eastin, & Gregg, 2001), lack of time to dedicate to new tasks, cultural barriers or simply lack of financial and technical resources that impede the adoption of complex technologies. Browsing online resources for e-research could be perceived as a less difficult task to accomplish compared to using online virtual simulators. Interestingly, we have not encountered any study reporting skeptical attitudes towards the use of e-research environments; this is another difference between E-LE and E-RE. Are some doctors simply too old to learn new tricks? Is there a technological–education divide? In reality, new E-LEs are already changing doctors' professional and private lives, giving to many of them—especially newer generations—the possibility to quickly acquire and transfer, to colleagues and patients, educational and research information (Murero, 2006) or perhaps just give headaches to their skeptical colleague.

Limits and Opportunities for Developing Countries

Disparities in medical information and education are a major determinant of health practice inequities in developing communities. Online medical education, training, and telementoring are opening new frontiers to medical knowledge and practice in remote areas of the planet. But enormous barriers to access and use still need to be overcome. From a more global view, adequate policies should help close the digicultural medical divide that exists in the international medical community to reduce disparities in information and education (Filho, 2002). From a technological standpoint, despite efforts to overcome bandwidth limitations (Yamey, 2004) most universities are severely limited from accessing e-learning resources and e-research international programs by totally inadequate connectivity systems, that are available to sister organizations in developed nations. Solutions that try to bypass technological problems include the Virtual Health Library (http://www.dse.de/zg/lernbibl/links/index.htm). The developers take advantage of the potential of ICTs to foster access to state-of-the-art medical information and democratization of knowledge in poor countries, to promote equity in health.

From a cultural and educational perspective, medical students with access to the Internet but with low abilities to use information technology or computer skills might not be able to access E-LEs and E-REs for education and training in developing countries (Ajuwon, 2003; Horna, Curioso, Guillen, Torres, & Kawano, 2002; Odusanya & Bamgbala, 2002). In this regard, a UK study has assessed the ICT skills of medical students in Tanzania (Samuel, Coombes, Miranda, Melvin, Joung, et al., 2004). Interestingly, a period of approximately 5 hours of peer (UK students) online mentoring training produced an approximate doubling of competence scores. Similarly, telementoring should be further developed to improve access to medical E-LE, once basic skills are acquired. This result shows that facilitating cultural agents can play a great role in Internet education.

However, in order to address convenient solutions, further research should clarify if developing countries are experiencing the same problems that occurred during the truly early stages of the diffusion of the Internet (i.e., lack of literacy skills among local teachers to identify quality information online, lack of professional development, gender imbalance in access, need of cultural agents). Policies should help close the medical digital—and cultural—divide, and sustain the development of offline and online environment to improve patients' care. Medical training on "real" patients should not be acceptable anymore in developing countries as well as in developed countries. New technologies could offer remarkable new opportunities to underdeveloped areas, if current barriers are overcome.

BRAIN FRAMES FOR THE FUTURE
OF MEDICAL RESEARCH

In the last decade, computers and more recently the Internet have revolutionized the way society and individuals operate in everyday life, including medical education and patients' care. The intersection of concomitant factors—technological as well as medical advances—is expected to further revolutionize the medical field in the next few years, including e-research and e-learning environments, with tremendous impacts on patients' health care. For example, molecular scale research like nanotechnology, or the creation of devices, materials, and systems through the control of matter on the nanometer scale, is believed to be the basis for a profound transformation of our society (see http://www .landesbioscience.com/iu/output.php?id=219). At the same time, the integration of computer and statistical sciences along with biometric and biomedical research is breaking new ground for e-researchers who are working to create a "truly virtual" patient, which they say could one day replace real people in clinical trials for the development of new drugs and the cure of severe diseases like multiple sclerosis (Cleaver, 2004).

New computer-based technologies applied to medicine are helping doctors take better care of patients. Pilot studies in neuroscience and Epigenetic research are already allowing technology to be integrated in the human body to help rehabilitation medicine offer invaluable care to severely motor-impaired individuals suffering spinal cord injury, muscular dystrophy or stroke. Individuals participating in clinical trials are regaining the ability to communicate and control their environment by using a sensor that is implanted on the motor cortex of their brain; moving a mouse with their thoughts is the gateway to a range of self-directed activities. These include communication on the Internet, or the control of objects in the environment such as a wheelchair, a telephone, a television and lights. At the moment, researchers recruit volunteer candidates for their experiment online, and exchange scientific findings in e-research environments (http://www.cyberkineticsinc.com/content/clinicaltrials/ braingate_trials.jsp).

New miniaturization technologies and media integration, along with increased quality of medical information available to physicians (but also to the general public; Murero, 2006) could facilitate the development of sophisticated virtual learning environments that will help accelerate the diffusion of medical education and discoveries all over the planet, bringing along new threats and opportunities for both health care providers and seekers. The next step in this evolution might allow for E-LEs providing access to libraries of VR scenarios as a likely form of distribution and use (Rizzo, Strickland, & Bouchard, 2004). In sum, the integration of new ICTs, biotechnologies, genetic engineering, nanomedicine, and new frontiers in medical achievements and access, is likely to radically transform medical education, research, and practice, and benefit health care and well-being. E-research and e-learning environments could play an increasing facilitating role, if actual and future barriers are overcome.

BUILDING THE INFORMATION SOCIETY: THE CENTRAL ROLE OF RESEARCH AND EDUCATION

At the present (beginning 2006) *both* e-research and e-learning environments designed for physicians—but accessible to anyone online—are highly convincing means to provide unprecedented access to and exchange of medical knowledge, and can help doctors take better care of patients.

It is important to develop online environments to enhance the learning experience, train the human infrastructure of the future, build a collective knowledge (Levy, 1997) and foster medical research and innovation that overcome traditional boundaries. Institutions for higher education have a central role in this process, as they make available online resources to health care providers and seekers. Policymakers, health care providers, organizations of patients and pharmaceutical companies, should help remove barriers to the access to online virtual learning environments for physicians and try to close the digital and cultural medical divide in the future.

New generations of students, but also new cohorts of entrepreneurs, technicians, and politicians formed in online and offline learning environments can make a difference in the future of patients' care, and have the potential to sustain the future developments of the information society.

REFERENCES

Ahlberg, G., Heikkinen, T., Iselius, L., Leijonmarck, C. E., Rutqvist, J., & Arvidsson, D. (2002). Does training in a virtual reality simulator improve surgical performance? *Surgical Endoscopy, 16*(1), 126–129.
Aiken, L. H., Clarke, S. P., Cheung, R. B., Sloane, D. M., & Silber, J. H. (2003). Educational levels of hospital nurses and surgical patient mortality. *Journal of the American Medical Association, 290,* 1617–1623.

Ajuwon, G. A. (2003). Computer and Internet use by first year clinical and nursing students in a Nigerian teaching hospital. *BioMed Center Informatics and Decision Making, 3*(1), 10.

Ali, M. R., Mowery, Y., Kaplan, B., & DeMaria, E. J. (2002). Training the novice in laparoscopy: More challenge is better. *Surgical Endoscopy, 16*(12), 1732–1736.

Brennan, P. F. (1995). Characterizing the use of health care services delivered via computer networks. *Journal of American Medical Informatics Association, 2*(3), 160–168.

Castells, M. (1996). *The rise of the network society: Vol. 1. The information age.* Cambridge, MA: Blackwell.

Cleaver, A. (2004). German researchers are building a database to predict the progression of MS. *The Scientist*. Retrieved November 6, 2004, from http://www.biomedcentral.com/news/20031015/02

D'Ancona, G., Murero, M., Bergsland, J., & Karamanoukian, H. (2001). Is the Internet a useful tool to educate cardiac surgery patients? *Heart Surgery Forum, 5*(2). Retrieved December 1, 2005, from http://www.hsforum.com/vol5/issue2/2001-4444.html

Daniel, J. K. (2004). Will e-learning improve clinical judgment? *BMJ, 328*, 1147–1148.

Dobkin, B. H. (2004). Strategies for stroke rehabilitation. *The Lancet Neurology, 3*(9), 528–536.

eEurope. (2002). *Quality criteria for health related websites*. Retrieved August 14, 2004, from http://www.hon.ch/HONcode/HON_CCE_en.htm#5

Epstein, D. (2004). *Global health leaders join the World Health Organization to announce accelerated efforts to improve patient safety*. Retrieved October 28, 2004, from http://www.who.int/mediacentre/news/releases/2004/pr74/en/

Filho, A. P. (2002). Inequities in access to information and inequities in health. *Panam Salud Publica, 11*(5–6), 409–412.

Freitas, R. A., Jr. (2004). *Webpage hosted by the Foresight Institute*. Retrieved November 12, 2004, from http://www.foresight.org/Nanomedicine/

Gabriel, B. (2000). Point and click CME: The future of continuing medical education. *AAMC Reporter, 9*(11). Retrieved May 2, 2005, from http://www.aamc.org/newsroom/reporter/aug2000/point.htm

Gallagher, A. G., & Cates, C. U. (2004). Virtual reality training for the operating room and cardiac catheterisation laboratory. *Lancet, 364*(9444), 1538–1540.

Gerson, L. B., & Van Dam, J. (2003). A prospective randomized trial comparing a virtual reality simulator to bedside teaching for training in sigmoidoscopy. *Endoscopy, 35*(7), 569–575.

Gomez-Arbones, X., Ferreira, A., Pique, M., Roca, J., Tomas, J., Frutos, J. L., Vinyas, J., Prat, J., & Ballester, M. (2004). A cardiological web as an adjunct to medical teaching: Prospective analysis. *Medical Teacher, 26*(2), 187–189.

Grantcharov, T. P., Kristiansen, V. B., Bendix, J., Bardram, L., Rosenberg, J., & Funch-Jensen, P. (2004). Randomized clinical trial of virtual reality simulation for laparoscopic skills training. *British Journal of Surgery, 91*(2), 146–150.

Grunewald, M., Gebhard, H., Jakob, C., Wagner, M., Hothorn, T., Neuhuber, W. L., Bautz, W. A., & Greess, H. R. (2004). Web-based training in radiology: Student course in the Virtual University of Bavaria. *Rofo, 176*(6), 885–895.

Hackbarth, S. (1996). *The educational technology handbook: A comprehensive guide.* Englewood Cliffs, NJ: Educational Technology Publications.

Harris Interactive. (2003). eHealth's influence continues to grow as usage of the Internet by physicians and patients increases. *Health Care News, 3*(6), 1–7.

Heer, I. M., Middendorf, K., Muller-Egloff, S., Dugas, M., & Strauss, A. (2004). Ultrasound training: The virtual patient. *Ultrasound in Obstetrics & Gynecology, 24*(4), 440–444.

Hiltz, S. R., & Goldman, R. (Eds.). (2004). *Learning together online: Research on asynchronous learning.* Mahwah, NJ: Lawrence Erlbaum Associates.

Honebein, P. C. (1996). Seven goals for the design of constructivist learning environments. In B. G. Wilson (Ed.), *Constructivist learning environments: Case studies in instructional design* (pp.). Englewood Cliffs, NJ: Educational Technology Publications.

Horna, P., Curioso, W., Guillen, C., Torres, C., & Kawano, J. (2002). Knowledge, abilities and characteristics of the Internet access in medical students of a Peruvian university. *Anales de la Facultad de Medicina, 63*(1), 32–39. Retrieved February 25, 2005, from http://www.waltercurioso.com/uw/internet.pdf

Jastrow, H., & Hollinderbaumer, A. (2004). On the use and value of new media. *Anat Rec. (The New Anatomist), 280B*(1), 20–29.

Jonassen, D., Mayes, T., & McAleese, R. (1993). A manifesto for a constructivist approach to uses of technology in higher education. In M. Duffy, J. Lowyck, & D. Jonassen (Eds.), *Designing environments for constructive learning* (pp. 231–247). Berlin: Springer-Verlag.

Kropf, R. (2003). How shall we meet online? Choosing between videoconferencing and online meetings. *Journal of Healthcare Information Management, 16*(4), 68–72.

Kumar, R. K., Velan, G. M., Korell, S. O., Kandara, M., Dee, F. R., & Wakefield, D. (2004). Virtual microscopy for learning and assessment in pathology. *Journal of Pathology, 204*(5), 613–618.

LaRose, R., Eastin, M. S., & Gregg, J. (2001). Reformulating the Internet paradox: Social cognitive explanations of Internet use and depression. *Journal of Online Behavior, 1*(2). Retrieved February 20, 2001, from http://www.behavior.net/JOB/v1n1/paradox.html

Leaders discuss nanotechnology market. (2003). *Technology Innovation, 11*(3). NASA, USA. Retrieved October 29, 2004, from http://ipp.nasa.gov/innovation/3-techtrans4.html

Levy, P. (1997). *L'intelligence collective: Pour une antropologie du cyberspace* [Collective intelligence: Towards an anthropology of cyberspace]. Paris: La Découverte.

Marchevsky, A. M., Relan, A., & Baillie, S. (2003). Self-instructional "virtual pathology" laboratories using web-based technology enhance medical school teaching of pathology. *Human Pathology, 34*(5), 423–429.

Marescaux, J., Soler, L., Mutter, D., Leroy, J., Vix, M., Koehl, C., & Clement, J. M. (2000). Virtual university applied to telesurgery: From teleeducation to telemanipulation. *Studies in Health Technology and Informatics, 70*, 195–201.

Masoni, M., Guelfi, M. R., Conti, A., Conti, A. A., & Gensini, G. F. (2004). Online accessible database of clinical cases of unknown origin. Published Letter [online version] in reply to Stephen Pincock (2004) Initiative to exchange cancer research information is launched. *BMJ, 328*, 728. Retrieved March 23, 2005, from http://bmj.bmjjournals.com/cgi/eletters/328/7442/728

Midiri, G., Papaspiropoulos, V., Coppola, M., Eleuteri, E., Tucci, G., Conte, S., Marino, G., Luzzatto, L., & Angelini, L. (2003). Telementoring in surgery. *Giornale di Chirurgia, 10*, 382–384.

Murero, M. (2006). E-learning environments for health care: Advantages, risks and implications. In J. Weiss, J. Nolan, J. Hunsinger, & P. Trifonas (Eds.), *International handbook of virtual learning environments* (pp.). Berlin: Springer.

Murero, M., & D'Ancona, G. (2001, June). *E-health: Internet access to cardiac surgery*. Proceedings of the International conference on interdisciplinarity: No sense of discipline. University of Queensland, Brisbane, Australia.

Murero, M., D'Ancona, G., & Karamanoukian, H. (2001). Use of the Internet in patients before and after cardiac surgery: An interdisciplinary survey. *Journal of Medical Internet Research*. Retrieved December 1, 2005, from http://www.jmir.org/2001/3/e27/

Odusanya, O. O., & Bamgbala, O. A. (2002). Computing and information technology skills of final year medical and dental students at the College of Medicine University of Lagos. *Nigerian Postgraduate Medical Journal, 9*(4), 189–193.

Ogan, K., Jacomides, L., Shulman, M. J., Roehrborn, C. G., Cadeddu, J. A., & Pearle, M. S. (2004). Virtual ureteroscopy predicts ureteroscopic proficiency of medical students on a cadaver. *Journal of Urology, 172*(2), 667–671.

Pande, R. U., Patel, Y., Powers, C. J., D'Ancona, G., & Karamanoukian, H. L. (2003). The telecommunication revolution in the medical field: Present applications and future perspective. *Current Surgery, 60*(6), 636–640.

Pincock, S. (2004). Initiative to exchange cancer research information is launched. *British Medical Journal, 328*, 728.

Rice, R. E., & Katz, J. E. (Eds.). (2001). *The Internet and health communication: Expectations and experiences.* Thousand Oaks, CA: Sage.

Riva, G., Bacchetta, M., Cesa, G., Conti, S., & Molinari, E. (2002). E-health in eating disorders: Virtual reality and telemedicine in assessment and treatment. *Studies in Health Technology and Informatics, 85*, 402–408.

Rizzo, A. A., Strickland, D., & Bouchard, S. (2004). The challenge of using virtual reality in telerehabilitation. *Telemedicine Journal and E Health, 10*(2), 184–195.

Ruderich, F., Bauch, M., Haag, M., Heid, J., Leven, F. J., Singer, R., Geiss, H. K., Junger, J., & Tonshoff, B. (2004). CAMPUS—A flexible, interactive system for web-based, problembased learning. *Health Care Medinfo, 2004*, 921–925.

Samuel, M., Coombes, J. C., Miranda, J. J., Melvin, R., Joung, E. J., & Azarmina, P. (2004). Assessing computer skills in Tanzania medical students: An elective experience. *BioMed Central Public Health, 4*(1), 37.

Semere, W. G., Edwards, T. M., Boyd, D., Barsoumian, R., Murero, M., Donias, H. W., & Karamanoukian, H. L. (2003). The world wide web and robotic heart surgery. *Heart Surgery Forum, 6*(6), E111–E119.

Seymour, N. E., Gallagher, A. G., Roman, S. A., O'Brien, M. K., Bansal, V. K., Andersen, D. K., & Satava, R. M. (2002). Virtual reality training improves operating room performance: Results of a randomized, double-blinded study. *Annuals of Surgery, 236*(4), 458–463.

Speedie, S. M., & Niewoehner, C. (2003). The Minnesota virtual clinic: Using a simulated EMR to teach medical students basic science and clinical concepts. *AMIA Annual Symposium Proceedings*, 1013. Washington, DC: American Medical Informatics Association.

Sprague, L. A., Bell, B., Sullivan, T., & Voss, M. (2003, December). Virtual reality in medical education and assessment. *Technology.*

Starfield, B. (2000). Is US health really the best in the world? *Journal of the American Medical Association, 284*(4), 483–485.

Taylor, H. (2002). The Harris Poll. Retrieved October 23, 2004, from http://www.harrisinteractive.com/news/allnewsbydate.asp?NewsID=464

Torkington, J., Smith, S. G., Rees, B. I., & Darzi, A. (2001). Skill transfer from virtual reality to a real laparoscopic task. *Surgical Endoscopy, 15*(10), 1076–1079.

Vozenilek, J., Huff, J. S., Reznek, M., & Gordon, J. A. (2004). See one, do one, teach one: Advanced technology in medical education. *Academic Emergency Medicine, 11*(11), 1149–1154.

Weiss, J., Nolan, J., Hunsinger, J., & Trifonas, P. (Eds.). (2006). *The international handbook of virtual learning environments.* Berlin: Springer.

Wilson, B. G. (1995). Metaphors for instruction: Why we talk about learning environments. *Educational Technology, 35*(5), 25–30. Retrieved March 20, 2005, from http://www.carbon.cudenver.edu/~bwilson/metaphor.html

Wilson, B. G. (Ed.). (1996). *Constructivist learning environments: Case studies in instructional design.* Englewood Cliffs, NJ: Educational Technology Publications.

Winn, W. D., & Jackson, R. (1999). Fourteen propositions about educational uses of virtual reality. *Educational Technology, 39*(4), 5–14.

Yamey, G. (2004). The professor of "telepreventive medicine". *BMJ, 328*, 1158.

Chapter 4

The State of E-Commerce in Health: An Examination, Diagnosis, and Prognosis

Pamela Whitten
Charles Steinfield
Lorraine Buis
Michigan State University

It is important to recognize the growing significance of the health care sector to our economy, both as a source of economic opportunity and as a drain on our resources. The Office of the Actuary at the Centers for Medicare & Medicaid Services (CMS) reports that the nation's total spending for health care will top $3.4 trillion by 2013 (CMS, 2004). The United States is fast approaching 20% of gross domestic product (GDP) being allocated for health. In addition to economic drivers, social priorities are also increasing the momentum for innovative solutions to address health disparities and access challenges. Given this financial context, it is no surprise that new communication technologies such as the Internet, which have the potential to increase efficiency in the sector, improve access, and provide a platform from which entrepreneurs can launch innovative products, are enjoying particular attention by health researchers.

Although a great deal of attention has been paid to e-health activity over the past decade, the term *e-health* itself is used in many different ways (Oh, Rizo, Enkin, & Jadad, 2005; Pagliani, Sloan, Gregor, Sullivan, Detmer, Kahan, Oortwijn, & MacGillivray, 2005). Pagliani et al. (2005) reviewed nearly 400 publications in health-related journals between 1997 and 2003 to determine the scope of usage of the term e-health. Their review demonstrates that there is no consistent usage of the term, but they do find that a majority of publications to date focus on the Internet as a source of information or as a tool for communicating health information. Not one of the reviewed articles dealt with the intersection of health and electronic commerce (e-commerce). However, usage of e-health outside of traditional medical publications does refer to commerce. Oh et al. (2005) scanned more than 1,200 abstracts and 1,158 Web sites identified in a Google search to find definitions of e-health. Out of the 51 unique definitions identified, 11 explicitly mentioned the word "commerce."

To address the relative lack of attention to health-related e-commerce in the academic literature, in 2001 two authors of this chapter (Whitten and Steinfield) attempted an examination of e-health from a commercial perspective (Whitten, Steinfield, & Hellmich, 2001). Specifically, they performed an analysis of e-health trends through 2000 and performed case studies on two health organizations—an online pharmacy and an online physician practice.

Their examination of e-health trends and the case studies demonstrated the potential for health-related commercial activity on the Internet. Accessibility to health services via the web added value beyond financial advantages. For example, the e-pharmacy case demonstrated the opportunity for more private and personal communication with an online pharmacist. The e-doctor case pointed out the prospect of immediate access to care, 24 hours a day, from anywhere in the world. However, this initial analysis also pointed out almost insurmountable barriers at the time, including state licensure laws, reimbursement mechanisms, and cultural expectations concerning responsibility. The authors ultimately concluded that a click and mortar approach, where a health organization has both a physical and virtual presence, might ultimately emerge as the optimal strategy for commercial e-health.

More than five years have passed since this original assessment of the commercial implications of online health services and the conducting of the two case studies. Since the initial case studies were conducted, the e-pharmacy site morphed into a Web site that simply serves as an intermediary for traditional pharmacies and the e-doctor Web site has gone out of business. Yet, Internet activity in general has grown at staggering levels. A recent report from the Pew Internet and American Life Project reports that on an average day near the end of 2004, more than 70 million Americans accessed the Internet. As compared to the 52 million Americans online in 2000, this marked a 37% increase (Rainie & Horrigan, 2005). Furthermore, it has been estimated that more than 12.5 million health-related searches are conducted each day across the world (Eysenbach, 2003) and this composes as much as 4.5% of all searches conducted on the Internet (Eysenbach & Kohler, 2002). In fact, several studies posit that searching for health information is one of the top three activities performed on the Internet (Fallows, 2004; Fox & Fallows, 2003; Rice, 2006).

This chapter seeks to revisit the state of online health activity for services that extend beyond the delivery of information. Online health-related commercial activity includes all products and services that directly or indirectly lead to revenue generation or cost efficiencies for a business or consumer. We begin with an overview of current utilization and commercial online applications as of 2005. We then overview the barriers confronting deployment of online health products and services and conclude with a diagnosis for the current state of online commercial health activities.

AN OVERVIEW OF E-COMMERCE
AND HEALTH CARE IN THE UNITED STATES

The sheer size of health care expenditures in the United States made health an attractive sector for new Internet-based entrants in the early years of the dot-com boom. In the first generation of e-commerce, Internet firms attacked both the business-to-consumer (B2C) and business-to-business (B2B) markets by pursuing presumed cost advantages and scale economies (Laudon & Traver, 2003). In the B2C health care arena, online intermediaries appeared in such areas as pharmacy retailing, alternative medicine sales, home medical equipment provision, and even online physician services (Whitten et al., 2001). In B2B health care markets, independent online intermediaries attempted to use the Internet to help reduce supply chain costs (e.g., costs to identify, qualify, and negotiate with suppliers, inventory holding costs, etc.) for hospitals and health maintenance organizations. Using brokerage business models, companies such as Neoforma sought to capitalize on the demand for reducing health supply costs by introducing auction formats for new and refurbished goods, especially for big-ticket medical devices such as imaging equipment (Nunes & Kirby, 2000). In both B2C and B2B markets, however, the promised value provided by third-party Internet intermediaries failed to materialize as Internet start-ups ran out of cash before achieving profitability. Whitten et al. (2001) discussed the likely trajectory of e-commerce in health care, predicting an integration between Internet and traditional health care delivery channels in order to overcome barriers raised by payment and reimbursement models, licensing and regulatory restrictions, and other patient need.

Today, despite the failure of many first-generation Internet-based health care intermediaries, the Internet is playing an increasingly prominent role in health care (Katz, Rice, & Acord, 2004). In this section, we briefly overview the major areas of current e-health activity in both the B2C and B2B arenas.

B2C E-COMMERCE IN HEALTH CARE

In B2C e-commerce, consumer use of online health information sites continues to grow, supported by revenues from health industry advertising and sales of related consumer products (Fallows, 2004). Most large pharmacy chains, and even smaller ones, now offer prescriptions online (FDA, 2005). There are even signs that physicians are engaging in e-mail exchanges on a paid basis with patients (Freudenheim, 2005; Rice & Katz, chap. 8, this volume). Additionally, many hospitals have improved their interaction with patients on their online sites, offering such services as appointment scheduling, e-mail access to physicians and nurses, prescription renewals, directory and other basic hospital information, and health-related content such as disease management (Anonymous, 2002).

Online Health Information and E-Commerce

From an e-commerce perspective, many content providers have attempted to create health portals, supported in large part by advertising revenue. In addition, although some information sites may not be motivated by commercial interests, many are sponsored by organizations that sell health-related products and services. Many drug companies, for example, offer rich online health content, profiting both from the public relations benefits, as well as the opportunity to refer to proprietary products where appropriate (Rice, Peterson, & Christine, 2002). Even hospitals and health maintenance organizations provide online health content as services to existing and potential customers. Moreover, well-known Internet portals such as Healthcare Central and WebMD have attempted to parlay their position as a popular source of health information into a range of new businesses directed at consumers, physicians, and payment providers (Southwick, 2004). WebMD, in particular, was able to survive the dot-com crash by complementing their industry-leading health care information site with traditional offline businesses performing such services as claims processing and medical management software provision. Other lines of business include the provision of a physician's portal (Medscape) offering information and educational services to doctors.

Online Pharmacies

A wave of online pharmacies appeared throughout the boom years of e-commerce prior to 2001. Whitten et al. (2001) described one case of an Internet pureplay pharmacy that hoped to compete by offering more convenient access for refills, regardless of location or time of day. Today, most of the Internet pureplay pharmacies have either gone out of business, moved into alternative medicines, or aligned themselves in some way with established offline pharmacy chains. Essentially, there appear to be three approaches to online prescription drug provision: (1) the true click and mortar model, (2) the online–offline alliance model, and (3) the commission model.

In the first approach, established pharmacy chains capitalize on their existing infrastructure and market presence in order to add a complementary e-commerce channel. Primarily, these services target existing customers, and try to build synergy between online and offline channels. For example, in many types of retailing, the combination of physical outlets with e-commerce creates synergies, by enabling companies to offer services such as online ordering with in-store pickup to customers that are not easily replicated by single channel firms (Steinfield, Bouwman, & Adelaar, 2002). Especially in the case of prescription drugs, having the opportunity to pick up and arrange payment for prescriptions immediately from a familiar and trusted source can be a powerful draw over pure online services where sensitive information has to be input and delays in delivery are implied. The simple act of obtaining refill orders online provides efficiency benefits to pharmacies, creating incentives for establishing an e-commerce channel for nearly all physical pharmacies. A good example of a well-known chain pursuing this type of e-commerce strategy is CVS (http://www.cvs.com).

In the second approach, an established offline pharmacy chain teams up with an online partner, with each using their specialized skills and assets to complement the other. The offline pharmacy has relationships with drug suppliers, industry-specific knowledge, and the physical presence in a market that might be needed by some patients with immediate refill requirements. On the other hand, the e-commerce company has the web development, database, and picking, packing, and shipping skills necessary for a good online presence. In this case, the offline pharmacy essentially outsources the online activities to the e-commerce firm. An example of this type of alliance can be seen in Rite Aid's partnership with Drugstore.com. Drugstore.com had attempted to be a stand-alone full-service online pharmacy, but found that it needed partners with physical stores in order to offer the necessary range of services to customers.

The third approach represents something of a last-ditch survival effort by former online pharmacies that failed to attract enough customers as a pureplay, but also were not able to secure the kind of partnership/outsourcing arrangement seen with Drugstore.com and Rite Aid. The former online pharmacy Rx.com illustrates the case where these firms no longer sell directly to customers, but provide referral services to many different offline pharmacy chains. Each of these chains may have their own e-commerce channels, but provide referral fees for customers that arrive at their site via Rx.com's portal. Indeed, clicking on a preferred pharmacy from the Rx.com site launches the destination pharmacy site in a frame under the Rx.com header, with a message informing web users that any transactions will be handled according to the terms of the destination pharmacy site.

Consumers are increasingly turning to the Internet for the purchase of medications, both over the counter and prescription. Sites that specialize in the sale of over the counter drugs can be convenient to consumers because they will typically deliver to the location of the consumer's choosing. For example, many brick and mortar pharmacies that have an online presence such as CVS (www.cvs.com) and Walgreens (www.walgreens.com), as well as many smaller local pharmacies, give consumers the ability to have prescriptions mailed directly to their home.

Online Physician Services

In their earlier review, Whitten et al. (2001) described the case of an online doctor service providing virtual consultations for a fee, mainly to people traveling who were not able to visit their regular doctor. This firm is no longer in business, reflecting the challenges of offering this type of service. Licensing requirements and difficulties obtaining reimbursement from payment providers are some of the reasons why online consultation has been such a difficult service to establish. However, today, there are some signs that health insurers may be willing to reimburse physicians for the time they spend corresponding with patients via e-mail (Freudenheim, 2005). This creates a type of e-commerce opportunity, albeit different from the online brokerage model represented years ago by the e-doctor case. Rather, hospitals and health maintenance organizations can offer an e-mail service that connects patients securely to their existing physicians on a fee-reimbursed basis. This enhances physician efficiency as well as improving patient access. It is unlikely to be a major revenue-generator from an e-commerce perspective, as patients mainly would connect with their own physicians. However, the cost savings from unnecessary patient visits could be significant.

Finding and Communicating With Health Providers

Because the Internet connects people with a wealth of information, it is not surprising that people are turning to the web to help locate health care providers and insurance companies. People can use the Internet to help locate physicians in their area, as well as across the country. Organizations and businesses such as the American Medical Association (AMA), WebMD, DoctorDirectory, and practically every insurance company, allow people to search for doctors by name, location, or specialization (Katz, Rice, & Acord, 2004).

Another use of e-health has been e-mail for doctor–patient communication. Recently, health care providers such as doctors and nurses have been under pressure to start communicating with patients through computer-mediated means (Wilson, 2003). In a 2000 survey of college health clinics in which 88 health centers responded, 63.6% used some form of computer-mediated means to communicate with student patients and 27% used e-mail and the Internet to give medical advice (Neinstein, 2000). Currently, there are few conventional providers who place an emphasis on computer-mediated forms of communication, but with current trends, this could change (Wilson, 2003; Rice & Katz, chap. 8, this volume).

Home Medical Supplies

Another B2C health care e-commerce area that can be found is in the area of the provision of home medical supplies. Online purchasing of medical supplies and equipment has evolved into a significant online business enterprise. The online sale of medical equipment and supplies is focused toward two types of clients; industry members (e.g., hospitals, clinics, nursing homes, medical labs, etc.) and care recipients (e.g., patient or caregiver; Whitten et al., 2001). From the B2C perspective, elderly and disabled people are a significant target market for a range of home medical devices and supplies, which can be fulfilled via e-commerce. Online channels are particularly appropriate for such niche products, as the local market may be too small to justify maintaining a local inventory in a retail outlet (Steinfield, Mahler, & Bauer, 1999). Traditional home and durable medical equipment suppliers, hospitals, and Internet firms all compete in this market, in which normal merchant and catalogue e-commerce models prevail. A key issue is the extent to which the online vendor is willing to accept third-party payments (e.g., from Medicare), which generally depends on the extent to which the desired device or supply is deemed medically necessary by an attending physician (Franklin, n.d.).

Hospital Web Sites for Improved Patient Access

Many hospitals have developed a web presence offering information and services to patients (Anonymous, 2002). Most of these sites provide health content as well as hospital directory information. However, they are also aimed at reducing costs associated with patient communications. In one example, administrators at Henry Ford Hospital in Detroit reported that their goal was to reduce costs associated with the nearly 15 million annual telephone calls their hospitals receive from patients for such requests as prescription renewals, appointment requests, and medical advice (Anonymous, 2002).

Health Insurance

The Internet has become a major reference point for consumers seeking health insurance. Although most health insurance providers maintain informational Web sites, many have added e-commerce features that allow consumers to obtain forms to speed up the process of purchasing insurance, allow agents to order policies for their clients, and some even allow end-consumers to purchase health insurance directly as opposed to dealing with independent agents. For example, in 2004, California insurer Health Net Life Insurance Company launched Net Saver, the first Internet-only health plan. The entire application process is completed online and no paperwork is ever exchanged between applicant and insurer. The elimination of paper allows the company to process applications faster and keep costs to a minimum (Biotech Week, 2004). In addition, Blue Cross and Blue Shield of North Carolina is now able to directly sign up 8% of its applicants through its online system (Babcock, 2004).

Alternative Medicine

The business of alternative medicine has found quite the home on the Internet. Alternative medicine is typically thought to be any type of health care treatment found outside the traditional realm of mainstream medicine. This includes practices such as chiropractic treatment, acupuncture, homeopathy, or natural healing. In 1997, it was estimated that 42.1% of adult Americans had utilized one of 16 different forms of alternative medicine including herbal medicine, chiropractics, folk remedies, homeopathy, and so on. It was further estimated that between $27 billion and $34.4 billion had been spent out of pocket on alternative medicine services by a practitioner, herbal products, high-dose vitamins, diet products, and therapy books, classes, and so on (Eisenberg, Davis, Ettner, Appel, Wilkey, Van Rompay, & Kessler, 1998). With the advent of the Internet, many people are seeking out alternative medicine options online. Not only is there a wealth of information regarding alternative medicine practices, but specialty e-commerce sites have been developed to connect consumers to herbalists, acupuncturists, chiropractors, and other alternative healers in addition to the purchase of vitamins, crystals, and herbal supplements.

Business-to-consumer (B2C) offers a means for individual consumers to purchase goods or services directly online. Business-to-business (B2B), discussed next, enables business entities to engage in commercial activities online with other businesses.

B2B E-COMMERCE IN HEALTH CARE

In B2B e-commerce, reducing hospital procurement costs and improving efficiency in the health care system remains a primary focus of Internet use (Houghton, 2002; Seror, 2002). Many of the Internet intermediaries that attempted to establish B2B e-marketplaces in the health care sector have repositioned themselves as software providers and transaction processing firms. Formerly, they sought to operate using a brokerage model, bringing together suppliers and buyers for a fee. Today, there is growing recognition that such third-party Internet marketplaces are difficult to establish in the B2B arena (Laudon & Traver, 2003). Private electronic networks, connecting firms in existing buyer–supplier relationships, have remained a persistent fixture in the B2B arena (Steinfield, Kraut, & Plummer, 1995). Today, the former would-be marketplace providers sell web development services and software solutions, mainly to large hospital networks. WebMD, through its Web Envoy business, for example, provides transaction processing services for physicians, hospitals, pharmacies, and insurers. Neoforma offers supply chain management software for hospitals and health care systems. All provide software that helps client firms use the Internet to rationalize the flow of transaction information, removing errors and reducing costs associated with re-keying and forms translation.

The practice of purchasing supplies online has become so prevalent in hospitals that some believe that it has reached critical mass (Anonymous, 2003). Critical mass is said to occur when a technology is used by enough firms or individuals to tip the adoption rate toward widespread usage. The use of online purchasing has shown to be an effective way for hospitals and clinics to cut costs. It has been estimated that approximately $6 billion can be saved on inefficient practices regarding supply chain management if hospitals were to switch to electronic commerce (Anonymous, 2001). A study commissioned by Novation, one of the leading medical supply services companies, and their e-commerce partner Neoforma, discovered that hospitals typically overpay their suppliers by 2% to 7%. In addition, they found that the utilization of e-commerce for purchasing can cut work created by errors in processing by up to 52% (Anonymous, 2001). In addition to savings on the part of the hospitals, reports also indicate that the use of online purchasing can also lead to big savings for medical supply manufacturers and distributors. Through e-commerce, general and administrative expenses could be cut by anywhere from 1% to 10% for distributors and the administrative load on sales representatives of manufacturers could be cut by 25% to 49% (Anonymous, 2001). Other countries have documented the benefits of using electronic commerce to automate pharmaceutical and other supplies to hospitals. More and McGrath (2001) highlighted the benefits of Australia's Project Electronic Commerce and Communication for Healthcare (PeCC), which include more efficient interaction among the pharmaceutical outlets (retail and hospital pharmacies), wholesalers, suppliers and manufacturers.

Beyond the procurement of medical supplies by hospitals and health systems, and payment/transaction processing among physicians, hospitals, insurers, and pharmacies, another target for B2B health care e-commerce is the use of the Internet by physicians to send prescription information to pharmacies. Security, conformance to HIPAA guidelines, authorization and authentication requirements, and privacy all make this a challenging application. However, the reduction in errors and convenience benefits make this an attractive target for e-commerce providers.

The business concerns of health-related e-commerce are a critical area for assessment. However, online health businesses operate within the parameters of health care in general. As a result, they face unique diffusion barriers and impediments outlined in the next section.

BARRIERS AND IMPEDIMENTS

In our 2001 review of e-health, we cited lack of reimbursement, legal issues, safety and standards, privacy and security concerns, and telecommunications infrastructure as being the major barriers to the provision of online health services. Over the course of the last 5 years, besides the addition of HIPAA and international concerns, very little has changed.

HIPAA

The Health Information Portability and Accountability Act of 1996 (HIPAA) was designed to help people retain their health insurance while in-between jobs. In addition, it included many provisions to aid in the protection and security of personal medical information. It has been the implementation of these protections that have caused barriers to the growth of e-health. Because of HIPAA, many providers of health services and supplies have become wary of offering online goods and services because of the potential for privacy violations. To date, what it means to be HIPAA compliant is still being explored. Though it is clear that privacy policies are a must under HIPAA regulations, research suggests that a great many of the privacy policies found on Web sites are full of legal jargon and are virtually impossible for a layperson to understand. In addition, it has also been found that Web sites do not do enough to notify consumers regarding changes to privacy policies. It has been suggested that in order for a consumer to fully protect their privacy, they are forced to reread a particular site's privacy policy on each visit in order to ensure that they the same policies are in effect (Jensen & Potts, 2004). Wallis and Rice (chap. 14, this volume) also show that the majority of consumers do not correctly know their legal medical privacy rights.

International Concerns

Due to the fact that the Internet knows no boundaries, there are many international concerns that e-health faces, especially in the area of online pharmacies. Due to the proximity of Canada and Mexico, concerns with the entry of Mexican and Canadian drugs are high. In fact, as of 2002, there were approximately 70 pharmacies shipping Canadian drugs to the United States (Manzer, 2002). Because of the large flow of Canadian prescription drugs flowing into the United States, it is feared that online prescriptions from U.S. consumers to Canadian-based pharmacies may create a manufactured drug shortage in Canada (Square, 2004). Estimates suggest that if 1% of the U.S. prescription drug market started receiving drugs from Canadian pharmacies, there could be as much as a 10% increase in the Canadian market. In addition, it has been estimated by the U.S. media that $1 billion in prescriptions have been sold by Canadian pharmacies to U.S. citizens in 2002. Lastly, the *Wall Street Journal* estimated that each year, approximately 1 million packages of prescription drugs are sent from Canada to the United States (Manzer, 2002). The implications of regulation and jurisdiction are further discussed in the following section.

Reimbursement Issues

Payment for goods and services purchased online operates within the national infrastructure of health reimbursement. On one hand, consumers have the option of employing a credit card to directly pay for online products (e.g., medication, durable medical equipment) or services (e.g., provider opinion). Direct online purchases for health products and services have enjoyed the same upward trend as has general online commercial activity. However, consumers of health often have different expectations for the provision of health care. In the United States, for example, members of third-party payer systems expect much of their health care costs to be borne by the payer. This is a universal expectation that transcends private payers (e.g., Blue Cross/Blue Shield) and public payers (e.g., Medicare, Medicaid). The expectation that consumers contribute more than simple co-pays for clinical services is simply outside the cultural norm for many consumers.

Pilot work is underway to develop payment schemas for online services. For example, some have estimated that a third of all physician visits could be handled in a manner other than a face-to-face visit such as e-mail correspondence. Some have even argued that online care may be superior for some contexts. Care instructions via e-mail, for example, would provide patients with a written record that could be shared with family members. Online care does not vary from traditional care in the requirement that physicians provide focused time for a specific patient. Yet, medicine is business and physicians are only able to devote significant time to care that is reimbursed. The vast majority of care plans do not reimburse for online care, due in large part to the need for a CPT (Current Procedural Terminology) code. Developed by the Health Care Financing Industry for reimbursement purposes, CPT codes describe different medical or psychiatric procedures that are performed by health care providers. In 2004, 0074T was approved as a Category III CPT code. Specifically, it defines an online consultation as comprising a substantive electronic communication between a physician and patient that is clinically relevant and carried out in the context of an existing relationship. Yet, the creation of a CPT code is not a quick fix. Payment for these online services is the prerogative of the payer. And, at this time, very few third-party payers are choosing to reimburse for online care, with or without a CPT code. Perhaps the most significant payer with no stated intention to provide reimbursement is CMS (Medicare and Medicaid).

However, a handful of projects are emerging that are embracing online consultative services via payment. For example, Blue Cross and Blue Shield of Florida (BCBSF) has introduced a plan to reimburse physicians for online medical consultations with established patients seeking non-urgent services (http://www.relayhealth.com). BCBSF has an agreement with RelayHealth, a California-based company, to provide its clients with a web platform that offers a clinically structured online process. BCBSF members will be able to use this electronic portal to consult with their physicians on non-urgent issues, receive lab results, submit prescription request for renewals or refills, schedule appointments, and request referrals to specialists.

In general, reimbursement for online goods and services has a long way to go before it even remotely resembles traditional care. Without a paradigm shift toward new cultural norms for payment, this will serve as a significant impediment to the growth in online commercial health activities.

Legal and Regulatory Issues

Cross-state and international licensure was a significant issue 5 years ago and remains an issue today. In essence, a health provider or pharmacy must be licensed in every state in which it serves clients. The paperwork, license fees, and variation in continued education requirements can be time consuming and expensive. In the United States, online pharmacies have been allowed to function on the same regulations that bricks and mortar pharmacies have (Arruñada, 2004). The problem arises when we enter the area of interstate commerce. In an interstate commerce situation, the questions of who gets to claim regulation rights, the location where the online pharmacy is based, and the location where the consumer is based become salient matters (Crawford, 2003).

Of particular interest to the federal and state governments has been the regulation of illegal pharmaceutical sales. Due to the nature of the Internet, it is quite easy for online pharmacies engaged in the sale of illegal pharmaceuticals, drugs without a prescription, or even fraudulent sales to reopen under a different name and location after being shut down by the authorities. In 1999, the Federal Trade Commission launched a program called Operation Cure-All whose aim is to stop bogus claims of cure-all drugs and "miracle cure" products on the Internet. In addition, at least 14 states including Arizona, California, Colorado, Connecticut, Illinois, Michigan, Kansas, Nevada, New Jersey, Ohio, Texas, Washington, Wisconsin, and Wyoming have taken action to stop physicians from prescribing drugs over the Internet. The FDA has been working closely with other agencies, including the Federation of State Medical Boards, the National Association of Attorneys General, and the National Association of Boards of Pharmacy in an effort to crack down on problems associated with online pharmacies (FDA, 2005).

There are different standards of practice that have allowed for the vast differences in quality of online pharmacies. Two factors are cited: (1) there are some countries that have allowed for the creation of licensed online pharmacies; and (2) due to the problems associated with controlling e-commerce, in all countries, the enforcement of stopping unlicensed online pharmacies to sell prescriptions is weak. This leads to very high- and very low-quality online pharmacies (Arruñada, 2004).

Privacy and Security

As with any Internet endeavor, issues of privacy, security, and confidentiality are always of great concern (Wallis & Rice, chap. 14, this volume). Although the use of passwords and firewalls are a step towards ensuring privacy and security, they are not always good enough (Crawford, 2003).

Identity theft is one of the fastest growing crimes in the United States and American citizens should not be complacent about issues such as these. Due to the need for expressing caution when dealing with e-commerce, privacy and security concerns have been impediments to the growth of e-health. Oftentimes, the perceived risk of privacy and security infringements is much greater than the actual risk associated with these issues.

THE BOTTOM LINE

This brief overview of health care e-commerce approaches reveals a few important trends. First, Internet pureplays have largely disappeared, and most successful e-commerce undertakings involve the active participation by established offline health care providers. Hence, the prediction by Whitten et al. (2001) that click and mortar approaches to e-commerce would become more common in health has been borne out. The Internet firms that survived have done so by acquiring offline businesses, forming alliances with offline companies, and redirecting their efforts towards the provision of business services aimed at traditional health care companies.

The focus of much of the e-health activity, in both B2C and B2B areas, now appears to be focused on two broad goals: (1) improving services and patient access, and (2) lowering costs. This is in stark contrast to the vision of e-commerce applied in many other sectors, which heavily emphasized expansion into new markets, growth of market share, pursuit of network effects—whereby the more customers a firm has, the more desirable it becomes to new customers—and the accompanying massive scale economies made possible by automation of transactions (Laudon & Traver, 2003). Many e-health services are simply not amenable to such effects—and more midrange efficiencies and service improvements represent a more feasible goal.

During the "gold rush" excitement of developing online businesses from 1998 to 2001, many entrepreneurs and established commercial entities assumed that they could apply traditional principles of online commerce to health services and products (Katz, Rice, & Accord, 2004). However, lessons from the early years indicate that the health industry is complex and ensconced in a complicated web of reimbursement, legal, and ethical constraints. Commercial health sites did not result in the immediate cost-saving avenue to sell products and services to an almost infinite population. However, developments over the past 5 years do offer reason for optimism. Business-to-business commercial activity has demonstrated important efficiencies for all concerned. Business-to-consumer activities hint that growing numbers of Americans expect the availability of certain health services online as they continue to walk in storefronts for other aspects of their care. With continuous changes in federal priorities and legislation, expanding opportunities are bound to emerge.

REFERENCES

Anonymous. (2001). Study: e-Commerce could save hospitals and suppliers $6 billion. *Hospital Materials Management, 26*(9), 17.

Anonymous. (2002). Untangling the web. *Health Leaders Magazine.* Retrieved March 20, 2005, from http://www.healthleaders.com/magazine/feature1.php?contentid=34949

Anonymous. (2003). Internet use for buying reaches 'critical mass'. *Hospital Materials Management, 28*(10), 2.

Arruñada, B. (2004). Quality safeguards and regulation of online pharmacies. *Health Economics, 13,* 329–344.

Babcock, C. (2004, September 20). Insurers turn to web to speed services. *Information Week,* p. 1006.

Biotech Week. (2004, April 28). Health Net, Inc.; Insurer launches first Internet-only health plan. *Biotech Week,* p. 200.

CMS. (2004, September 17). *National healthcare expenditures projections: 2003–2013.* Retrieved February 23, 2005, from http://www.cms.hhs.gov/statistics/nhe/projections-2003/highlights.asp

Crawford, S. (2003). Internet pharmacy: Issues of access, quality, costs, and regulation. *Journal of Medical Systems, 27*(1), 57–65.

Eisenberg, D. M., Davis, R. B., Ettner, S. L., Appel, S., Wilkey, S., Van Rompay, M., & Kessler, R. C. (1998). Trends in alternative medicine use in the United States, 1990–1997: Results of a follow-up national survey. *Journal of the American Medical Association, 280*(18), 1569–1575.

Eysenbach, G. (2003). The impact of the Internet on cancer outcomes. *CA Cancer Journal for Clinicians, 53,* 356–371.

Eysenbach, G., & Köhler, C. (2002). How do consumers search for and appraise health information on the world wide web? Qualitative study using focus groups, usability tests, and in-depth interviews. *British Medical Journal, 324,* 573–577.

Fallows, D. (2004). *The Internet and daily life.* The Pew Internet & American Life Project. Washington, DC: Pew Charitable Trusts. Retrieved November 19, 2004, from http://www.pewinternet.org/PPF/r/132/report_display.asp

FDA. (2005). *U.S. Food and Drug Administration frequently asked questions.* Retrieved March 1, 2005, from http://www.fda.gov/oc/buyonline/faqs.html

Fox, S., & Fallows, D. (2003). *Internet health resources: Health searches and e-mail have become more commonplace, but there is room for improvement in searches and overall Internet access.* The Pew Internet & American Life Project. Washington, DC: Pew Charitable Trusts. Retrieved October 29, 2004, from http://www.pewinternet.org/PPF/r/95/report_display.asp

Franklin, M. B. (n.d.). Home medical devices a draw for scam artists. *Senior-Inet Online.* Retrieved March 20, 2005, from http://www.senior-inet.com/articles/article16.htm

Freudenheim, M. (2005, March 2). Digital Rx: Take two aspirins and e-mail me in the morning. *New York Times,* Electronic Edition. Retrieved March 2, 2005, from http://www.nytimes.com/2005/03/02/technology/02online.html

Houghton, J. (2002). *Information technology and the revolution in healthcare* (No. 4). Melbourne, Australia: Centre for Strategic Economic Studies. Retrieved March 20, 2005, from http://www.cfses.com

Jensen, C., & Potts, C. (2004). Privacy policies as decision making tools: An evaluation of online privacy notices. *Proceedings of the 2004 Conference on Human Factors in computing systems, 6*(1), 471–478.

Katz, J. E., Rice, R. E., & Acord, S. (2004). E-health networks and social transformations: Expectations of centralization, experiences of decentralization. In M. Castells (Ed.), *The network society: A cross-cultural perspective* (pp. 293–318). London: Edward Elgar.

Laudon, K., & Traver, C. (2003). *ECommerce: Business, technology, society* (2nd ed.). Boston: Addison-Wesley.

Manzer, J. (2002). Is Canada America's favourite drugstore? *Medical Post, 38*(46), 1.

More, E., & McGrath, G. M. (2001). Competitive collaboration in Australia's pharmaceutical industry. In R. E. Rice & J. E. Katz (Eds.), *The Internet and health communication: Experiences and expectations* (pp. 329–350). Thousand Oaks, CA: Sage.

Neinstein, L. (2000). Utilization of electronic communication (e-mail) with patients at university and college health centers. *Journal of Adolescent Health, 27*(1), 6–11.

Nunes, P., & Kirby, J. (2000). What goes around comes around. *Accenture Outlook Online Journal.* Retrieved March 20, 2005, from http://www.accenture.com/xd/xd.asp?it =enweb&xd=ideas\outlook\1.2000\over_whatgoes.xml

Oh, H., Rizo, C., Enkin, M., & Jadad, A. (2005). What is eHealth (3): A systematic review of published definitions. *Journal of Medical Internet Research, 7*(1), e1. Retrieved April 11, 2005, from http://www.jmir.org/2005/1/e1/

Pagliani, C., Sloan, D., Gregor, P., Sullivan, F., Detmer, D., Kahan, J., Oortwijn, W., & MacGillivray, S. (2005). What is eHealth (4): A scoping exercise to map the field. *Journal of Medical Internet Research, 7*(1), e9. Retrieved April 11, 2005, from http://www .jmir.org/2005/1/e9/

Rainie, L., & Horrigan, J. (2005). *Trends 2005.* The Pew Internet & American Life Project. Washington, DC: Pew Charitable Trusts. Retrieved February 23, 2005, from http://pewresearch.org/trends/trends2005.pdf

Rice, R. E. (2006). Influences, usage, and outcomes of Internet health information searching: Multivariate results from the Pew surveys. *International Journal of Medical Informatics, 75*(1), 8–28.

Rice, R. E., Peterson, M., & Christine, R. (2002). A comparative features analysis of publicly accessible commercial and government health database Web sites. In R. E. Rice & J. E. Katz (Eds.), *The Internet and health communication: Expectations and experiences* (pp. 213–231). Thousand Oaks, CA: Sage.

Seror, A. (2002). Internet infrastructures and healthcare systems: A qualitative comparative analysis on networks and markets in the British National Health Service and Kaiser Permanente. *Journal of Medical Internet Research, 4*(3). Retrieved March 20, 2005, from http://www.jmir.org/2002/3/e21/

Southwick, K. (2004). Diagnosing WebMD: Ultimate dot-com survivor faces new challenges. *CNET News.Com.* Retrieved March 20, 2005, from http://news.com.com/Diagnosing+WebMD/2009-1017_3-5208510.html

Square, D. (2004). Group says Internet pharmacies will create manufacturing drug shortage. *Medical Post, 40*(14), 5.

Steinfield, C., Bouwman, H., & Adelaar, T. (2002). The dynamics of click and mortar eCommerce: Opportunities and management strategies. *International Journal of Electronic Commerce, 7*(1), 93–119.

Steinfield, C., Kraut, R., & Plummer, A. (1995). The effect of networks on buyer–seller relations. *Journal of Computer Mediated Communication, 1*(3). Available from http://www .ascusc.org/jcmc/vol1/issue3/steinfld.html

Steinfield, C., Mahler, A., & Bauer, J. (1999). Electronic commerce and the local merchant: Opportunities for synergy between physical and web presence. *Electronic Markets, 9*(1/ 2), 51–57.

Whitten, P., Steinfield, C., & Hellmich, S. (2001). EHealth: Market potential and business strategies. *Journal of Computer Mediated Mass Communication, 6*(4). Retrieved March 20, 2005, from http://jcmc.indiana.edu/vol6/issue4/whitten.html

Wilson, E. V. (2003). Asynchronous healthcare communication. *Communications of the ACM, 46*(6), 79–84.

Chapter 5

Media Use Theory and Internet Use for Health Care

Mohan J. Dutta-Bergman
Purdue University

The rapid growth of new communication technologies and the increasing public participation in issues of health have led to a surge in both scholarly and practitioner interest in the health uses of the Internet (Dutta-Bergman, 2004a; Rice, 2001). In a survey conducted by the Pew Internet and American Life Project in 2003, 66% of Internet users reported having gone online for health or medical information compared to 54% of Internet users in 2000 (Fox & Fallows, 2003). The dramatic rise in the use of the Internet for health care has been propelled by (a) increasing consumer interest in health care (Carlsson, 2000; Dutta-Bergman, 2004b); (b) increasing analytical sophistication of the new consumer (Mittman & Cain, 2001); and (c) growing accessibility of health information on the Internet (Dutta-Bergman, 2004b). The critical role of the Internet as a health information resource has shifted traditional patterns of consumer health information use, physician–patient relationship, health services delivery, and health care policy (Dutta-Bergman, 2003b; Rice, 2001). This new paradigm in health communication triggered by the advent of the Internet calls for a theoretical examination of how consumers use the Internet for health care purposes.

Based on reviews of articles (Cline & Hayes, 2001; Napoli, 2001) that point out that the empirical examination of consumer health information uses should drive scholarly and policy discussions of e-health, this chapter examines the theories explaining the different uses of the Internet for health communication. Central to these theories are the role of consumer motivation in shaping the selection of health information channels, the processing of information from such channels, and the subsequent behavioral outcomes that result from information processing. Motivation refers to the underlying interest in an issue or topic. The health communication literature points out that consumers systematically differ in their motivations in health-related issues, and that such motivations are shaped by both dispositional and situational factors (Dutta-Bergman, 2004b; Napoli, 2001). This chapter reviews the key theories of motivation surrounding media use and health, establishing the role of human motivation in the realm of media use, followed by a discussion of motivation in the realm of health, with particular attention to Internet health information.

FUNCTIONAL APPROACH TO MEDIA USE

The functional approach to media use is built on the notion that the consumption of any medium is a heterogeneous process. The medium (such as the Internet) performs a variety of functions for different audience segments under a variety of circumstances (Atkin, 1993; Dutta-Bergman, 2004d; Lin & Jeffres, 1998). Challenging the techno-deterministic conceptualization of a monolithic experience of a medium, it accentuates the diversity of media experiences driven by the different functions served by the medium. The function served by a particular medium emerges from the communicative needs of the audience, which in turn are determined by the disposition of the user and the specific situation that triggers the media consumption within larger systems of media access and control (see Ball-Rokeach & DeFleur, 1976). For instance, the Internet is sometimes used by the consumer for the purposes of finding information about a treatment, whereas at other times it is used for seeking reinforcement regarding a health behavior (such as weight loss support groups). An impressive collection of media effects theories captures the functional approach to media use: uses and gratifications, selective processing, dual processing, and channel complementarity theories, each discussed in turn.

Uses and Gratifications Perspective

Reflecting a functional approach to media use, the uses and gratifications perspective is founded on the conceptualization of audience initiative and activity (Rubin, 1994). Uses and gratifications research examines the purposes or functions served by the medium for audiences of media programs. Located in the realm of audience choice of media stimuli, this line of research explores the purposes, functions, or uses of mass media as driven by the choice patterns of receivers (Rubin, 1994, 2002). The emphasis here is on the uses of mass media in meeting the felt needs of the audience. Uses and gratifications research seeks to explain how people use media to satisfy their needs, to understand motives underlying media behavior, and to identify functions or consequences that emerge from the intersection of needs, motives, and behaviors.

The goals that consumers bring to the media landscape shape the media types that are selected, and the subsequent processing of media content. According to Rubin (1994), five key points establish the framework for uses and gratifications research:

1. communication behavior is goal-directed;
2. individuals select and use communication channels to satisfy felt needs;
3. individual communication behavior is mediated by a plethora of social and psychological factors;
4. media compete with other forms of communication; and
5. although individuals are typically more influential than the media in the relationship, this is not always the case.

The motives that have been systematically investigated under the rubric of uses and gratifications research include information, surveillance, entertainment, habit, social interaction, escape, pass time and relaxation.

The uses and gratifications framework has been widely applied in the context of new communication technologies. In a national random digit-dialing telephone survey conducted in 1994, Perse and Dunn (1998) reported that the use of home computers was typically associated with ritualistic uses such as keeping busy and passing time. On a similar note, Parker and Plank (2000) reported that university students were primarily using online sources for relaxation and escape. Ferguson and Perse (2000) observed the salience of entertainment as a motive for visiting the World Wide Web among college students. The most visited Web sites were sports and entertainment Web sites. Also, another important motive for using the web in the college sample was acquisition of information. Kargaonkar and Wolin (1999) reported that web usage was positively correlated with social escapism, information, interactive control, and socialization motivations. Papacharissi and Rubin (2000) similarly demonstrated that information seeking and entertainment were the most salient motives for using the Internet.

One of the functional categories that emerges from the uses and gratifications research is surveillance (Rubin, 1994). Uses and gratifications researchers posit that instrumental needs involve the use of media for knowledge seeking; these needs most often are expressed in the form of environment scanning and specific information seeking (Ferguson, 1992). This surveillance function, however, is quite broad in scope and does not capture the variance in different kinds of information seeking. This is especially the case in the realm of health information gathering.

The Internet is used for a wide variety of information-seeking purposes and these purposes are qualitatively different from one another. For instance, it may be argued that gathering information for learning about preventative healthy behaviors is fundamentally different from gathering health information for the purpose of detecting a disease. Gathering health information for choosing a treatment option is fundamentally different from the habitual consumption of medical news. It is important to sketch out this variance in consumer health information search on the Internet because of its possible impact on consumer information processing. The cues that the consumer will attend to will perhaps differ by the different types of health information gathering the consumer engages in. Also, consumer expectations of information quality and his or her satisfaction with the health information are likely to vary with the specific function. Dutta-Bergman (2004d) suggested the following health-related information functions of the Internet: (a) gathering medical news; (b) looking for information about medical services; (c) searching for information about drugs and medications; (d) gathering disease-specific information; (e) searching for information about healthy lifestyle; and (f) looking for, and participating in, discussion groups (see also Rice, 2006).

Selective Processing Theories

Selective processing theories also reflect the functional approach to media use (Atkin, 1985). Central to the articulations of selective processing theories is the idea that individuals orient their attention to specific stimuli in their environment, selecting and processing information that is consistent with existing attitudes and beliefs, and avoiding information that is discrepant. Selective processing of media messages plays out in the realms of selective exposure, interpretation, and memory (Oliver, 2002). Selective exposure theory articulates that individuals select media messages that match their existing attitudes and beliefs based on the notion that individuals seek consistency in their cognitions. The stimuli that receive focused attention are dependent on the underlying motivations and dispositions of the individual (Oliver, 2002; Webster & Wakshlag, 1985).

That audience members systematically differ in their media choices and that these choices are driven by dispositional differences have been extensively investigated in the domain of audience exposure to violent television material (Atkin, 1985), indicating that individual aggressiveness is associated with the viewership of violent television programming. Selective exposure effects documenting the link between a particular predisposition and the exposure to media content that matches the disposition are also observed in the area of prosocial behavior, political, and moral values (Atkin, 1985). For instance, Sweeney and Gruber (1984) observed that interest in, and attention to, the McGovern hearings was lowest among Nixon supporters, moderate among undecided citizens, and highest among McGovern supporters. Similarly, Capella, Turow, and Jamieson (1996) observed that listeners of Rush Limbaugh were politically conservative as compared to the listeners of liberal and moderate radio shows. At the crux of selective exposure theory is the role of consumer motivation that drives the use of media outlets. Selective perception theory suggests that readers and viewers ascribe meanings to, and judgments of, media messages that are consistent with their existing values and beliefs. For instance, Vidmar and Rokeach (1974) demonstrated that highly prejudiced individuals who watched *All in the Family* were likely to interpret the program as sympathetic to the bigoted main character whereas low-prejudiced individuals tended to interpret the program as sympathetic to the politically liberal main character. In the realm of political attitudes, similar results have been observed, with individuals being more likely to perceive their own candidates more favorably than the opponents (Bothwell & Brigham, 1983). In addition to influencing message *perception*, preexisting beliefs and attitudes also influence what is *remembered* (Oliver, 2002). Eagly and Chaiken (1993) observed that existing beliefs and cognitions influence memory by shaping attention and elaboration at the time of encoding and by affecting retrieval and reconstruction of information subsequent to exposure. In other words, the accurate or inaccurate recall of media information reflects the existing values and beliefs.

Selective processing effects are also documented in the realm of health information processing. Dutta-Bergman (2004a, 2004b) demonstrated that health-active individuals, those who are highly engaged in health-related issues, are more likely to seek out health-specialized media content as compared to the individuals who are not involved in issues of health. Researchers studying health information uses on the Internet point out that audience members selectively orient their attention to certain Web sites that match their dispositional orientation. The searchability of the Internet allows the consumer to selectively choose those Web sites that match his or her information needs. Compared to traditional media such as television and the radio, the interactivity of the Internet facilitates selective processing of information such that the visit to a particular site by an Internet user is predicated on the underlying motivation of the user in the information content of the site.

Dual-Processing Theories

Dual-processing theories (the elaboration likelihood model and the heuristic systematic model) further add to the notion of the functional construction of media use. This stream of research, primarily originating from psychology, articulates two distinct routes of information processing: central and peripheral (Petty & Cacioppo, 1986, 1990). When processing messages centrally because of salience/involvement of message, consumers attend to the arguments of a message (Petty & Cacioppo, 1986). Peripheral processing, however, involves decision making based on heuristic or affective cues (Petty & Cacioppo, 1986). Under such situations, the consumer searches for cognitively nonintensive cues for decision making such as source attractiveness, price heuristics, and so on.

The decision-making route followed by the consumer is a function of his or her level of involvement with the issue or subject area and his or her ability to process a message (Petty & Cacioppo, 1986, 1990). The involvement of the consumer in a topic/issue depends on the relevance of the issue to his or her information-processing needs. Whereas high levels of involvement lead to central processing, low involvement levels lead to peripheral processing. Therefore, consumers who are motivated in a particular issue are more likely to seek out information about the issue and process the arguments present in that information as compared to individuals who are not motivated in a specific issue.

Extrapolation to the realm of health-oriented content on the Internet suggests that health-involved individuals would be more likely to consume health-oriented content on the Internet and centrally process information presented in such outlets as compared to low involvement individuals. In addition, the level of involvement of the consumer may be used as a variable for message tailoring, such that audience members receive prevention messages oriented toward central or peripheral processing ("elaboration") depending on their level of involvement in the issue/topic. For example, messages with strong salient arguments would be available to highly involved audience members, whereas messages that appeal to popularity or social acceptance would be made available to low-involved audiences.

In addition to the motivation of the consumer in processing information related to a specific issue, individuals must also possess the ability to process the message (Petty & Cacioppo, 1986). Knowledge about the cognitive ability of the audience member allows health message designers to develop messages that match the cognitive capacity of the receiver. Developers of health-related web materials need to take into account the cognitive ability of the receiver and incorporate multiple communication channels such as graphics, photo, animations, audio, and video in addition to text-based messages (Bernhardt & Cameron, 2003). For instance, newspapers require higher cognitive processing levels and are typically consumed by educated consumers, whereas television presents information through video and audio, and is more likely to be effective in delivering comprehensible information for less-educated consumers and consumers with lower cognitive processing abilities.

Theory of Channel Complementarity

Reflecting the motivation-based approach to media choice, the theory of channel complementarity provides a framework for understanding the relationship between the use of different channel types that share similar functions (Dutta-Bergman, 2004e; Stempel, Hargrove, & Bernt, 2000). The theory draws its conceptual foundation from selective exposure, uses and gratifications, and dual-processing theories, articulating the existence of complementarity among channel types that offer similar functions for the consumer. For instance, Stempel, Hargrove, and Bernt (2000) observed that Internet users were also more likely to be newspaper readers and radio news listeners. The researchers used an information-seeking model to explain the greater newspaper use of Internet users, suggesting that they may turn to their newspapers or newspaper readers may go the Internet to retrieve more information on a topic. In this case, the information-seeking behavior through the different media complement each other in fulfilling the individual's information needs. LaRose and Atkin (1992) observed that the use of local audiotext information services was complementary with the use of similar information technologies such as videotexts, ATMs, 800 numbers, and telephone answering services that shared the function of providing information on demand to the user. Similarly, Rice and Case (1983) documented the use of e-mail in the context of other organizational media, concluding that new media were often complementary rather than substitutional in their relationship with traditional media. Rice (1993) observed "clusters" of complementary media in organizational settings. The concept of complementarity is also related to "innovation clusters," whereby people are likely to adopt new innovations that fit in with preexisting clusters of adopted technologies (Atkin, 1993; Perse & Courtright, 1993; Rogers, 1995).

The theory of channel complementarity posits that audience members actively participate in the consumption of media types, choosing those media forms that are most likely to serve the relevant functions driven by enduring involvement in a specific content area. This enduring involvement in a specific content area is a product of the disposition and the situation surrounding media consumption, and systematically varies within the population such that whereas some individuals are intrinsically interested in health information, others are not interested in seeking out and processing health-related information.

The theory of channel complementarity argues that channels that perform similar functions are likely to demonstrate complementarity among each other (Dutta-Bergman, 2004e; Rice, 1993). In other words, the individual who feels the functional need to consume a specific channel in a certain content area is also likely to consume other, even new, channels that perform the same function in the content domain. For instance, the health-motivated consumer who is intrinsically interested in issues of health is not only likely to read health magazines such as *Prevention* and *Health*, but is also likely to watch health television, and surf health-related Web sites to gather health information. The enduring interest in health in this case prompts the use of multiple media types (magazines, television, Internet) in the specific content domain of health. The specific medium chosen for retrieval of health information at any particular time depends on what is available and convenient (Ball-Rokeach & DeFleur, 1976). The individual is loyal to the content and uses different media types that serve this need for content; content drives the relationship among different media types. As a consequence, the theory of channel complementarity states that media use demonstrates congruence across media types within specific content domains. Dutta-Bergman (2004e) demonstrated that use of the Internet for science and health information was congruent with the use of traditional media for science and health information. In other words, individuals who went online to get science and health news were also more likely to follow such news in radio, television and print as compared to those individuals who did not go online to seek science and health news. Channel complementarity may also be driven by other characteristics such as modality, accessibility, quality, and so on.

MOTIVATION AND HEALTH

The previous section investigates the general issue of motivations to use complementary media, and sets the stage for exploring the role of motivations to use health information specifically. In the theories of health behavior discussed in the next few sections, motivation is a key determinant of the sources of health information, amount of health information, and quality of health information sought by the consumer (see Napoli, 2001). In addition, motivation shapes the subsequent processing of health messages and engagement in health behaviors (Dutta-Bergman, 2004a, 2004d). The central role of motivation in information seeking, message processing and health behavior change offers the template for designing health information systems that respond to the different levels and types of motivation in the population.

Health Orientation

Health orientation is a motivation-based construct, reflecting systematic individual-level differences within a population with respect to the extent to which individuals are motivated in health-related issues and are willing to process health-related information (Dutta-Bergman, 2004a, 2004b; MacInnis, Moorman, & Jaworski, 1991; Moorman & Matulich, 1993). It is defined as "a goal-directed arousal to engage in preventive health behaviors" (Moorman & Matulich, 1993, p. 210).

Motivation is the subject of a large body of research in psychology and is treated as an antecedent to subsequent information processing and decision making. It triggers an individual's interest in a particular issue or topic, subsequently leading to active engagement in issue-relevant thoughts and actions (Petty & Cacioppo, 1986), which, as just reviewed, then influences preferences for and use of individual and complementary media. Motivation in the domain of health, therefore, suggests an active consumer participation in issues of personal health and an active search for relevant health information (MacInnis, Moorman, & Jaworski, 1991). It influences the individual's health preventive and health maintenance behaviors.

Consumers who seek out medical news on the Internet are more health conscious and health information oriented, hold stronger health beliefs, and are more likely to engage in healthy activities (Dutta-Bergman, 2004a, 2004b, 2004d). Consumers who seek out information about drugs and medications on the Internet are also more health information oriented, hold stronger health beliefs, and are more likely to engage in healthy activities. The search for disease-specific information is also positively correlated with health orientation. Further, the search for information about a healthy lifestyle is positively associated with health consciousness, health information orientation, health beliefs, and healthy activities. Finally, individuals who seek out discussion groups on the Internet are more health information oriented.

In addition to its influence on health information-seeking and processing strategies on the Internet, health orientation also influences the processing of persuasive health prevention messages. Highly health-motivated respondents are more likely to comprehend health messages, learn from such messages, and follow the guidelines of the message as compared to those audience members who are less motivated in health-related issues. In an examination of audience segmentation based on motivation, Dutta-Bergman (2005) demonstrated that health-motivated audience members are more likely to comprehend and respond to health messages embedded in media programming. Also, extant research documents the preference of different message types among the high health-involved segment as compared to the low-involvement segment.

Personality

Personality refers to within-population differences with respect to certain systematic characteristics in the population. Harnessing the power of new media technologies, the personality-based approach has been applied by health communication scholars to develop tailored health communication strategies addressing the personality traits of individual audience members (Dutta-Bergman, 2003d; Lieberman, 2001). This literature on personality and health demonstrates that the personality of the audience member influences the type of message he or she responds to. Among the different personality variables applied in message design strategy, sensation seeking, self-monitoring, and idiocentrism-allocentrism have received considerable attention in audience response to health intervention messages (Dutta-Bergman, 2003d; Lieberman, 2001; Palmgreen, Donohue, Lorch, Hoyle, & Stephenson, 2001).

Sensation seeking is a personality trait with high biochemical correlates and taps into the need for novel, complex and emotionally intense stimuli and the willingness to take risks in order to obtain such stimulation (Palmgreen et al., 2001). The trait has been systematically examined in the context of drug use, demonstrating that it is a strong predictor of use of more, and greater variety of, drugs (Donohew, Lorch, & Palmgreen, 1991; Rice, Donohew, & Clayton, 2003). The need for novel and unusual experiences also drives high sensation seekers toward the consumption of high sensation value messages that are typically novel, dramatic, arousing, fast-paced, graphic, and unconventional. In addition, high sensation seekers are more likely to attend to a public service announcement when it is placed in high sensation value television programming as compared to low sensation value television programming (Lorch, Palmgreen, Donohew, Helm, Baer, et al., 1994). The behavioral patterns of high sensation seekers accompanied by the message preference of the group has led to the SENTAR (sensation-seeking targeting) approach that employs sensation seeking as a segmentation variable, develops high sensation value messages based on formative research with high sensation seekers, and delivers such messages in high sensation value contexts.

Self-monitoring is a personality index that is based on the extent to which an individual is likely to monitor and control his or her expression in situations that contain reliable cues to social appropriateness (Snyder

& DeBono, 1985). Therefore, high self-monitors are typically concerned with projecting social images that allow them to meet the varying needs of different social situations. On the other hand, low self-monitors are more concerned with being consistent with their internal feelings and preferences rather than with social appropriateness (Dutta-Bergman, 2003d; Snyder & DeBono, 1985). Thus image-based messages, focusing on impressions created by using the product, are especially effective for high self-monitors (Snyder & DeBono, 1985) whereas low self-monitors are particularly responsive to utilitarian messages that feature appeals to a product quality (Dutta-Bergman, 2003d; Snyder & DeBono, 1985).

Another trait that has received considerable attention in health message design is *idiocentrism* (Dutta-Bergman, 2003d). Idiocentrism pertains to people's tendency to value personal and individual time, freedom, and experiences. High idiocentrics view self as a relatively autonomous, self-sufficient entity independent from its surrounding interpersonal context. Low idiocentrics are more focused on maintaining harmony with others by coming to terms with their needs and expectations. Extant research on health interventions documents that high idiocentrics respond positively to functional appeals that focus on quality whereas low idiocentrics prefer social appeals that emphasize social acceptance (Dutta-Bergman, 2003d).

Health Belief Model

According to the health belief model, health information processing is determined by six key components: perceived severity, perceived susceptibility, benefits, barriers, cues to action and self-efficacy (Rosenstock, 1974). These six components situate the preventive behavior in the realm of a certain health outcome such as HIV infection, cancer, heart disease, and so on. Perceptual processes filter how the individual evaluates the proposed preventive behavior and the outcomes associated with it. In addition, the combination of the six factors shapes the information-processing strategies of the consumer.

Whereas *perceived severity* refers to the individual's assessment of the outcome associated with the preventive behavior, *perceived susceptibility* focuses on the individual's assessment of the extent to which he or she is likely to succumb to the negative outcome. Both perceived severity and perceived susceptibility have to be sufficiently high for the individual to pay attention to health information related to a certain preventive behavior. For instance, the target audience of an HIV/AIDS campaign has to perceive the severity of HIV/AIDS and his or her susceptibility to the disease in order to process health information related to HIV/AIDS.

Benefits are the individual's beliefs regarding the effectiveness of the proposed preventive behavior (Rosenstock, 1974). Formative research often demonstrates that individuals in the target group are unaware of the benefits associated with a self-protective action; in such instances, action can be promoted by highlighting the benefits associated with it (Valente, Paredes, & Poppe, 1998). *Barriers* decrease the individual's ability to engage in the preventive behavior and are described as the evaluation of potential negative consequences that might result from the enactment of the espoused health behavior (Rosenstock, 1974). Health information messages often seek to initiate behavior change by addressing the barriers to a particular behavior. The interactive technology offered by the Internet facilitates the segmentation of the audience based on the different barriers to action, accompanied by differential messages that may be tailored to address these different barriers in different audience segments. The benefits of the behavior need to outweigh the barriers related to the behavior for the behavior to be performed. The audience's perceptions of benefits and barriers related to a particular health behavior are also important in determining health information seeking strategies.

Self-efficacy is the amount of confidence individuals have in their ability to perform the health behavior and positively predicts the adoption of the preventive behavior (Bandura, 2002). It is the perceived ability to exert personal control. Self-efficacy influences the likelihood of health information seeking and health information processing. Rimal (2001) combined perceived risk and self-efficacy to suggest a segmentation strategy for examining the differential motivation to seek information about heart disease. Cues to action are the specific stimuli that are needed to trigger the appropriate health behavior.

Another widely used health communication model, the *extended parallel process* model (Witte, 1992), is based on a similar conceptualization of risk and efficacy: the evaluation of perceived threat and perceived efficacy related to a specific intervention determine the pathway taken by the target audience. When exposed to a health threat and both perceived threat and efficacy are high, the individual attempts to control the danger by adhering to the recommendations of the message; when the perceived threat is high but efficacy is low, individuals are motivated to control the fear through defensive avoidance or denial, not adopting the recommended action.

The health belief model has been used by Johnson and Meischke (1993) to develop the *comprehensive model of health information seeking* with respect to cancer. The authors highlighted the role of demographics, direct experience, salience, and beliefs in shaping information-seeking strategies (Johnson & Meischke, 1991, 1993). The individual's degree of direct experience with the disease, either through symptoms or in one's personal network, influences cancer-related information seeking. Johnson, Meischke, Garu, and Johnson (1992) reported that the strongest predictor of cancer-related information seeking was the respondent's personal experience with cancer. Salience refers to the personal significance of health information to an individual and is related to the perceived risk associated with a behavior or condition. A higher level of salience leads to a greater degree of health information seeking related to the specific topic or issue. Health information seeking is also influenced by the individual's belief in the efficacy of various available procedures in dealing with his or her situation. Therefore, information seeking is positively related to the extent to which individuals believe they can control their future and that there are efficacious options of prevention and control available to him or her.

Transtheoretical Model

The transtheoretical model is the most widely used theory in the area of health campaigns that harnesses the power of interactive technology in delivering appropriate messages to the target audience, depending on the underlying motivation to change a health behavior (Prochaska, DiClemente, & Norcross, 1992; Witherspoon, 2001). For instance, smoking cessation campaigns have frequently used the transtheoretical model (Prochaska et al., 1992). Other areas of implementation of the stages of change model include information delivery on HMO Web sites, physical activity, diet, and HIV/AIDS prevention.

According to the transtheoretical model, individuals can be categorized into groups based on their readiness to change their health behaviors (Prochaska et al., 1992). The five stages of readiness for behavior change are precontemplation, contemplation, preparation, action and maintenance. Individuals who are least ready to make the behavior change are categorized into the precontemplation stage. Contemplation involves thinking about changing the behavior in the next 6 months. The next stage, preparation, refers to an intention to quit, combined with taking active steps to change. Action refers to the stage where the individual has adopted the behavior over a short term. The maintenance stage captures those individuals who have already made the change to their behavior and are consistently engaging in the behavior over a period of time.

Through the use of interactive technologies, the individual's readiness to change is measured and subsequent messages are delivered based on the stage of the audience member (Witherspoon, 2001). Tailored message campaigns have systematically used the interactive technology of the World Wide Web to deliver messages to the audience based on segmentation principles derived from the transtheoretical model. In addition, the stage of change of a consumer with respect to a behavior is likely to influence his or her information-seeking and -processing strategies on the Internet. For instance, the individual in the contemplation and preparation stages is likely to seek out health information on the Internet related to the behavior.

INTERNET AND HEALTH COMMUNICATION: KEY ISSUES

Figure 5.1 presents an integrative model of health information usage based on a summary of the key findings of the published literature reviewed in this chapter. Personality and situation-specific factors contribute to the motivation to process health-related information on the Internet, which, in turn, interacts with consumer efficacy to shape the health uses of the medium. For instance, high perceived severity and perceived susceptibility toward a health risk are likely to trigger motivation in processing health-related information. Individuals who perceive themselves at great risk of HIV/AIDS are more likely to seek out and process HIV/AIDS-related information as compared to individuals who perceive themselves to be at lower risks of contracting HIV/AIDS. In addition, health orientation—an indicator of intrinsic consumer interest in issues of health—contributes to the motivation to search for health information. Therefore, health-oriented consumers are more likely to seek out health information on the Internet compared to their less health-oriented counterparts. The transtheoretical model also captures this motivation by documenting the specific stage of change of the consumer with respect

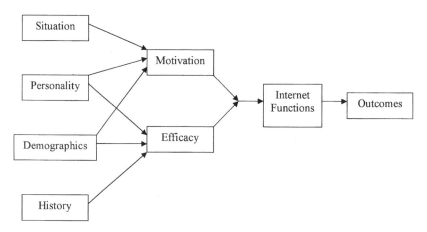

FIG. 5.1.   An integrative model explaining e-health use.

to a specific behavior. Beyond the role of situational and dispositional factors, motivation is also shaped by demographic variables. For instance, Dutta-Bergman (2004d) demonstrated that motivation in health-related issues increases with education and income.

In addition to the motivation for health information seeking, the consumer needs to have access to the Internet, and the ability to use the Internet for health information processing. The concept of efficacy taps into the consumer's belief in his or her ability to engage in a behavior. The greater the efficacy, the stronger the relationship between motivation and the likelihood of health information seeking. Efficacy is shaped by the dispositional orientation of the consumer, his or her experience with the medium (Internet), and his or her demographic characteristics. Of particular relevance are the demographic correlates of access and efficacy, given the technology-related gaps in the population. Consumer uses of the Internet for health care purposes influence a variety of outcomes such as accessibility of care, quality of care, patient satisfaction, physician–patient relationship, and the effectiveness of health care policy.

Access and Equity

One of the key concerns facing the health care industry is one of accessibility. Whereas health care is accessible for some population segments, such care and its benefits are typically inaccessible to the marginalized groups of society. These patterns of inaccessibility are also replicated on the World Wide Web. People with preventable health problems and without insurance coverage are least likely to have access to the necessary technologies (Eng, Maxfield, & Gustafson, 1998). Published research on the digital divide point out significant differences between the higher and lower socioeconomic status (SES) groups in the realm of access to the Internet, with the lower SES groups facing a variety of barriers such as cost, location, illiteracy, physical ability and capacity (Rice, 2001).

Research on the knowledge gap documents that public information campaigns typically improve overall outcome levels, and simultaneously increase the gaps between the higher and lower SES groups of society (Viswanath & Finnegan, 1995). Health information systems on the Internet are likely to contribute to such gaps. Motivation serves an important role as a mediating variable because higher SES groups are typically more health motivated as compared to lower SES groups (Dutta-Bergman, 2004d, 2004e; Johnson & Meischke, 1999). As a result, higher SES groups are more likely to seek out health information resources on the Internet, process information from such resources, and adopt healthy behaviors as compared to lower SES groups (Dutta-Bergman, 2004d). This suggests the need for public and governmental efforts that are specifically targeted at reducing the gaps between the health "haves" and "have nots" in society (Freimuth, Stein, & Kean, 1989). Such efforts need to highlight both issues of access and motivation. Eng, Maxfield, and Gustafson (1998) recommend steps such as providing public and residential access, increasing health and technology literacy, and integrating universal access into health planning. Technology such as multimedia kiosks, information portals, and Internet-equipped computers need to be made available in publicly accessible spaces. One such attempt in bridging the digital divide is the creation of Community Technology Centers (CTCs) that are public access computer facilities located in low-income neighborhoods (Breeden, Cisler, Guilfoy, Roberts, & Stone, 1998).

In addition, schools and worksites in lower SES sectors need to specifically incorporate health-oriented programs that seek to build health orientation in the underprivileged sectors. Such programs also need to include components of self and response efficacy to increase the perceived ability of the underprivileged segments in using the Internet for health care purposes. Targeted workshops and training sessions are needed that teach technology literacy skills related to the effective and efficient use of the Internet, especially for health uses (Cameron, Salazar, Bernhardt, Burgess-Whitman, Wingood, & DiClemente, 2005). For instance, Salovey, Mowad, Pizarro, Edlund, and Moret (2002) developed two community technology centers affiliated with two Head Start early-childhood education programs in New Haven, Connecticut, one of the three poorest cities in the state of Connecticut. The program trained Head Start staff members to become technology coaches, and offered training programs for Head Start parents as well as other individuals in the neighborhood who desired training.

In the realm of prevention, the interactivity of the Internet and other new media technologies may be used for developing tailored health prevention campaigns that address the barriers of the at-risk groups, and deliver communication messages that match the stage of change of the receiver of the message (Rimer & Glassman, 1998). Such message tailoring might be particularly relevant for the underserved sectors of the population because of the uniqueness of the barriers experienced in such segments.

Quality

With the exponential growth in the use of the Internet in consumer segments, one of the important concerns regarding e-health relates to the quality of health information retrieved by patients (Dutta-Bergman, 2003a, 2003b, 2004c; Eysenbach, 2000; Rice, 2001). Quality of health information influences the quality, cost, and effectiveness of care received by the patient. This line of work points out that the quality of health information is intertwined with a plethora of consumer outcomes. Published criteria in the area of Internet use for health care include source credibility, accuracy, completeness, relevance, and applicability. The motivation-driven framework suggests that the evaluation of quality of health information on the Internet varies with the type of function being served by the medium. In other words, the evaluation of quality is a heterogeneous process that varies with the information needs of the consumer. Whereas certain quality criteria might be particularly relevant for consumer decision making in the domain of certain Internet functions, other quality criteria become critically relevant when the consumer uses the Internet for other functions. For instance, the consumer using the Internet for purchasing medicines might be more likely to evaluate the privacy policy of the Web site as compared to the consumer who is simply surfing the web for health information. The motivation-driven approach to quality provides a framework for addressing the relevant aspects of quality based on the needs of the segment.

In summary, the intersection of the Internet and health communication offers a theoretically and pragmatically important field of study that holds important social, political, and economic implications for the health of the public. The examination of motivations in the realm of uses of the Internet for health-related purposes provides a rich entry point into the exploration of this intersection.

REFERENCES

Atkin, C. (1985). Informational utility and selective exposure. In D. Zillman & J. Bryant (Eds.), *Selective exposure to communication* (pp. 63–82). Hillsdale, NJ: Lawrence Erlbaum Associates.

Atkin, D. (1993). Adoption of cable amidst a multimedia environment. *Telematics and Informatics, 10,* 51–58.

Ball-Rokeach, S. J., & DeFleur, M. L. (1976). A dependency model or mass-media effects. *Communication Research, 3,* 3–21.

Bandura, A. (2002). Social cognitive theory of mass communication. In J. Bryant & D. Zillman (Eds.), *Media effects: Advances in theory and research* (pp. 121–154). Mahwah, NJ: Lawrence Erlbaum Associates.

Bothwell, R. K., & Brigham, J. C. (1983). Selective evaluation and recall during the 1980 Reagan-Carter debate. *Journal of Applied Social Psychology, 5,* 427–442.

Breeden, L., Cisler, S., Guilfoy, V., Roberts, M., & Stone, A. (1998). *Computer and communications use in low-income communities: Models for the neighborhood transformation and family development initiative.* Baltimore, MD: Annie E. Casey Foundation.

Cameron, K. A., Salazar, L. F., Bernhardt, J. M., Burgess-Whitman, N., Wingood, G. M., & DiClemente, R. J. (2005). Adolescents' experience with sex on the web: Results from on-line focus groups. *Journal of Adolescence, 28*(4), 535–540.

Capella, J. N., Turow, J., & Jamieson, K. H. (1996). *Call-in political talk radio: Background, content, audiences, portrayal in mainstream media* (Report Series No. 5). Philadelphia: University of Pennsylvania, Annenberg Public Policy Center.

Carlsson, M. (2000). Cancer patients seeking information from sources outside the health care system. *Supportive Care in Cancer: Official Journal of the Multinational Association of Supportive Care in Cancer, 8*(6), 453–457.

Cline, R. J., & Hayes, K. M. (2001). Consumer health information seeking on the Internet: The state of the art. *Health Education Research, 16*(6), 671–692.

Donohew, L., Hoyle, R., Clayton, R., Skinner, W., Colon, S., & Rice, R. E. (1999). Sensation seeking and drug use by adolescents and their friends: Models for marijuana and alcohol. *Journal of Studies on Alcohol, 60*(5), 622–631.

Donohew, L., Lorch, E. P., & Palmgreen, P. (1991). Sensation seeking and targeting of televised anti-drug PSAs. In L. Donohew, H. E. Sypher, & W. J. Bukoski (Eds.), *Persuasive communication and drug use prevention* (pp. 209–226). Hillsdale, NJ: Lawrence Erlbaum Associates.

Dutta-Bergman, M. (2003a). Health communication on the web: The roles of web use motivation and information completeness. *Communication Monographs, 70,* 264–274.

Dutta-Bergman, M. (2003b). Trusted online sources of health information: Differences in demographics, health beliefs, and health-information orientation. *Journal of Medical Internet Research, 5,* e21. Retrieved June 2, 2004, from http://www.jmir.org/2003/3/e21/index.htm

Dutta-Bergman, M. (2003c). Demographic and psychographic antecedents of community participation: Applying a social marketing model. *Social Marketing Quarterly, 9,* 17–31.

Dutta-Bergman, M. (2003d). The linear interaction model of personality effects in health communication. *Health Communication, 15,* 101–115.

Dutta-Bergman, M. (2004a). Developing a profile of consumer intention to seek out health information beyond the doctor. *Health Marketing Quarterly, 21,* 91–112.

Dutta-Bergman, M. (2004b). Primary sources of health information: Comparison in the domain of health attitudes, health cognitions, and health behaviors. *Health Communication, 16,* 273–288.

Dutta-Bergman, M. (2004c). The impact of completeness and web use motivation on the credibility of e-health information. *Journal of Communication, 54,* 253–269.

Dutta-Bergman, M. (2004d). Health attitudes, health cognitions and health behaviors among Internet health information seekers: Population-based survey. *Journal of Medical Internet Research, 6,* e15. Retrieved June 2, 2004, from http://www.jmir.org/2004/2/e15/index.htm

Dutta-Bergman, M. (2004e). Complementarity in consumption of news types across traditional and new media. *Journal of Broadcasting and Electronic Media, 48,* 41–60.

Dutta-Bergman, M. (2005). Psychographic profiling of fruit and vegetable consumption: The role of health orientation. *Social Marketing Quarterly, 11,* 1–17.

Eagly, A., & Chaiken, S. (1993). *The psychology of attitudes.* Fort Worth, TX: Harcourt Brace Jovanovich.

Eng, T. R., Maxfield, A., & Gustafson, D. (1998). Access to health information and support: A public highway or private road? *Journal of the American Medical Association, 280,* 1371–1375.

Eysenbach, G. (2000). Consumer health informatics. *British Medical Journal, 24,* 1713–1716.

Ferguson, D. A. (1992). Channel repertoire in the presence of remote control devices, VCRs, and cable television. *Journal of Broadcasting and Electronic Media, 36,* 83–91.

Ferguson, D., & Perse, E. (2000). The World Wide Web as a functional alternative to television. *Journal of Broadcasting and Electronic Media, 44,* 155–168.

Fox, S., & Fallows, D. (2003). *Internet health resources*. Washington, DC: Pew Internet and American Life Project. Retrieved December 18, 2004, from http://www.pewinternet .org/pdfs/PIP_Health_Report_July_2003.pdf

Freimuth, B. S., Stein, J. A., & Kean, T. J. (1989). *Searching for health information: The Cancer Information Service model*. Philadelphia, PA: University of Pennsylvania Press.

Johnson, J. D., & Meischke, H. (1991). Cancer information: Women's sources and content preferences. *Journal of Health Care Marketing, 11,* 37–44.

Johnson, J. D., & Meischke, H. (1993). A comprehensive model of cancer-related information seeking applied to magazines. *Human Communication Research, 19,* 343–367.

Johnson, J. D., Meischke, H., Garu, J., & Johnson, S. (1992). Cancer-related channel selection. *Health Communication, 4,* 183–196.

Kargaonkar, P. K., & Wolin, L. (1999, March). A multivariate analysis of web usage. *Journal of Advertising Research, 39*(2), 53–68.

LaRose, R., & Atkin, D. (1992). Audiotext and the reinvention of the telephone as a mass medium. *Journalism Quarterly, 69,* 413–421.

Lieberman, D. A. (2001). Using interactive media in communication campaigns for children and adolescents. In R. E. Rice & C. K. Atkin (Eds.), *Public communication campaigns* (pp. 373–388). Thousand Oaks, CA: Sage.

Lin, C. A., & Jeffres, L. W. (1998). Factors influencing the adoption of multimedia cable technology. *Journalism and Mass Communication Quarterly, 75,* 341–352.

Lorch, E., Palmgreen, P., Donohew, L., Helm, D., Baer, S., & Dsilva, M. (1994). Program context, sensation seeking, and attention to televised anti-drug public service announcements. *Human Communication Research, 20,* 390–412.

MacInnis, D. J., Moorman, C., & Jaworski, B. (1991). Enhancing and measuring consumers' motivation, opportunity, and ability to process brand information from ads. *Journal of Marketing, 55,* 32–53.

Mittman, R., & Cain, M. (2001). The future of the Internet in health care: A five-year forecast. In R. E. Rice & J. Katz (Eds.), *The Internet and health communication* (pp. 47–73). Thousand Oaks, CA: Sage.

Moorman, C., & Matulich, E. (1993). A model of consumers' preventive health behaviors: The role of health motivation and health ability. *Journal of Consumer Research, 20,* 208–228.

Napoli, P. (2001). Consumer use of medical information from electronic and paper media: A literature review. In R. E. Rice & J. E. Katz (Eds.), *The Internet and health communication: Experiences and expectations* (pp. 79–98). Thousand Oaks, CA: Sage.

Oliver, M. B. (2002). Individual differences in media effects. In J. Bryant & D. Zillman (Eds.), *Media effects: Advances in theory and research* (pp. 507–524). Mahwah, NJ: Lawrence Erlbaum Associates.

Palmgreen, P., Donohew, L., Lorch, E. P., Hoyle, R. H., & Stephenson, M. T. (2001). Television campaigns and adolescent marijuana use: Tests of a sensation seeking targeting. *American Journal of Public Health, 91,* 292–296.

Papacharissi, Z., & Rubin, A. (2000). Predictors of Internet use. *Journal of Broadcasting and Electronic Media, 44,* 175–196.

Parker, B. J., & Plank, R. E. (2000). A uses and gratifications perspective on the Internet as a new information source. *American Business Review, 4,* 43–49.

Perse, E. M. (1990). Media involvement and local news effects. *Journal of Broadcasting and Electronic Media, 34*(1), 17–36.

Perse, E. M., & Courtright, J. A. (1993). Normative images of communication media: Mass and interpersonal channels in the new media environment. *Human Communication Research, 19,* 485–503.

Perse, E., & Dunn, D. (1998). The utility of home computers and media use: Implications of multimedia and connectivity. *Journal of Broadcasting and Electronic Media, 42,* 435–456.

Petty, R. E., & Cacioppo, J. T. (1986). *Communication and persuasion: Central and peripheral routes to attitude change.* New York: Springer-Verlag.

Petty, R. E., & Cacioppo, J. T. (1990). Involvement and persuasion: Tradition versus integration. *Psychological Bulletin, 107*(3), 367–374.

Prochaska, J. O., DiClemente, C., & Norcross, J. (1992). In search of how people change: Applications to addictive behaviors. *American Psychologist, 47,* 1102–1114.

Rice, R. E. (1993). Media appropriateness: Using social presence theory to compare traditional and new organizational media. *Human Communication Research, 19,* 451–484.

Rice, R. E. (2001). The Internet and health communication: A framework of experiences. In R. E. Rice & J. Katz (Eds.), *The Internet and health communication* (pp. 5–46). Thousand Oaks, CA: Sage.

Rice, R. E. (2006). Influences, usage, and outcomes of Internet health information searching: Multivariate results from the Pew surveys. *International Journal of Medical Informatics, 75*(1), 8–28.

Rice, R. E., & Case, D. (1983). Electronic message systems in the university: A description of use and utility. *Journal of Communication, 33,* 131–152.

Rice, R. E., Donohew, L., & Clayton, R. (2003). Peer network, sensation seeking, and drug use among junior and senior high school students. *Connections, 25*(2), 32–58.

Rimal, R. (2001). Perceived risk and self-efficacy as motivators: Understanding individuals' long-term use of health information. *Journal of Communication, 51,* 633–654.

Rimer, B. K., & Glassman, B. (1998). Tailoring communication for primary care settings. *Methods of Information in Medicine, 37,* 1610–1611.

Rogers, E. M. (1995). *Diffusion of innovations* (5th ed.). New York: Free Press.

Rosenstock, I. M. (1974). The health belief model and preventive health behavior. *Health Education Monographs, 2,* 354–386.

Rubin, A. (1994). Media uses and effects: A uses and gratifications perspective. In J. Bryant & D. Zillman (Eds.), *Media effects: Advances in theory and research* (pp. 417–436). Hillsdale, NJ: Lawrence Erlbaum Associates.

Rubin, A. (2002). The uses and gratifications perspective of media effects. In J. Bryant & D. Zillman (Eds.), *Media effects: Advances in theory and research* (pp. 525–548). Mahwah, NJ: Lawrence Erlbaum Associates.

Salovey, P., Mowad, L., Pizarro, J., Edlund, D., & Moret, M. (2002). Developing computer proficiency among Head Start parents: An in-progress case study of a New England CIS digital divide project. *Electronic Journal of Communication, 11,* 3. Retrieved October 9, 2002, from http://www.cios.org/getfile/saolvey_v11n3

Snyder, M., & DeBono, K. G. (1985). Appeals to image and claims about quality: Understanding the psychology of advertising. *Journal of Personality and Social Psychology, 49,* 586–597.

Stempel, G., Hargrove, T., & Bernt, J. (2000). Relation of growth of use of the Internet to changes in media use from 1995 to 1999. *Journalism and Mass Communication Quarterly, 77,* 71–79.

Sweeney, P. D., & Gruber, K. L. (1984). Selective exposure: Voter information preferences and the Watergate affair. *Journal of Personality and Social Psychology, 46,* 1208–1221.

Valente, T. W., Paredes, P., & Poppe, P. R. (1998). Matching the message to the process: The relative ordering of knowledge, attitudes and practices in behavior change research. *Human Communication Research, 24,* 366–385.

Vidmar, N., & Rokeach, M. (1974). Archie Bunker's bigotry: A study in selective perception and exposure. *Journal of Communication, 24,* 36–47.

Viswanath, K., & Finnegan, J. R. (1995). The knowledge gap hypothesis: Twenty-five years later. In B. Burleson (Ed.), *Communication Yearbook 19* (pp. 187–228). Thousand Oaks, CA: Sage.

Webster, J. G., & Wakshlag, J. (1985). Measuring exposure to television. In D. Zillmann & J. Bryant (Eds.), *Selective exposure to communication* (pp. 35–62). Hillsdale, NJ: Lawrence Erlbaum Associates.

Witherspoon, E. (2001). A pound of cure: A content analysis of health information on websites of top-ranked HMOs. In R. E. Rice & J. E. Katz (Eds.), *The Internet and health communication* (pp. 189–212). Thousand Oaks, CA: Sage.

Witte, K. (1992). Putting the fear back into fear appeals: The extended parallel process model. *Communication Monographs, 59,* 329–349.

III

SEARCHING, DISCUSSING, AND EVALUATING ONLINE HEALTH INFORMATION

Singapore Internet Users' Health Information Search: Motivation, Perception of Information Sources, and Self-Efficacy*

Evelyn Tang
Waipeng Lee
Nanyang Technological University

Modern technology has facilitated the creation, dissemination, and reception of information. In the last two decades, the Internet has emerged to be the new medium, complementing, expanding on, integrating, and in some cases replacing television, radio, and print media. The Internet's popularity has led to the repositioning and reconceptualization of various sectors, including commerce, government, and education.

One of the growing online sectors is e-health. An estimated 74% of American Internet users have searched for health information at one time or another (Taylor & Leitman, 2004), and millions of Germans, Japanese, and French people are looking up health information online (Taylor & Leitman, 2002). Given the importance of health in people's lives, it is not surprising to see a boom in health-related online services, which range from telemedicine to online pharmacies.

Unfortunately, information on Singapore's e-health scene is limited. However, it is reasonable to speculate that many Singaporeans have access to online health sites—either within or outside Singapore. In fact, Singapore is one of the most wired countries in the world. It has 62.2 computers per 100 persons; and the figure is just slightly behind the United States, which has the highest computers per capita (International Telecommunication Union [ITU], 2004). Singapore's Internet penetration

---

*The Singapore Internet Project funded this study.

rate is one of the highest in the world, with more than half of its population being Internet users (ITU, 2001). According to Internet World Stats' (2005) compilation of worldwide penetration rates, the global average is only 13.9%, but Singapore is ranked 13th at 60.2%.

In addition to a high Internet penetration rate, the Singapore government has been a significant promoter of applying information technology in health care (ITU, 2001; Tay-Yap & Al-Hawamdeh, 2001). This social and political environment encourages health care organizations to join the e-health bandwagon. In fact, Singapore's Ministry of Health (MOH) is one of the greatest promoters of e-health (ITU, 2001). Portals and systems are set up to facilitate communication and education among health care professionals, and between health care providers and patients. Online access to archiving and retrieving of health and medical records is also available. Many public and private health care providers, such as clinics and hospitals, have their own Web sites. Health care providers have gone beyond posting introductions to their organizations, and are supplying health-related content on the Internet (e.g., Changi General Hospital and Alexandra Hospital). Some even have e-pharmacies (e.g., Changi General Hospital and Tan Tock Seng Hospital). Nonprofit health-related organizations, ranging from the Breast Cancer Foundation to the Singapore Medical Council, also have online presence. However, e-health raises many questions, including the credibility of information providers, privacy issues, and veracity of health claims.

AIMS

Because e-health encompasses many aspects, this study is limited to health information searching. To limit the scope further and for meaningful comparison, this study focuses on Internet users only. Understandably, not all Internet users will ever, or always, go online to search for health information. Our intention is to examine why some Internet users will go online for health information, whereas other users will not. To avoid cumbersome terminologies, we refer to Internet users who go online to search for health information as "e-health seekers," and Internet users who do not, as "nonseekers."

The approach is to use the focus group method to explore how Singapore Internet users search for health information. Specifically, we are interested in knowing (a) how they use the various sources; (b) what motivates them to search for health information; (c) their perception of the Internet and other health information sources, including mass media and interpersonal contacts; and (d) the role of self-efficacy.

Uses and Gratifications Approach and Motivations

The uses and gratifications approach has been applied in the investigation of various communication technologies, such as network and cable television (Heeter & Greenberg, 1985; Miyazaki, 1981; Rubin, 1983), newspapers (Elliot & Rosenberg, 1987), magazines (Towers, 1986), and videocassette recorders (Levy, 1987; Rubin & Bantz, 1987). More recently, researchers have also examined telephone/cellular telephones (Dimmick, Kline, & Stafford, 2000; Leung & Wei, 2000) and the Internet (Dimmick et al., 2000; Kaye & Johnson, 2002; Papacharissi & Rubin, 2000) with this perspective (see also Dutta-Bergman, chap. 5, this volume).

At the emergence of any communication technology, one of the questions that researchers commonly pose is why do people use the technology. Therefore, despite the criticism that the uses and gratification approach is atheoretical, it still has its appeal and its place (Kaye & Johnson, 2002; Ruggiero, 2000). It is even more attractive considering its emphasis on an active audience. The idea of an active user is more apparent with the Internet than with traditional mass media. This is because Internet users decide what they want to do online and which site and information to search. This gives the impression of active gatekeeping. In contrast, traditional mass media users seem passive as they receive prepackaged information from journalists and editors.

According to uses and gratifications, people have different needs: cognitive, affective, personal integrative, social integrative, and escapist (Katz, Blumler, & Gurevitch, 1974; Katz, Gurevitch, & Haas, 1973). Their needs influence their expectations of a source, which in turn affect how much they will use a particular source (Rubin, 1986). In the case of the Internet, research shows that people use it for interpersonal utility, passing time, entertainment, information, and convenience (Papacharissi & Rubin, 2000). Another study shows that Internet users seek online political information for four reasons: guidance on decision-making, surveillance, entertainment, and interpersonal utility (Kaye & Johnson, 2002).

In the context of health, the Pew Internet and American Life Project discovers that people search for online health information because of: a new diagnosis on others or self, new treatments or medications, the need to cope with health problems, and unanswered questions after visiting doctors (Fox & Rainie, 2002; Rice, 2006). Another study shows that HIV/ AIDS patients use the Internet to gain knowledge, learn about coping strategies, and acquire social support (Kalichman, Benotsch, Wienhardt, Austin, Luke, & Cherry, 2003). However, health information is available not only on the Internet, but also through other sources.

Although people have access to a plethora of information sources— ranging from the mass media to interpersonal contacts—they do not use the mass and interpersonal sources in the same manner (on health information-seeking behaviors, see Dutta-Bergman, chap. 5, this volume; Napoli, 2001; Wilson, 1997). Nonetheless, mass media and interpersonal channels are not in competition; although there may be some displacement, they serve complementary functions (Chaffee, 1982). Moreover, people have different needs and they derive different levels of gratifications from the use of particular information sources. As Dimmick and his associates (2000) have pointed out, it is useful if we are able to compare a new medium with established sources, and see how each satisfies its users. This allows researchers to understand if these sources displace or complement each other.

According to uses and gratifications, people have expectations about information sources, and those expectations influence usage (Katz et al., 1974). Logically, if people hold a positive perception of a source, they should use it more, and vice versa. However, when it comes to the Internet and its trustworthiness, this notion may not be true. For example, many Internet users have expressed their skepticism toward online information (Murero, D'Ancona, & Karamanoukian, 2001; Newport & Saad, 1998), yet they have not terminated their Internet usage.

Because health, in some situations, is a matter of life and death, it is not surprising that e-health raises questions about quality and credibility of information, along with privacy and confidentiality issues. Studies reveal that objective and accurate online health information is rare (Lissman & Boehnlein, 2001; Rice, 2003; Sacchetti, Zvara, & Plante, 1999; Seidman, chap. 10, this volume), and users do not always trust presumably credible Web sites, such as government-sponsored ones (Bernhart, Lariscy, Parrott, Silk, & Felter, 2002). Even the completeness of information on a health site can affect perception of credibility (Dutta-Bergman, 2004).

Although research shows that people are concerned about online information, are they equally worried about information from other sources? Although mass media have gatekeepers, this does not guarantee good quality information either. Health care practitioners have accused the mass media of sensationalism, reporting out of context, and omitting vital information (Stamm, Williams, Noël, & Rubin, 2003). In Singapore, the mass media enjoy a high level of trust (Kuo, Choi, Arun, Lee, & Soh, 2002); a majority of the people trust the news found in newspaper, television, and radio. Therefore, it is plausible that the same trust is applicable to health coverage.

Mass media aside, people do turn to their family and friends, coworkers, and doctors for health advice. Clearly, some of these interpersonal sources are not health experts. However, people trust that their family and friends will not intentionally harm them. Therefore, we are interested in comparing the Internet to traditional mass media and interpersonal sources, which include both experts and non-experts.

Past research on Internet use has examined socioeconomic and psychological factors to explain why some people embrace the new medium readily whereas others lag behind. Among them is Bandura's (1986) self-efficacy, or the confidence of one's ability in performing a task. When people have confidence in doing something, they are more likely to succeed. Although people can exude confidence in many settings, self-efficacy is task specific. A 2001 study shows that media self-efficacy is related to media uses and exposure (Hofstetter, Zuniga, & Dozier, 2001). Self-efficacy is a characteristic that purportedly differentiates Internet users and non-users (Eastin & LaRose, 2000); that is people's confidence in their own ability to use computer and the Internet. In another study, the reverse is also true—that is, the more people use the Internet, the more confident they become (LaRose, Eastin, & Gregg, 2001). In other words, self-efficacy and usage influence each other. Therefore, we are interested in understanding:

RQ1: How do e-health seekers and nonseekers use various information sources?

RQ2: What motivates e-health seekers and nonseekers to search for health information on various sources?

RQ3: How do e-health seekers and nonseekers perceive mass media, the Internet, and interpersonal sources in terms of (a) information quality, and (b) source credibility?

RQ4: What is the role of self-efficacy in using, discerning, and verifying the Internet mass amount of information to differentiate e-health seekers from nonseekers?

METHODS

To examine the four research questions, we conducted a series of focus group sessions in April 5–12, 2003, at the Nanyang Technological University's Executive Center on Orchard Road, Singapore. We used the snowballing technique to recruit participants. We asked friends to recommend their acquaintances. Our selection criteria were that participants must be Internet users, conversant in English, and 18 years old and above. As mentioned earlier, our intention was to examine Internet users only. By focusing on this group, we were able to investigate why some would seek online information, whereas others would not. This helped us rule out digital divide-related issues on unequal access to new technology (see Katz & Rice, 2002). Although non-Internet users could provide insights as to why people did not adopt the technology in general, they might not be helpful in the discussion of e-health due to a lack of access, relevant literacy, or online experience.

In total, we recruited 38 adults to participate in the discussions. We scheduled six discussion groups—three for e-health seekers and three for nonseekers. Participants could choose one that suited their schedules. At the end, four groups had six participants each, and the other two had seven each. Both researchers moderated three discussion groups each; and while they were not moderating, they assisted in taking notes and recording. Each discussion lasted about 1½ hours, and participants received $30 (Singapore; = US$18) incentive. With the consent of the participants, we tape-recorded all conversations. We asked participants to compare their experiences with traditional mass media, the Internet, and interpersonal sources. Specifically, they discussed their use of the sources; and perceived importance, credibility, relevance, ease of use, and convenience for each source. Overall, the participants shared some demographic characteristics, which gave us two advantages. First, perceived similarity could foster disclosure and allowed participants to be more candid in their discussion. Second, we could rule out alternative reasons that might differentiate the e-health seekers from nonseekers.

We then transcribed all six discussions for coding. Open-ended data were coded along two aspects—use of information sources and motivation of use. For the first aspect, we coded for the advantages/disadvantages of (a) traditional media; (b) the Internet; and (c) interpersonal contacts; and source credibility, and search pattern (i.e., how they use information sources in a sequential or parallel fashion). For the second aspect, we coded for curiosity, personal health management, control/uncertainty reduction, social support, and interpersonal utility (i.e., for conversational purposes).

RESULTS

Demographic results showed that 21 of the 38 participants were in the 25- to 45-year-old age group. All except seven participants had earned a university degree; and the remaining seven had at least O-Level (equivalent to 10th grade in the American education system). All, except five, held full-time employment.

USE OF INFORMATION SOURCES (RQ1)

We asked participants to compare their experiences with traditional mass media, the Internet, and interpersonal sources. Specifically, they discussed their use of the sources; and perceived importance, credibility, relevance, ease of use, and convenience for each source.

We did not ask participants to explain the sequence of their information-seeking behavior. However, their discussion on information sources actually elucidates three distinct dimensions of information-seeking behavior, which may or may not occur in sequence: scanning or monitoring, understanding, and confirming.

Information Sources: Surveillant, Excavator and Verifier

Information sources play three roles: surveillant, excavator, and verifier. As the term implies, *surveillants* are information sources who are constantly observing the environment. They can act as beacons and inform participants of new and developing health concerns. *Excavators* allow people to dig deep into health issues and retrieve detailed and complex information, whereas *verifiers* help them confirm the veracity and accuracy of information. Participants rely on surveillants to obtain information, usually requiring little effort on the part of the users. However, surveillants' information may not be satisfactory so people are typically required or stimulated to do more. Therefore, people turn to excavators, sources that can provide specific and in-depth information. Unfortunately, details are not always enough. People still need to determine the veracity of their information, and to confirm or disconfirm their beliefs about health-related matters. As such, they seek out sources that function as verifiers.

E-health seekers and nonseekers in our study manifest different behavioral patterns. The former uses television and newspaper as surveillants; the Internet and books as excavators; and interpersonal sources as verifiers. Of the 19 e-health seekers, eight rely on television and newspapers as surveillants; 12 use the Internet and books as excavators; and 12 turn to interpersonal sources for confirmation. As for the nonseekers, 11 out of 19 use television and newspaper as surveillants. However, despite their access to the Internet, the new medium is not their excavator. They prefer books or doctors for specific information. Even then, they seem to be less proactive in searching for health information regardless of source. Thirteen out of 19 nonseekers seem to use interpersonal sources as both their excavators and verifiers.

These findings parallel certain aspects of Wilson's (1997) proposed information behavior model. Wilson's model includes four characteristics: passive attention, passive search, active search, and ongoing search. Passive attention refers to unintentional acquisition of information. When our participants say that they use traditional mass media (except books) to search for information, they are in fact describing this process. For example, they may come across information about health while watching the news. To our participants, the use of mass media for health purposes is an ongoing-search strategy. They realize that the mass media do highlight important health information and issues. When something captures their attention, they may decide to pursue with an active search, such as looking up medical books, talking to friends and health care professionals, or searching the Internet. People can also acquire information when they are searching for something unrelated, and this process is called *passive search*.

Ellis and Haugan (1997) studied how scientists and engineers conducted their information searches. The components include: surveying (i.e., identifying relevant sources); chaining (i.e., following through with the identified sources); monitoring (i.e., checking the sources for updates); browsing (i.e., scanning source features, such as table of contents, for relevance); distinguishing (i.e., ranking the importance of information sources); filtering (i.e., screening for relevant information, such as using keyword search); extracting (i.e., retrieving information); and ending the search. Our study does not address microlevel information-seeking behaviors, such as filtering and extracting, and therefore we cannot map our findings to Ellis' model. However, we notice that our participants have a predetermined idea as to which information sources are useful (i.e., surveying) and important (i.e., distinguishing) for health information.

Internet Health Seekers

As just mentioned, e-health seekers appeared to rely on television and newspaper for surveillance purposes. This is because, in Singapore, the two media are ubiquitous, and they bring breaking news, discoveries, and ongoing health debates to the audience. In other words, little effort is required on the part of the audience.

Moreover, television and newspaper prompt e-health seekers to look for more information. That is, if health news on television or newspaper triggers their curiosity, e-health seekers will turn to the Internet or books for more specific or in-depth information. As L.P., one of the focus group participants, says, "Because of my busy schedule, the most immediate source will be the mass media. . . . If I feel I need more in-depth information, then I'll go to the Internet or bookshop. But the most immediate source is the mass media." However, television and newspaper are not the only triggers for deeper search. Other forms of mass-communicated messages, such as government campaign posters, magazines, and pamphlets at clinics, can also set them off to find out more.

Interestingly, although eight out of 19 e-health seekers use the television and newspaper to scan their environment, only two say that the Internet is their choice of surveillance tool. These few e-health seekers often miss television broadcasts or have little time for reading newspaper. As such, they surf the Internet first, and then turn to health or medical books for details.

In general, e-health seekers do not rely on interpersonal sources for new health information. Undeniably, health care professionals, and family and friends are able to provide health tips, but they are less important to e-health seekers, who treat interpersonal sources as verifiers. E-health seekers may have found information through other means, and they approach interpersonal sources to verify such information. Health care professionals are experts and are in the position to confirm the validity of information, especially on treatments or diagnoses, found elsewhere. In fact, e-health seekers often label health care professionals as their "advisors" or "consultants." On the other hand, non-expert interpersonal contacts are helpful in providing testimonies on the success of treatments. As participant Jane says, "People are important because they would be the ones who have gone through it, and can give you a first-hand experience." Nonetheless, e-health seekers can be discerning. If they have a reason to doubt their interpersonal contacts—regardless of expertise—they will revert to the Internet for more.

Internet Health Nonseekers

Our findings show that nonseekers, too, regard television and newspaper as surveillants. However, when compared to e-health seekers, they seem less keen on finding out more for themselves. Nonseekers are less patient with large quantities of information. A few have gone online to search for health information, but it is because their family members have asked them to do so. In contrast, e-health seekers are likely to volunteer to search for their family and friends.

For in-depth information, a minority of nonseekers will turn to books or health magazines. However, 14 out of 19 nonseekers will simply ask health care professionals, or family and friends. As participant Ganesh said, "When you want to know more, ask people who are in the know because it's their job to know." Now, contrast Ganesh with an e-health seeker like Nicholas. "I'm very inquisitive. Each time when I go for medical check-up, I'll talk to the doctor," explains Nicholas. "But before I go, I read up so that I will know what questions to ask him. And for things I don't know, I even want him to spell them out, and I'll write them down. When I go back, I'll go straight to the Internet or some of the [medical] directories that I have."

Overall, nonseekers seem to prefer a passive approach and rely on others—be it media gatekeepers or interpersonal sources—for digested information. They place a premium on trust, which acts as their heuristic in health decision making. If e-health seekers seem more proactive, then nonseekers appear more efficient.

MOTIVATIONS OF USE (RQ2)

In our sample, when people search for health information, it is often because of personal or social support needs. The third reason, interpersonal utility—that is, to use health information they have collected from mass media (including the Internet) for conversations with others—is limited to a minority. E-health seekers and nonseekers seem to share similar needs.

Personal Needs

According to our findings, three types of personal needs seem to prevail: curiosity, health management, and sense of control.

Often people come across a particular medical jargon, condition, or treatment, and *curiosity* to understand this material motivates them to search for more. Eight out of 38 participants have cited curiosity or the need to know as a reason. For example, one of the participants, Adrian, has a friend, who was diagnosed with AIDS. He describes his searching:

> That same night, I just went onto the Net to find out more. I read the whole history of it . . . and found the cocktails [remedies] and their effects. There were so many message boards, with people writing about their own experiences after taking the cocktails. . . . Just within 3 hours, I was so well informed with HIV, and I actually knew what it was. I can't imagine going to the library and finding a book, or calling up 10 people to find out.

The second category of personal need is *health management*. This can be as simple as keeping fit or learning to cope with critical illnesses, and 16 out of 38 participants have mentioned it. Often, people need to understand a diagnosis or a treatment, compare the effectiveness and side effects of treatments, keep abreast of medical developments that have implications on their health, seek clarification or answers, and to some extent, self-diagnose (see also Murero et al., 2001).

The third type of personal need is a *sense of control*. Knowing reduces uncertainty, which can be distressing. Information seeking is a way to deal with unpredictability (Berger, 1987; Brashers, Neidig, Haas, Dobbs, Cardillo, et al., 2000). Overall, 11 out of 38 participants have alluded to this. As participant Raphael says, motivation to search for information and severity of a condition are related. That is, a mild and common condition is not alarming. However, an unusual or serious one will prompt him to take charge, and gaining more information is a way to be control and be independent. As participant Adlinah puts it, "I think it's a responsibility to your own health. . . . You can't always assume what the doctor says [is true]. I think you should have a bigger say in your health."

Social Support Needs

People also feel responsible for family and friends' well-being, and it is not surprising that they will search for information on behalf of others. In fact, 13 of the 38 participants have volunteered to do so. Social support needs parallel personal needs. People are willing to help family and friends to satisfy their curiosity about a condition or treatment. They also help manage their family and friends' health. Certainly, by providing information to their loved ones, they are also conferring a sense of control. Participants are able to provide many anecdotes to illustrate these aspects. For example, one participant has searched for information to help his mother, who has undergone four surgeries. Another has tried to help an infertile friend, and a third has created a concoction of Chinese herbs to treat her friend's gastrointestinal problem. This is consistent with the literature that people do facilitate their family and friends' acquisition of health information (Wyatt, Henwood, Hart, & Smith, 2005). In fact, social support comes in different forms, such as provision of information and emotional support. Patients resort to information seeking as a means to cope with their conditions and to reduce uncertainty, and their family and friends do support by passing on information to them (Brashers et al., 2000; Brown, Koch, & Webb, 2000; Wright, 2002).

Interpersonal Utility Needs

They are not widespread among the participants. Only three participants say that they need to find out more about health so that they can have intelligent conversations with health care professionals. Indeed many may look up information to help others, and as a result, they have to communicate with their family or friends. However, the driving force is to provide social support and not to use the information as conversational topics.

INFORMATION QUALITY (RQ3a)

E-health seekers and nonseekers in this study agree that television and newspapers are good for overviews, whereas the Internet and books provide specifics and depth. Both groups also agree that the Internet carries an unfathomable amount of information. However, this is where the similarity ends.

To e-health seekers, television and newspaper lack depth, and may not carry useful or relevant information. Therefore, health or medical books become good companions to them. Daniel's response illustrates this point, "I have this thousand-page book called *Prevention of Diseases*, which I read. I also go to the Internet. I rank traditional mass media like TV, radio, and newspaper as not relevant because, to me, they're very basic."

Despite the complexity of Internet search—including handling information overload, navigating through hundreds of relevant and irrelevant hits, and separating veracious from dubious health tips—e-health seekers are keen to use the technology. Of the 19 e-health seekers, 12 have explicitly said that believe they can find online health information that is specific and detailed, new, and relevant. In fact, e-health seekers recognize the shortcomings of the Internet, but they do not shun the medium at all.

"In the Internet, you do get [varying views]. And a lot of times, some of them are controversial. And I think that's great, as it forces you to think about it yourself, and it forces you to go and find out even more and ask even more people," says June. "So, you get a clearer picture in the end—not just one view you get from the newspaper, especially ours."

June does not avoid complexities. She also realizes that in Singapore, media are tightly controlled and therefore they may simply provide a single perspective.

In contrast, nonseekers favor television and newspaper because they are easy to understand. Simplicity seems to be an advantage, and specifics are unattractive. Meanwhile, the mixture of good and misleading information on the Internet bothers nonseekers, who repeatedly complain that there is too much information and too many sites; even reputable health sites provide conflicting views; it takes too much time and effort to sort out the information; and online health information is not always accurate.

As for interpersonal sources, both e-health seekers and nonseekers place little emphasis on quality. As highlighted earlier, e-health seekers treat interpersonal sources as verifiers that can help them confirm or dispel health tips. Therefore, it is not necessary for interpersonal contacts to provide them with new ideas or details. On the other hand, nonseekers single out trust as an important decision-making rule. Fourteen of the 19 nonseekers will listen to trusted interpersonal sources, and there is no evidence that quality of information is an issue.

SOURCE CREDIBILITY (RQ3b)

As just noted, both e-health seekers and nonseekers reported their belief that the Singapore mass media are credible sources. To them, the Singapore government has tight control over the media. As such, they perceived that reporters provide accurate coverage. In addition, the Singapore government is perceived as trustworthy, and a credible health information source (e.g., the Ministry of Health). Eight participants believe government control keeps health coverage in Singapore credible; no participants oppose this view. However, at least two e-health seekers think that there is a disadvantage to this. Tight control translates to limited information and perspective. As Daniel says, "My view is that the newspapers are rather sanctified and general. They do not want to go in depth in case there may be some things that attract controversy. So, they tend to be very careful."

Similarly, both e-health seekers and nonseekers share the view that users have to exercise discretion with online health information. They agree that users should look for credible institutional sites, verify online information with that from other sources and sites, remain open-minded, and use common sense. Although nonseekers believe it is possible to distinguish good and bad online health information, they offer fewer suggestions on how to do so. On the other hand, e-health seekers are able to articulate their strategies in detail and provide examples. Participant Linda describes her method:

> If [the information] is university or hospital related, and if articles are written by a physician or vetted by a healthcare professional or a panel of medical professional or nurse, then you know it's reliable. Nevertheless, if the article is written by someone who is not attached to a university, I can still use the information and verify [it] against another Web site.

Like Linda, Nicholas examines the credibility of the Web site as well. He even checks out the "about us" and "contact us" sections. These provide hints as to whether the health information can be trusted or not.

When it comes to interpersonal sources, both e-health seekers and nonseekers are selective. They understand that interpersonal sources, experts and non-experts, may offer conflicting or inaccurate information. However, e-health seekers are more willing to listen to a variety of interpersonal sources, but are less likely to trust any blindly. To them, health care professionals can make mistakes, do not necessary know enough, or may lack the skills to explain medical jargons to patients. Yet, this does not mean e-health seekers hold a negative perception toward health care professionals. E-health seekers recognize health care professionals' vulnerabilities and when it comes to seeking information and advice, they are careful. As for non-expert interpersonal sources, e-health seekers only trust those who have extensive health knowledge, and those who share a particular medical or treatment experience with them. Even then, they seem to be tentative.

In contrast, nonseekers seem to place great trust on health care professionals, especially physicians, despite their shortcomings, such as inconsistent diagnoses and aversive to alternative ideas. Nonseekers believe that every information source has its imperfections, but health care professionals seem most dependable. Seven of the 19 nonseekers have expressed a high level of trust on health care professionals (as opposed to two e-health seekers). Nonseekers also hold ambiguous feelings toward non-experts.

SELF-EFFICACY (RQ4)

The three research questions just discussed explore the differences between e-health seekers and nonseekers in terms of their motivations and perceptions of information sources. However, self-efficacy may also play a role in distinguishing e-health seekers and nonseekers.

All participants—seekers and nonseekers—agree that the Internet carries a lot of information, and some sites are dubious and cannot be trusted. Whereas nine out of 19 e-health seekers have openly discussed how they can handle information overload, only four out of 19 nonseekers are able to do so. Overall, e-health seekers exude confidence in handling large amounts of online information, discerning, and verifying it. They seem to welcome the challenge. They claim that common sense is necessary and important. In contrast, nonseekers are less sure if they can cope with the complexity of e-health. The prior sections on the perception of information quality and credibility sections also revealed some aspects of the importance of self-efficacy in distinguishing e-health seekers from nonseekers. Participant Shireen does not use the Internet for health purposes because it is "too vast," and she feels frustrated having to spend time sieving through layers of information and still not find what she needs.

"I'm not very IT savvy," she says. "I don't know which sites to go to. With the Internet, you don't know what's right and what's wrong. The written stuff on medical issues is so technical that you don't understand."

Table 6.1 summarizes the primary differences between e-health seekers, and nonseekers, across the four research questions.

CONCLUSION

Overall, this study confirms the uses and gratification model that people use information sources for different reasons. These information sources play different roles in health information seeking. The differentiation is clear for e-health seekers—who seem to use television and newspapers as their main surveillants; the Internet and books for uncovering deeper information; and interpersonal contacts for verification purposes. Nonseekers also use television and newspapers as surveillants. However, they are not keen on digging deeper for information themselves. Instead, they rely on trusted interpersonal contacts for proven tips.

Although the uses and gratification model takes into account motivation, it does not include factors that may facilitate or hinder the use of certain information sources. In this study, e-health seekers and nonseekers differ little in terms of their motivation in health information search, and their perception of mass media, the Internet, and interpersonal contacts. However, the two groups seem to differ in self-efficacy. E-health seekers are comfortable with large quantities of inconsistent information, welcome conflicting views, and like to decide good and bad information themselves. However, nonseekers prefer to use trust and expert role as heuristics for decision making. They generally complain about information overload and inconsistent suggestions. As such, a more comprehensive perspective, such as Wilson's (1997) information behavior model, which includes psychological to environmental factors, and Ellis' (1997) information-seeking model, which describes the processes of search, can expand our understanding.

This study shows that the motivations behind health information search are relatively predictable. People are curious and want to know more, they need the information to manage their own health, they want some sense of control due to uncertainty, and they want to provide support to others. In general, traditional mass media, such as television and newspaper, act as surveillants, which help people scan the environment for any interesting health issues or information. However, for details and

TABLE 6.1
Summary of Differences Between E-Health Seekers and Nonseekers

Research Questions	E-Health Seekers	Nonseekers
RQ1: How do e-health seekers and nonseekers use various information sources?	• Use television and newspaper to monitor health-related issues • Use the Internet and books to find specific information • Use interpersonal sources to verify information	• Use television and newspaper to monitor health-related issues • Use books and interpersonal sources to find specific information • Use interpersonal sources to verify information
RQ2: What motivates e-health seekers and nonseekers to search for health information on various sources?	• Curiosity • Personal health management • Control • Provide social support	• Curiosity • Personal health management • Control • Provide social support
RQ3a: How do e-health seekers and nonseekers perceive mass media, the Internet, and interpersonal sources in terms of information quality?	• Television and newspaper: has breadth, lacks depth, not useful, irrelevant • Books: detailed and specific, useful, relevant • Internet: mixture of right and wrong information, detailed and specific, carries useful and relevant information • Interpersonal sources: mixed—can be useful and relevant, or misleading and wrong	• Television and newspaper: has breadth, easy to comprehend • Books: detailed and specific, useful, relevant • Internet: mixture of useful and misleading information, confusing • Interpersonal sources: mixed—can be useful and relevant, or misleading and wrong
RQ3b: How do e-health seekers and nonseekers perceive mass media, the Internet, and interpersonal sources in terms of source credibility?	• Mass media in Singapore: credible • Internet: not all credible • Interpersonal sources: not all credible, cannot fully trust health care professionals	• Mass media in Singapore: credible • Internet: not all credible • Interpersonal sources: not all credible, more likely to trust health care professionals
RQ4: What is the role of self-efficacy in using, discerning, and verifying the Internet mass amount of information to differentiate e-health seekers from nonseekers?	• Confident in handling conflicting information, investigating source reputation/credibility, discerning misinformation	• Feel overwhelmed by information, do not wish to handle or lack the confidence in handling conflicting information or discerning misinformation

verification purposes, people will switch to a different type of information sources. This shows that health care promoters can leverage on traditional mass media to highlight health issues. Although traditional mass media content is easily accessible and comprehensible, it cannot carry all relevant details due to various constrains. As long as people are interested, they will switch to other information sources to find out more. Recognizing this, health promoters should attempt to include access information to alternative sources (such as the specific Web sites and health care professionals) in their mass media content.

As mentioned in an earlier section, both e-seekers and nonseekers are aware of the large amount and diverse information on the Internet. They also do not trust all online health information. However, health promoters can enhance e-health experience by establishing credibility and improving comprehensibility and navigation. According to our participants, they seem to prefer reputable institutions (such as hospitals and universities) to sponsor the sites. Therefore, it is important to include a section about the institutions, as well as contact information. This raises the need for reputable sites to disassociate themselves from dubious ones. Highlighting the authors' credentials will also improve the image. Because health matters can be complicated and technical, and yet the people searching for health information may not have the relevant background, health promoters should make a point not to use jargons. Because Web sites can have multilayer of links, a design that facilitates navigation and ease of accessing information will be ideal. A handful of our e-health participants say that they do not always use search engines, which can turn up hundreds and thousands of hits. Instead, they go directly to sites that they have found to be informative, such as the Mayo Clinic or World Health Organization. Once a site is perceived to be useful and reputable, people will return to them when needs arise.

Our study shows that interpersonal sources—both health care professionals and nonprofessionals—play a major role in verifying the accuracy of information and effectiveness of a recommended treatment. Health care professionals are experts and therefore asking them for verification seem logical. Families and friends are equally important, as people need confirmation from those they can trust or with similar experiences. On the other hand, people also search for information for their families and friends. In our study, none of the participants are caregivers, and yet they do pass on health information to others. Perhaps health promoters can consider mobilizing interpersonal networks for health purposes.

In conclusion, this study finds that information sources play complementary roles. We find that uses and gratifications theory, which originates from the discipline of communication, emphasizes the differential use of information sources, but leaves out processes and other predictors of use. Incorporating ideas from information science models, which emphasize processes, can be useful.

REFERENCES

Bandura, A. (1986). *Social foundations of thought and action: A social cognitive theory*. Englewood Cliffs, NJ: Prentice Hall.

Berger, C. R. (1987). Communicating under uncertainty. In M. E. Roloff & G. R. Miller (Eds.), *Interpersonal processes: New directions in communication research* (pp. 39–62). Newbury Park, CA: Sage.

Bernhart, J. M., Lariscy, R. A., Parrott, R. L., Silk, K. J., & Felter, E. M. (2002). Perceived barriers to Internet-based health communication on human genetics. *Journal of Health Communication, 7*(4), 325–340.

Brashers, D. E., Neidig, J. L., Haas, S. M., Dobbs, L. K., Cardillo, L. W., & Russell, J. A. (2000). Communication in the management of uncertainty: The case of persons living with HIV or AIDS. *Communication Monographs, 67*(1), 63–84.

Brown, M., Koch, T., & Webb, C. (2000). Information needs of women with non-invasive breast cancer. *Journal of Clinical Nursing, 9*(5), 713–722.

Chaffee, S. H. (1982). Mass media and interpersonal channels: Competitive, convergent, or complementary. In G. Gumpert & R. Cathart (Eds.), *Intermedia: Interpersonal communication in a media world* (pp. 57–77). New York: Oxford University Press.

Dimmick, J., Kline, S., & Stafford, L. (2000). The gratification niches of personal e-mail and the telephone: Competition, displacement, and complementarity. *Communication Research, 27*(2), 227–248.

Dutta-Bergman, M. J. (2004). The impact of completeness and web use motivation on the credibility of e-health information. *Journal of Communication, 54*(2), 253–269.

Eastin, M. S., & LaRose, R. (2000). Internet self-efficacy and the psychology of the digital divide. *Journal of Computer Mediated Communication, 6*(1). Retrieved January 26, 2004, from http://www.ascusc.org/jcmc/vol6/issue1/eastin.html

Elliott, W. R., & Rosenberg, W. L. (1987). The 1985 Philadelphia newspaper strike: A uses and gratifications study. *Journalism Quarterly, 64*(4), 679–687.

Ellis, D., & Haugan, M. (1997). Modeling the information seeking patterns of engineers and research scientists in an industrial environment. *Journal of Documentation, 53*(4), 384–403.

Fox, S., & Rainie, L. (2002). *Vital decisions: How Internet users decide what information to trust when they or their loved ones are sick*. Retrieved August 30, 2004, from the Pew Internet and American Life Project Web site: http://www.pewinternet.org/pdfs/PIP_Vital_Decisions_May2002.pdf

Heeter, C., & Greenberg, B. (1985). Cable and program choice. In D. Zillmann & J. Bryant (Eds.), *Selective exposure to communication* (pp. 203–224). Hillsdale, NJ: Lawrence Erlbaum Associates.

Hofstetter, C. R., Zuniga, S., & Dozier, D. (2001). Media self efficacy: Validation of a new concept. *Mass Communication and Society, 4*(1), 61–76.

International Telecommunication Union. (2001). *The e-city: Singapore Internet case study*. Retrieved August 28, 2004, from http://www.itu.int/ITU-D/ict/cs/singapore/material/Singapore.pdf

International Telecommunication Union. (2004). *Information technology*. Retrieved August 28, 2004, from http://www.itu.int/ITU-D/ict/statistics/at_glance/Internet03.pdf

Internet World Stats. (2005). *Top 24 countries with the highest Internet penetration rate.* Retrieved May 26, 2005, from http://www.internetworldstats.com/top25.htm

Kalichman, S. C., Benotsch, E. G., Wienhardt, L., Austin, J., Luke, W., & Cherry, C. (2003). Health-related Internet use, coping, social support, and health indicators in people living with HIV/AIDS: Preliminary results from a community survey. *Health Psychology, 22*(1), 111–116.

Katz, E., Blumler, J. G., & Gurevitch, M. (1974). Utilization of mass communication by the individual. In J. G. Blumler & E. Katz (Eds.), *The uses of mass communications: Current perspectives on gratification research* (pp. 19–32). Beverly Hills, CA: Sage.

Katz, E., Gurevitch, M., & Haas, H. (1973). On the use of the mass media for important things. *American Sociological Review, 38,* 164–181.

Katz, J. E., & Rice, R. E. (2002). *Consequences of Internet use: Access, involvement and interaction.* Cambridge, MA: The MIT Press.

Kaye, B. K., & Johnson, T. J. (2002). Online and in the know: Uses and gratifications of the web for political information. *Journal of Broadcasting & Electronic Media, 46*(1), 54–71.

Kuo, E. C. Y., Choi, A., Arun, M., Lee, W., & Soh, C. (2002). *Internet in Singapore: A study on usage and impact.* Singapore: Times Academic Press.

LaRose, R., Eastin, M. S., & Gregg, J. (2001). Reformulating the Internet paradox: Social cognitive explanations of Internet use and depression. *Journal of Online Behavior, 1*(2). Retrieved May 27, 2005, from http://www.behavior.net/JOB/v1n2/paradox.html

Leung, L., & Wei, R. (2000). More than just talk on the move: Uses and gratifications of the cellular phone. *Journalism and Mass Communication Quarterly, 77*(2), 308–320.

Levy, M. (1987). VCR use and the concept of audience activity. *Communication Quarterly, 35,* 267–275.

Lissman, T. L., & Boehnlein, J. K. (2001). A critical review of Internet information about depression. *Psychiatric Services, 53*(8), 1046–1050.

Miyazaki, T. (1981). Housewives and daytime serials in Japan: A uses and gratifications perspective. *Communication Research, 8*(3), 323–341.

Murero, M., D'Ancona, G., & Karamanoukian, H. (2001). Use of the Internet in patients before and after cardiac surgery: An interdisciplinary study. *Journal of Medical Internet Research, 3*(3). Retrieved May 30, 2005, from http://www.jmir.org/2001/3/e27

Napoli, P. (2001). Consumer use of medical information from electronic and paper media: A literature review. In R. E. Rice & J. E. Katz (Eds.), *The Internet and health communication: Experiences and expectations* (pp. 79–98). Thousand Oaks, CA: Sage.

Newport, F., & Saad, L. (1998, July/August). A matter of trust. *American Journalism Review.* Retrieved August 30, 2004, from http://www.ajr.org/article.asp?id=352

Papacharissi, Z., & Rubin, A. M. (2000). Predictors of Internet use. *Journal of Broadcasting & Electronic Media, 44*(2), 175–196.

Rice, R. E. (2006). Influences, usage, and outcomes of Internet health information searching: Multivariate results from the Pew surveys. *International Journal of Medical Informatics, 75*(1), 8–28.

Rice, R. E. (2003). The Internet and health communication: An overview of issues and research. In P. Lee, L. Leung, & C. So (Eds.), *Impact and issues in new media: Toward intelligent societies* (pp. 173–204). Cresskill, NJ: Hampton Press.

Rubin, A. M. (1983). Television uses and gratifications: The interactions of viewing patterns and motivations. *Journal of Broadcasting, 27*(1), 37–51.

Rubin, A. M. (1986). Uses, gratifications, and media effects research. In J. Bryant & D. Zillmann (Eds.), *Perspectives on media effects* (pp. 281–301). Hillsdale, NJ: Lawrence Erlbaum Associates.

Rubin, A. M., & Bantz, C. R. (1987). Utility of videocassette recorders. *American Behavioral Scientist, 30,* 471–485.

Ruggiero, T. E. (2000). Uses and gratifications theory in the 21st century. *Mass Communication and Society, 3*(1), 3–37.

Sacchetti, P., Zvara, P., & Plante, M. K. (1999). The Internet and patient education—resources and their reliability: Focus on a select urologic topic. *Urology, 53*(6), 1117–1120.

Stamm, K., Williams, J. W., Jr., Noël, P. H., & Rubin, R. (2003). Helping journalists get it right: A physician's guide to improving healthcare reporting. *Journal of General Internal Medicine, 18*(3), 138–145.

Tay-Yap, J., & Al-Hawamdeh, S. (2001). The impact of the Internet on healthcare in Singapore. *Journal of Computer-Mediated Communication, 6*(4). Retrieved January 20, 2004, from http://www.ascusc.org/jcmc/vol6/issue4/tayyap.html

Taylor, H., & Leitman, R. (Eds.). (2002, May 28). Four-nation survey shows widespread but different levels of Internet use for health purpose. *Health Care News, 2*(11). Retrieved August 25, 2004, from http://www.harrisinteractive.com/news/newsletters/healthnews/HI_HealthCareNews2002Vol2_Iss11.pdf

Taylor, H., & Leitman, R. (Eds.). (2004, April 12). No significant change in the number of "cyberchondriacs"—those who go online for health care information. *Health Care News, 4*(7). Retrieved August 25, 2004, from http://www.harrisinteractive.com/news/newsletters/healthnews/HI_HealthCareNews2004Vol4_Iss07.pdf

Towers, W. M. (1986). Uses and gratifications of magazine readers: A cross-media comparison. *Mass Communication Review, 13*(1–3), 44–51.

Wilson, T. D. (1997). Information behavior: An interdisciplinary perspective. *Information Processing & Management, 33*(4), 551–572.

Wright, K. (2002). Social support within an online cancer community: An assessment of emotional support, perceptions of advantages and disadvantages, and motives for using the community from a communication perspective. *Journal of Applied Communication Research, 30*(3), 195–209.

Wyatt, S., Henwood, F., Hart, A., & Smith, J. (2005). The digital divide, health information and everyday life. *New Media & Society, 7*(2), 199–218.

Chapter 7

Patients' Online Information-Seeking Behavior

Ulrika Josefsson
Göteborg University, Sweden

Lately patients' online activities have been the subject of substantial research efforts covering various aspects. Studies have concerned how patients become informed and empowered through online medical information (Dolan, Iredale, Williams, & Ameen, 2004; Morahan-Martin, 2004) and how this contributes to patients challenging the medical expertise (Hardey, 1999) and creating new demands on health care providers (Rice & Katz, 2001). Other studies are directed towards specific features of online activities such as patients' use of cyber-doctor services (Umefjord, Petersson, & Hamberg, 2003) or self-help groups (Josefsson, 2005; Preece & Ghozati, 2001). Additional examples of scholarly work involve the influence of Internet use on the patient–doctor relationship (Anderson, Rainey, & Eysenbach, 2003; Rice & Katz, chap. 8, this volume). Further, issues related to information-seeking behavior of online medical information have been explored. For instance, some have focused on information seeking among health care professionals (Zhang, Zambrowicz, Zhou, & Roderer, 2004) whereas others have considered strategies for online information seeking among health consumers (Eysenbach & Köhler, 2002; Warner & Procaccino, 2004). Some studies have considered the risks of such activities and directed our attention towards issues of how to deal with unreliable medical information online (Adams & Berg, 2004; Eysenbach & Jadad, 2001).

However, there are few studies that focus on patients themselves and their information-seeking behavior (Anigbogu & Rice, 2001; Leydon,

Boulton, Moynihan, Jones, Mossman, Boudioni, & McPherson, 2000; Morahan-Martin, 2004; Murero, Ancona, & Karamanoukian, 2001; Napoli, 2001; Tang & Lee, chap. 6, this volume). Capturing how patients pursue their seeking activities online is motivated by the requirements for developing Internet use in the patient–health care relationship. The Internet is often pictured as an underused resource in this area (Rice & Katz, 2001) and the increasing demands from patients for online contact with health care and doctors has been pointed out (Wullianallur & Tan, 2002). To support the design of Internet use in this relationship, the patient perspective as prospect user must be taken seriously (Van't Riet, Berg, Hiddema, & Sol, 2001). Studying patients' online behavior is thus believed to be a fruitful way to increase our knowledge about the patients' situation, needs, and demands when adopting and using online medical resources. Consequently, the purpose of this chapter is to capture important characteristics of patients' search patterns and, in a wider perspective, support the design of emergent forms of Internet-based health care resources. It accomplishes this by taking the perspective of the patient, involving respondents with different diagnosis and search patterns.

Discussions on patients' use of the Internet have been criticized for being one-sided, often emphasizing the benefits of these online activities. Among others, Henwood, Wyatt, Hart, and Smith (2002) pointed out the need for a more balanced discussion that "map out a more complex picture of both information handling and Internet use" (p. 89). Therefore, the chapter aims to provide a nuanced discussion, derived from the empirical data about the consequences related to patients' online information seeking.

To accomplish this, the work is informed by lessons from information science on human information-seeking behavior. More specifically, Wilson's (1997) formulation of information seeking and acquisition is used as presented in his general model of information behavior. Building on the work by Kuhlthau (1991) and Ellis (1989), the proposed model is believed to be useful in an effort to capture patients' active, as well as passive, search patterns.

RELATED RESEARCH

Several research studies have been performed focusing how Internet users seek out health information. For instance, Eysenbach and Köhler (2002) studied the methods used by health consumers to search the Internet for medical information and how the information is appraised. The study was performed using a qualitative approach in a laboratory setting with focus groups and follow-up interviews. The authors conclude that, in spite of the rather inefficient search techniques, the participants were successful in finding online health information and that the use of search engines was the most common behavior to reach relevant Web sites.

Mainly focusing on online information, Warner and Procaccino (2004) studied women's health information-seeking behavior. They address issues of why, where, and how women access health information and their awareness of different information sources. Using a survey method (119 respondents) the authors found women being active information seekers, mainly using search engines to access health-related Web sites. However, the study also showed low awareness among the participants about the sources as well as concerns about the reliability of the information found. Anigbogu and Rice (2001) provided an in-depth, over-time summary of one woman's progress toward learning how to use computers, the Internet, as well as health information Web sites to learn more about infertility, eventually leading to a more empowered relation with both her physician and husband.

Murero et al. (2001) studied Internet use among patients undergoing medical treatment. Using a semistructured questionnaire, 82 telephone interviews were conducted with patients before and after cardiac surgery. Approximately 20% of the participants had experiences of retrieving online medical information; the study concluded that a main problem among these participants was interpreting and understanding the information found. The study also highlights the fact that some patients might avoid using the Internet for medical information. Referring to the field of social science and the work by Festinger (1957) on the theory of cognitive dissonance, the authors find that: "Avoidance of using the Internet to retrieve information related to medical diseases could be interpreted, in part, as an attempt by patients to defensively prevent anxiety, since, being highly involved with a problem, the patients tend to avoid other sources of stimuli that could generate further dissonance, anxiety, and stress" (p. 4).

Some patients' deliberate avoidance of medical information is further developed in a study by Leydon et al. (2000) that captures important variations in patients' information-seeking behavior (without specific focus on online information). Based on 17 in-depth interviews with cancer patients, the study found that, due to different coping strategies, patients have different needs for information during the development of their disease.

MODELS OF INFORMATION-SEEKING BEHAVIOR

Several models have been presented focusing on various aspects of information-seeking behavior (cf. Napoli, 2001; Rice, McCreadie, & Chang, 2001; Wilson, 1999). For example, in the field of information science,

Kuhlthau (1991) and Ellis (1989) illustrated the information-seeking process, which has influenced Wilson's (1997) formulation of his general model introduced in the next section.

Kuhlthau's (1991) stepwise model is based on theories and ideas of the user's cognitive processes. As an example, the stage of *initiation* is about the initial development of awareness about the existing problem and this phase is often characterized by feelings of uncertainty. This is followed by a phase of *selection* where the person, often optimistically, takes on the task to identify a general topic to investigate. The further investigation of that general topic is then pursued during the stage of *exploration*. Again, feelings of uncertainty increase as the person tries to extend his or her personal understanding of the topic. Kuhlthau (1991) described the next phase (*formulation*) as "the turning point of the ISP (Information Search Process) when feelings of uncertainty diminish and confidence increases" (p. 367). During the formulation phase the person goes to find a more specific subject that becomes the starting point for the stage of *collection* where relevant information related to that specific subject is gathered. Finally, *presentation* ends the search process and involves the task "to present or otherwise use the findings" (p. 368).

The model by Ellis (1989) is based on studies of information seeking performed by social scientists. The model captures six characteristics or features of the seeking pattern: *starting* (activities characteristic of the initial search for information), *chaining* (follows chains of citations or other forms of referential connection between material), *browsing* (semi-directed searching in an area of potential interest), *differentiating* (using differences between sources as filters on the nature and quality of the material examined), *monitoring* (maintaining awareness of developments in a field through the monitoring of particular sources), and *extracting* (systematically working through a particular source to locate material of interest; Ellis, 1989, p. 178).

THEORETICAL APPROACH

With the objective to propose a *general* model of information behavior, Wilson (1997) brings together ideas from different models while also investigating a variety of disciplines beside information science (such as psychology, consumer behavior, health communications studies, and information systems design). Such interdisciplinary approach to understanding information access and browsing have also been applied by Rice et al. (2001), and Murero et al. (2001), who combined communication science, cardiothoracic surgery, psychology, and sociology of consumption.

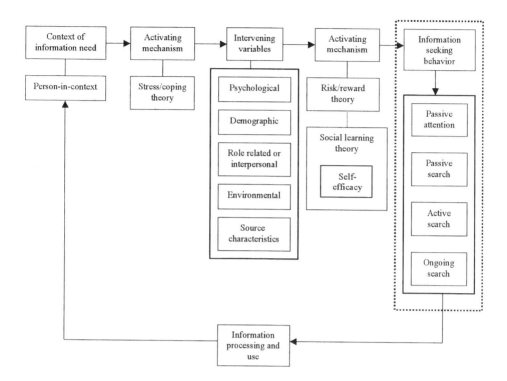

FIG. 7.1. General model of information behavior (Wilson, 1997); applied features of information seeking marked.

The present studies apply the features of Wilson's (1997) general model covering information-seeking behavior (see Fig. 7.1). This part of the model is related to the ideas of Kuhlthau (1991) and Ellis (1989), as just presented, although Wilson added the passive modes of information "seeking," sometimes also termed *acquisition*. The model is based on the idea that the information seeker has personal characteristics and is acting in a specific context of information need. The person is triggered by some activating mechanism to search for information on how to resolve the problem. Along the way there are various intervening variables affecting the person's ability to search for information. Other activating mechanisms exist that help the person to overcome the barriers. The person then uses different search modes (*passive attention, passive search, active search*, and *ongoing search*) describing their information-seeking behavior. This is followed by a stage where the information found is processed and used.

The model illustrates four types of search modes (Wilson, 1997, p. 562):

- *Passive attention*: such as listening to the radio or watching television programs, where information acquisition may take place without intentional seeking;
- *Passive search*: signifies those occasions when one type of search (or other behavior) results in the acquisition of information that happens to be relevant to the individual;
- *Active search*: where an individual actively seeks out information; and
- *Ongoing search*: where active searching has already established the basic framework of knowledge, ideas, beliefs, or values, but where occasional continuing search is carried out to update or expand one's framework.

These modes serve as tools for presenting the empirical data of patients' search for online medical information. This means that the data is organized around various *features* of the search process in contrast to following the entire search process. Before presenting the empirical data, the overall research approach is outlined.

RESEARCH APPROACH

This research is based on semistructured interviews with patients active on the Internet. This means that the interviewees are using the Internet in various ways as means to cope with illness and their overall situation as a patient. During the interviews we went through issues of how they started to use computers and the Internet, their strategies for adopting the Internet for medical information, and their experiences and ideas of the pros and cons of searching and using online medical information. The interviews were conducted as a conversation between the respondent and the interviewer. A few specified question areas were used to guide the performance of the interviews. The question areas served as means to ensure that all topics were covered, as well as to control the scope of the interviews, as contrasted with completely open-ended interviews (Mc-Cracken, 1988).

The researcher conducted a total of 18 interviews in two related studies. Each interview lasted for 40–75 minutes and was transcribed. The participants were guaranteed anonymity and the names used in the presentation of the data are fictitious. Also, because the interviews were conducted in Swedish, the quotes presented have been translated. To ensure that the overall meaning of each statement is captured and to avoid translation bias, the extracts has been discussed and double-checked with research colleagues.

The first study involved 10 patients sharing the experience of initiating and running patient-managed self-help groups on the Internet. The self-help groups offer a set of web pages containing a variety of medical information about a specific disease together with interactive facilities such as discussion boards and/or e-mail lists. The purpose of the self-help groups is mainly to provide patients with medical information and the possibility to get contact with fellow patients for exchange of experiences on a peer-to-peer basis. The idea was to capture "patients in action" on the Internet, meaning that the pattern of information seeking, as well as the interaction and communication performed, was central. Therefore, the selection of patients as initiators and managers of self-help groups was guided by the interactive facilities provided and the "patient activity" that occurred in the self-help groups. In addition, to get a broad patient perspective, the goal was to select patients representing several diseases and health conditions (involving multiple sclerosis, thyroid problems, whiplash injury, chronic prostatitis, fibromyalgia, endometriosis, poly-cystic ovary syndrome, panic disorder, and chronic fatigue syndrome/myalgic encephalomyelitis).

In order to provide a deeper example of how patients make their way on the Internet and search for online medical information, the second study focused on patients with a shared diagnosis. As a result, this study involved interviews with patients suffering from prostate cancer. Prostate cancer is cancer of the prostate gland. In Sweden, there are about 7,600 new cases each year. Slightly more than one third of all cancer in men is prostate cancer, which make this type of cancer the most common cancer among men. Prostate cancer mostly strikes elderly men, with more than two thirds of patients over 70 years old (Swedish Cancer Society, 2004). In United States prostate cancer is the second leading cause of cancer death in men—230,900 new cases in 2004—exceeded only by lung cancer (American Cancer Society, 2004). The incidence of this type of cancer makes these patients an important group to follow when it comes to Internet use and the specific needs and demands for on-line activities and medical information related to the diagnosis. Cooperating with the Department of Oncology at the Sahlgrenska University Hospital in Göteborg (Sweden), contacts with prostate cancer patients were established. During November 2003 to March 2004, eight men were interviewed who had been diagnosed between 1995 and 2003. Three of the patients were recently diagnosed and treatment options were under investigation. Five of the men had undertaken various forms or combinations of treatments such as surgery, radiation therapy, and hormone therapy.

PATIENTS' ONLINE
INFORMATION-SEEKING BEHAVIOR

The patients provided rich descriptions of how they approach the Internet to search for information about their disease and overall situation as a patient. In order to capture this picture the results are presented using concepts from Wilson's (1997) general model as just presented. This provides the possibility to capture aspects of *active* as well as *passive* search. Figure 7.2 illustrates the main scope of information-seeking behavior identified among the patients in the two studies.

Passive Attention

In Wilson's (1997) model, *passive attention* is when individuals accidentally get relevant and useful information. Although this does not represent active search efforts, these occasions are important to recognize as a part of patients' overall information-seeking behavior. Mary's story from her self-help group for women suffering from PCO (Polycystic

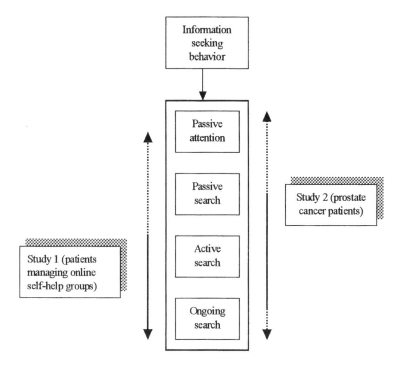

FIG. 7.2. Main patterns of information-seeking behavior observed in the performed studies.

Ovarie Syndrome) provides an example of the role of passive attention for patients' online information seeking:

> There were some articles published in Swedish newspapers that made people go out on the Internet and they found my Web site and the number of members increased a lot during 1999 and even more in the year 2000. . . . There was an article in *Aftonbladet* [Swedish evening paper] in January (2003) and one in *Expressen* [Swedish evening paper] 2 weeks ago and I notice that at once. When there has been an article published my mailbox is full! As soon as newspapers draw attention to it [PCO] there are many patients contacting me.

Also in the study, David, a prostate cancer (PC) patient, describes how he, besides his active search efforts online, has come across web addresses by coincidence by reading evening papers online: "*Aftonbladet* [Swedish evening paper] has had some online articles that I have read and they end with 'read more here' and then I follow the links."

Passive Search

Passive search occurs when relevant information is encountered unintentionally *during other search efforts*. In the studies, this is exemplified by patients being provided online resources by a third party, such as family, friends, health care providers/doctors or books and brochures, and so on. John, a PC patient, exemplifies such a passive search mode. He is familiar with the Internet and he reported regularly using online facilities. He has searched for information about PC in various sources, but when he was diagnosed, he did not turn to the Internet at once. Instead, his offline search efforts provided him with information about online resources: "In the beginning I didn't search online. I bought a few books in English that gave me some input and after that I really started to search online." This differs from passive attention, as John was involved in actual search efforts as he encountered relevant information.

Further, passive search can be described as an additional way to find guidance to online resources in general. Among the participants, this is exemplified by Mark, a PC patient recently diagnosed and scheduled for surgery. He is familiar with computers from his office work, although he has limited experience with the Internet. This reduces his search for online medical information, although he uses a few specific Web sites. Some of the web addresses were provided through a brochure about PC that Mark received during a visit at the doctor's office. Other addresses he found in a book about PC written by a PC patient. However, he finds his abilities to reach online information beyond the given Web sites limited:

"I know that there is a lot to learn about PC out there (on the Internet) but I am not really sure where to go or how to search."

Similarly, Richard illustrates passive search as he describes how his online information seeking was limited to the Web sites provided in a leaflet about PC. At the time of the interview, Richard was discussing surgery as a possible treatment option: "I didn't search online—instead it was through the leaflet that I found the information about these Web sites."

In the studies, patients report searching for information in Swedish, yet ending up on foreign (mostly English/American) Web sites where they encountered relevant information. As an example, for Charles, who organizes a self-help group for patients with chronic prostatitis, this has influenced the content on his web pages, as well as the number of international contacts he has today and the valuable information with which they have provided him: "I wouldn't have had all this information if it wasn't for these Internet contacts from all over the world." Also, the initiation of the self-help group was affected by contacts he accidentally made as he searched the Internet. Initially he "happened to find an American newsgroup" where he made contacts with other Swedish patients with whom he has cooperated in order to start the self-help group.

Active Search

The participants' use of *active search* mode is characterized by patients entering the Internet on their own looking for information and support triggered by an information void. Mary (cited earlier) pictures this as: "When I was diagnosed I didn't get enough information from the doctors. At first I thought I was well informed but they (the doctors) were only talking about a small part of it all. So I was left to do some readings in books and I found almost nothing there. Then I went on the Internet and I discovered that there was so much I didn't know about this (PCO)."

A common method among the participating patients for entering the Internet was to perform broad searches using search engines. This strategy takes patients to a variety of Web sites and put demands on the patient's ability to choose among the hits and to judge the information found. Tom (PC patient), being a frequent Internet user and familiar with information-seeking procedures online, describes how he first entered the Internet looking for medical information about PC: "Well, I used a search engine and went for 'prostate cancer' and then I made my way from one site to the other following links back and forth." On the question of how he chose between the many hits that were generated, he replied: "I believe it was randomly. I clicked until I found something that seemed reasonable and then I followed the links from that." When asked about what made him decide what could be considered "reasonable," he described this as an effort of trust-building mainly on his personal references about credibility: ". . . there must be knowledge represented and hospitals and doctors behind—not just private individuals who believe they have the solution to everything." As a complementary strategy to judge online information, Tom also compares the sources with each other. He explains: "I compare the information from various sources . . . if you do that the picture will get more balanced. Perhaps you will never get the whole truth but at least you will get rid of the more extreme forms of medical advices."

In addition, active search mode can be described as an exhaustive way of exploring the Internet for medical information. One example from the first study is Maria. She is a sufferer of multiple sclerosis (MS) and an organizer of an online self-help group for patients with MS. She describes her initial search behavior as: "I wanted to find out as much as I could . . . I read everything online . . . everything there was to know about MS."

Similarly, Eric (PC patient) searched extensively online as he realized that there was a lot more to know about prostate cancer than he first expected and that he himself had to find that out: "It was after the surgery that I realized that there was so much that I was not informed about. One evening I decided to start (to search online) and when you start you find so much . . . so many threads you just have to follow."

Ongoing Search

According to Wilson (1997), active search might grow into an *ongoing search* mode where the individual uses, tests, and elaborates a personal frame of reference including knowledge, experiences, and viewpoints derived from earlier search efforts. Consequently, the individual uses the results of previous information seeking but occasionally makes new searches to further develop the frame of reference. An example of ongoing search is the use of "favorites" which are Web sites that the users keep returning to, so are kept and listed in the user's Internet browsers for easy access. In the studies, such Web sites were regarded as trustworthy, relevant, and updated. For example, David (PC patient) often returns to the "state-of-the-art" page about prostate cancer produced by the Swedish National Board of Health and Welfare: "I went to the page for the 'state-of-the-art' in an early stage and I have read those papers at least 10–15 times. Maybe it has become my 'bible' so to speak."

Another example of ongoing search and the use of favorite Web sites is provided by Sara, a thyroid patient running an online self-help group and a Web site with extensive information about thyroid problems. In the work with her disease and the self-help group, she has often returned to an American Web site about thyroid that has become a model both for herself and for many of the members of her group:

> Thyroid.about.com is an American Web site about thyroid and . . . well, there is so much information! It was started by a patient who wrote a book some years ago about thyroid problems. At first the Web site was quite limited but now it has grown and presents huge amount of information. We have discussed that perhaps our group should now become a Swedish corresponding Web site . . . and many members want that too.

Further, participation in online discussions with fellow patients is an additional form of ongoing search providing the opportunity for patients to further develop and test their knowledge and personal frame of reference. Irene, who is managing a self-help group for patients with endometriosis, provides her thoughts on such interchanges: ". . . all the girls on the mailing list have something to give. They have knowledge and experiences and they have been through things or taken certain medications . . . it spreads to others and they give back . . . everything they have been through can be used for good things."

DISCUSSION

The participating patients applied a variety of online search modes where some modes might be considered more beneficial than others. However, when carefully considering the consequences of the online information-seeking behavior, numerous aspects should be taken into account revealing a complexity that cannot easily be reduced to the dichotomy of pros and cons (Morahan–Martin, 2004; Warner & Procaccino, 2004). Recognizing this multifaceted picture, the following discussion aims to give voice to patients themselves. Firstly, the discussion will be centered on three themes: accessing online medical information, social support, and information accuracy and applicability. The themes summarize important consequences of the participants' online information-seeking behavior. Secondly, the discussion considers three balancing factors deriving from the interviews also: coping strategy, resource requirements, and online information-seeking assistance. These factors capture circumstances important to consider in order to deepen and nuance the picture of the participants' online information-seeking behavior. To support the discussion, Fig. 7.3 summarizes the search modes, identified themes, consequences and balancing factors.

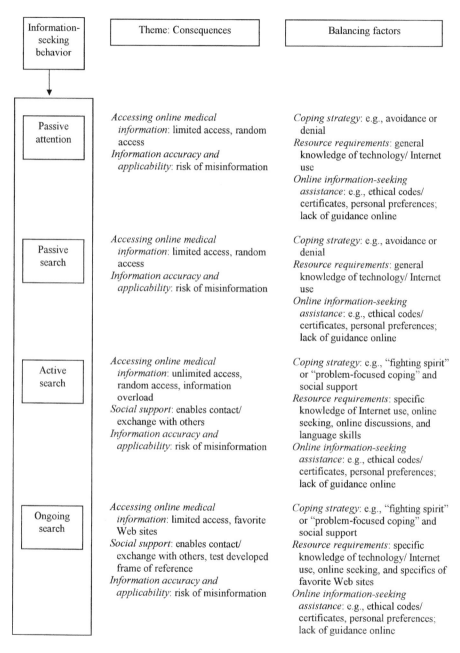

Information-seeking behavior	Theme: Consequences	Balancing factors
Passive attention	*Accessing online medical information*: limited access, random access *Information accuracy and applicability*: risk of misinformation	*Coping strategy*: e.g., avoidance or denial *Resource requirements*: general knowledge of technology/ Internet use *Online information-seeking assistance*: e.g., ethical codes/ certificates, personal preferences; lack of guidance online
Passive search	*Accessing online medical information*: limited access, random access *Information accuracy and applicability*: risk of misinformation	*Coping strategy*: e.g., avoidance or denial *Resource requirements*: general knowledge of technology/ Internet use *Online information-seeking assistance*: e.g., ethical codes/ certificates, personal preferences; lack of guidance online
Active search	*Accessing online medical information*: unlimited access, random access, information overload *Social support*: enables contact/ exchange with others *Information accuracy and applicability*: risk of misinformation	*Coping strategy*: e.g., "fighting spirit" or "problem-focused coping" and social support *Resource requirements*: specific knowledge of Internet use, online seeking, online discussions, and language skills *Online information-seeking assistance*: e.g., ethical codes/ certificates, personal preferences; lack of guidance online
Ongoing search	*Accessing online medical information*: limited access, favorite Web sites *Social support*: enables contact/ exchange with others, test developed frame of reference *Information accuracy and applicability*: risk of misinformation	*Coping strategy*: e.g., "fighting spirit" or "problem-focused coping" and social support *Resource requirements*: specific knowledge of technology/ Internet use, online seeking, and specifics of favorite Web sites *Online information-seeking assistance*: e.g., ethical codes/ certificates, personal preferences; lack of guidance online

FIG. 7.3. Information seeking, themes, consequences, and balancing factors.

139

Accessing Online Medical Information

Wilson (1997) included passive search modes as a part of individuals' information-seeking behavior as an attempt to illustrate that "other modes of 'searching' do take place" (p. 562) adding to ideas of information seeking as solely active (see also Rice et al., 2001). The participating patients' use of passive attention and passive search naturally generate a limited and random set of medical information. Usually the consequences of limited access to medical information online are viewed against issues of computer literacy and general knowledge of Internet use (Morahan-Martin, 2004). As we discuss in the following paragraphs, patients' need for such competencies is undoubtedly essential to their online information-seeking behavior. However, the passive search modes that limit the amount of information obtained should also be considered in relation to the fact that some patients do not *want* additional information (Henwood et al., 2003; Murero et al., 2001).

Although there might be several reasons for patients to limit their information seeking, this is fruitful to consider from the perspective of coping strategies (Johnson, 1997; Wilson, 1997) as a balancing factor. Applying a well cited definition, coping is ". . . the persons' constantly changing cognitive and behavioral efforts to manage specific external and/or internal demands that are appraised as taxing or exceeding the person's resources" (Lazarus & Folkman, 1984, p. 141).

Facing illness is an example of a stressful (external and/or internal) demanding situation characterized by high level of uncertainty (Johnson, 1997). Various strategies to deal with such situations have been identified (cf. Festinger, 1957; Lazarus & Folkman, 1984). For instance, some patients' reluctance to seek additional information could be explained as a coping strategy characterized by avoidance (Lazarus & Folkman, 1984) or denial (Sullivan & Reardon, 1986). In the study Ian (a PC patient) illustrates such avoiding strategy as he expresses: "I am not really sure if I want to find anything more on this (prostate cancer) . . . it shouldn't get too much."

Limited access to online information is a consequence of ongoing search as well. For instance, in applying this search mode, participants in the studies limited their search to web pages that could be described as their "favorites." Such limitation of the information seeking is, however, a result of earlier active search efforts where the person has developed a clear focus and is able to perform targeted information searches (Ellis, 1989; Kuhlthau, 1991). However, returning to the resource requirements as an important balancing factor, patients need competencies such as how to manage the Internet and online information-seeking procedures in order to develop this mature way of online seeking (Henwood et al., 2003). In addition, patients must be able to handle the specifics of their favorite Web site, such as search methods in certain databases or how to participate in discussion boards, and so on.

As a contrast to limited search efforts, the active search mode results in a considerable and almost unlimited amount of information (cf. Eysenbach & Jadad, 2001; Hardey, 1999; Morahan-Martin, 2004). However, a broad and extensive way of approaching the Internet creates advantages as well as less desirable consequences. On the one hand, this means a possibility to access a variety of information sources such as medical databases and journals as well as web pages of patient associations, health portals, cyber-doctors, and so on, providing patients the opportunity to get additional information and different views of their problems. On the other hand, the access of such vast amount of medical information increases the risk of "information overload" (Reeves, 2000), causing patients to experience confusion, frustration and disempowerment (Henwood et al., 2002). In the study Steve, a PC patient, offered a comment on information overload that illustrates the view of several of the participants: "You can't read everything. It is hopeless since there is so much. You have to sort out what to read and that is difficult."

Additionally, active search can be considered from the perspective of coping strategies as a balancing factor. For instance, contrasting avoidance or denial is what Sullivan and Reardon (1986) called "Fighting spirit." This coping strategy is characterized by highly optimistic attitudes, active search for information, desire to know as much as possible, and low levels of distress (Johnson, 1997, p. 116). Similarly, Lazarus and Folkman (1984) termed such behavior *problem-focused coping*. This way of coping was highlighted in the studies as several of the interviewees described their active search efforts online as a form of therapy. David (PC patient) illustrates this as he describes: "I felt good being on the Internet. There was so much. I could surf, search, and go through stuff and print it out. I copied things to my own computer so I had several hundred pages about prostate cancer."

The consequences of active search are thus both positive and negative. In order to deal with the problems and to make the most of the good parts, the requirements for particular resources as a balancing factor become important once more: here, with an emphasis on language skills and knowledge about information seeking. In the second study Tom, a PC patient, describes some of the barriers for active online information seeking: "The first thing is language skills. You have to know English . . . well, first you have to know how to handle a computer and how to use the Internet but then you really must have language skills in order to access Web sites other than Swedish."

Social Support

The active search mode brings not only medical facts but also an increased opportunity for patients to find their way to online spaces (such as discussion boards, e-mail lists, and/or self-help groups) for contact with fellow patients for support and empathy (Ferguson, 2002; Preece & Ghozati, 2001). Ongoing search provides the opportunity for this support on a peer-to-peer basis, also. For instance, through revisits to favorite Web sites providing such interactions, patients are able to test and further develop their knowledge or personal frame of references developed through previous information seeking (Preece, 2000).

The usefulness of this type of contact with fellow patients has been pointed out (cf. Ferguson, 2002; Josefsson, 2005; Rice & Katz, 2001). In the study, Mary (managing a self-help group for women with PCO) gives a good example of this:

> The best thing is that I have got in contact with so many other women. We have exchanged many common experiences and this has really meant a lot to me. And I feel that I know so much more from the things I have learned from others. We have shared our experiences and when I go to see my doctor I know my rights in a completely new way. The contact with others in the same situation have made me stronger and helped me put new demands on my health care provider that I probably wouldn't have done otherwise.

Additionally, Mary's statement illustrates the two-sided benefit of patient-to-patient support, meaning that the activities offer patients an opportunity to receive as well as *provide* social support. This is captured also in a study by Reeves (2000) on HIV-positive individuals where the coping effects of online support were emphasized as concerning both the possibility to get help, but just as much as an opportunity to be able to help others.

Further, it should be noted that online interactive forums provide patients the possibility to seek information in an indirect way. This so-called "lurking" (Nonnecke & Preece, 2001), where individuals follow online discussions without posting or commenting their own comments, is an additional strategy to find others' stories, knowledge, and experiences. Among the participants this is well-known and Linda (running an online self-help group for patients with panic disorders) expresses this as: "Some simply want to read. On the page 'Others' stories,' they can read about this (panic disorders) happening to other people as well. It is very comforting since you feel as the loneliest person in the world and you think that 'this happens only to me.' "

To deepen our understanding and to balance the picture of patients' search for contact with others, ideas of coping are once again believed to be helpful. In the coping literature, the seeking of social support is a well-known strategy to meet the challenges of facing illness (cf. Lazarus & Folkman, 1984; Reeves, 2000; Sullivan & Reardon, 1986). Social support involves several forms of support beneficial for the patient. For instance, referring to the work by Schaefer, Coyne, and Lazarus (1982), Lazarus and Folkman (1984, p. 250) described the seeking of social support as including "informational" support (like providing information or advice and feedback) as well as "tangible" (involving direct forms of aid) and "emotional" support (including attachment and reassurance). These forms of support are also illustrated in Mary's statement just discussed.

To further balance the picture, it is necessary to again consider the specific resources and qualifications required in order to participate and benefit from social and human supportive activities online (Henwood et al., 2002). Besides the earlier mentioned skills on language, Internet use, and information management, patients also require proficiency in how to (technically and socially) act in discussion boards or on e-mail lists (Preece, 2000).

Information Accuracy and Applicability

The third theme is connected to all four search modes and involves issues of information accuracy and applicability and the risk of becoming misinformed when pursuing online seeking for medical information. The risk concerns medical facts (Eysenbach & Jadad, 2001), as well as the information obtained through online personal support (Ferguson, 2002). In addition, problems of becoming misinformed include the risk of misinterpreting otherwise correct medical information and difficulties of judging the usefulness of the information in relation to the personal case of illness (Klein-Fedyshin, 2002). An example of this is patients entering Web sites directed towards health care professionals. John, suffering from prostate cancer, illustrated this as he refers to the difficulty of accessing "doctors' Web sites where the information is on a deeper medical level and since I'm not a doctor I quickly lose track of what I read."

The issues of online information accuracy and applicability are often viewed against the background of patients' individual abilities of assessing the information. Currently, high demands are put on patients to accomplish the task and to further develop their competencies (Eysenbach & Jadad, 2001). This means that besides the technical and social skills discussed earlier, patients must further develop their knowledge concerning information uncertainty. This is highlighted by Henwood et al. (2002) as the authors emphasized the "need for information literacy skills to be developed more widely so that the public are able to be aware of the relevance of information sources, to ask critical questions about information they access and to make judgments about the validity and quality of the information accessed" (pp. 88–89).

As a balancing factor, issues of online information accuracy and applicability should also be discussed in the light of online information-seeking assistance supporting information assessment. So far, much of this work has involved the use of online certificates or ethical codes (Adams & Berg, 2004) as instruments to find reliable online information. Other forms of guidance have, hitherto, been rare, leaving online medical information seekers to rely on their personal preferences about how to judge the information (Eysenbach & Köhler, 2002). However, recently several studies have emphasized the need for more direct forms of guidance on the Internet to reliable and relevant information sources (cf. Morahan-Martin, 2004; Murero et al., 2001; Salo, Perez, Lavery, Malankar, Borenstein, et al., 2004; Seidman, chap. 10, this volume). Also, these studies call for an increased responsibility and participation by health care providers to support this development. The patients in the reported studies confirm the lack of online guidance as they have been more or less left on their own, without support from health care providers to find trustworthy and timely online information. For instance, none of the participating patients had *directly* been advised about online sources for additional information by their doctor or health care provider (see also Rice & Katz, chap. 8, this volume).

LIMITATIONS AND FUTURE WORK

This chapter is an initial attempt to take a broad perspective on patients' information-seeking behavior. By means of the participants' experiences, the analysis has focused on a number of opportunities and challenges associated with patients' online information seeking. The features of information-seeking behavior employed from Wilson's (1997) general model have well served the illustrative purpose and supported the idea to capture actual search patterns. However, to illuminate further complexities such as patients' *shift* between and/or their *mix* of different search modes, the model requires some modification as well. Such development would enhance the utility of the model, although this calls for additional exploration of patients' online information behavior on issues such as frequency of online information seeking and development over time.

In addition, the analysis provided briefly reviews a number of dimensions of patients' online information-seeking behavior; but each should be explored in greater detail. For instance, the studies only touch on patient characteristics influencing their search behavior, although issues of education, income, sex, type of diagnosis, and so on, are important factors that should be considered profoundly in future work.

Finally, the studies use a qualitative approach and are based on a limited number of interviews and self-reported experiences of information seeking online. In order to get a more comprehensive picture future work should acknowledge the use of quantitative approaches as well.

CONCLUSIONS

Informed by ideas from information science, this chapter illustrates patients' different ways of seeking online information. The research findings discussed here give voice to patients' experiences and deriving from the empirical data the analysis focus on three themes related to consequences of the observed search behavior: accessing online medical information, social support, and issues of information accuracy and applicability. In order to provide a nuanced picture, the findings further suggest that the search mode applied and the amount and type of information obtained should be viewed against the background of balancing factors. Stemming from the participants' experiences the balancing factors considered here are related to patients' coping strategies, resource requirements, and online information-seeking assistance available.

REFERENCES

Adams, S., & Berg, M. (2004). The nature of the Net: Constructing reliability of the health information on the Web. *Information, Technology & People, 17*(2), 150–170.

American Cancer Society. (2004). Home page. Retrieved August 30, 2004, from http://www.cancer.org/docroot/home/index.asp

Anderson, J. G., Rainey, M. R., & Eysenbach, G. (2003). The impact of cyberhealthcare on the physician–patient relationship. *Journal of Medical Systems, 27*(1), 67–84.

Anigbogu, J., & Rice, R. E. (2001). Expectations and experiences of seeking infertility information via the Internet and telephone directory. In R. E. Rice & J. E. Katz (Eds.), *The Internet and health communication: Expectations and experiences* (pp. 121–143). Thousand Oaks, CA: Sage.

Dolan, G., Iredale, R., Williams, R., & Ameen, J. (2004). Consumer use of the Internet for health information: A survey of primary care patients. *International Journal of Consumer Studies, 28*(2), 147–153.

Ellis, D. (1989). A behavioural approach to information retrieval system design. *The Journal of Documentation, 45*(3), 171–212.

Eysenbach, G., & Jadad, A. R. (2001). Consumer health informatics in the Internet age. In A. Edwards & G. Elwyn (Eds.), *Evidence-based patients choice* (pp. 289–308). Oxford, UK: Oxford University Press.

Eysenbach, G., & Köhler, C. (2002). How do consumers search for and appraise health information on the world wide web? Qualitative study using focus groups, usability tests, and in-depth interviews. *British Medical Journal, 324,* 573–577.

Ferguson, T. (2002). From patients to end users. Quality of online patient networks needs more attention than quality of online health information. *British Medical Journal, 324*(7337), 555–556.

Festinger, L. (1957). *A theory of cognitive dissonance.* Stanford, CA: Stanford University Press.

Hardey, M. (1999). Doctor in the house: The Internet as a source of lay health knowledge and the challenge to expertise. *Sociology of Health and Illness, 21*(6), 820–835.

Henwood, F., Wyatt, S., Hart, A., & Smith, J. (2002). Turned on or turned off? Accessing health information on the Internet. *Scandinavian Journal of Information Systems, 14*(2), 79–90.

Henwood, F., Wyatt, S., Hart, A., & Smith, J. (2003). "Ignorance is bliss sometimes": Constraints on the emergence of the "informed patient" in the changing landscape of health information. *Sociology of Health and Illness, 25*(6), 589–607.

Johnson, J. D. (1997). *Cancer related information seeking.* Cresskill, NJ: Hampton Press.

Josefsson, U. (2005). Coping with illness online: The case of patients' online communities. *The Information Society, 21*(2), 143–153.

Klein-Fedyshin, M. S. (2002). Consumer health informatics—Integrating patients, providers, and professionals online. *Medical Reference Services Quarterly, 21*(3), 35–49.

Kuhlthau, C. (1991). Inside the search process: Information seeking from the user's perspective. *Journal of the American Society for Information Science, 42*(5), 361–371.

Lazarus, R. S., & Folkman, S. (1984). *Stress, appraisal, and coping.* New York: Springer.

Leydon, G. M., Boulton, M., Moynihan, C., Jones, A., Mossman, J., Boudioni, M., & McPherson, K. (2000). Cancer patients' information needs and information seeking behavior: In depth interview study. *British Medical Journal, 320,* 909–913.

McCracken, G. (1988). *The long interview.* Newbury Park, CA: Sage.

Morahan-Martin, J. M. (2004). How Internet users find, evaluate, and use online health information: A cross-cultural review. *CyberPsychology & Behavior, 7*(5), 497–510.

Murero, M., Ancona, G. D., & Karamanoukian, H. (2001). Use of the Internet by patients before and after cardiac surgery: Telephone survey. *Journal of Medical Internet Research, 3*(3), e27. Retrieved January 13, 2004, from www.jmir.org/2001/3/e27/

Napoli, P. M. (2001). Consumer use of medical information from electronic and paper media. In R. E. Rice & J. E. Katz (Eds.), *The Internet and health communication: Experiences and expectations* (pp. 79–98). Thousand Oaks, CA: Sage.

Nonnecke, B., & Preece, J. (2001, August). Why lurkers lurk: Paper presented to Americas Conference on Information Systems. In D. Strong & D. Straub (Eds.), *Proceedings of the Seventh Americas Conference on Information Systems* (pp. 1521–1531). Boston, MA: Omnipress.

Preece, J. (2000). *Online communities: Designing usability, supporting sociability.* New York: Wiley.

Preece, J., & Ghozati, K. (2001). Experiencing empathy online. In R. E. Rice & J. E. Katz (Eds.), *The Internet and health communication: Experiences and expectations* (pp. 237–260). Thousand Oaks, CA: Sage.

Reeves, P. M. (2000). Coping in cyberspace: The impact of Internet use on the ability of HIV-positive individuals to deal with their illness. *Journal of Health Communication, 5,* 47–59.

Rice, R. E., & Katz, J. E. (Eds.). (2001). *The Internet and health communication: Experiences and expectations.* Thousand Oaks, CA: Sage.

Rice, R. E., McCreadie, M., & Chang, S.-J. (2001). *Accessing and browsing information and communication.* Cambridge, MA: The MIT Press.

Salo, D., Perez, C., Lavery, R., Malankar, A., Borenstein, M., & Berstein, S. (2004). Patient education and the Internet: Do patients want us to provide them with medical Web sites to learn more about their medical problems? *The Journal of Emergency Medicine, 26*(3), 293–300.

Schaefer, C., Coyne, J. C., & Lazarus, R. S. (1982). The health-related functions of social support. *Journal of Behavioral Medicine, 4,* 381–406.

Sullivan, C. F., & Reardon, K. K. (1986). Social support satisfaction and health locus of control: Discriminators of breast cancer patients' styles of coping. In M. L. McLaughlin (Ed.), *Communication Yearbook 9* (pp. 707–722). Beverly Hills, CA: Sage.

Swedish Cancer Society. (2004). Home page. Retrieved August 30, 2004, from http://www.cancerfonden.se/

Umefjord, G., Petersson, G., & Hamberg, K. (2003). Reasons for consulting a doctor on the Internet: Web survey of users of an ask the doctor service. *Journal of Medical Internet Research, 5*(4), e26. Retrieved January 13, 2004, from www.jmir.org/2003/4/e26/

Van't Riet, A., Berg, M., Hiddema, F., & Sol, K. (2001). Meeting patients' needs with patient information systems: Potential benefits of qualitative research methods. *International Journal of Medical Informatics, 64,* 1–14.

Warner, D., & Procaccino, J. D. (2004). Toward wellness: Women seeking health information. *Journal of the American Society for Information Science and Technology, 55*(8), 709–730.

Wilson, T. D. (1997). Information behavior: An interdisciplinary perspective. *Information Processing & Management, 33*(4), 551–572.

Wilson, T. D. (1999). Models in information behavior research. *The Journal of Documentation, 55*(3), 249–270.

Wullianallur, R., & Tan, J. (2002). Strategic IT applications in health care. *Communications of the ACM, 45*(12), 56–61.

Zhang, D., Zambrowicz, C., Zhou, H., & Roderer, N. K. (2004). User information seeking behavior in a medical web portal environment: A preliminary study. *Journal of the American Society for Information Science and Technology, 55*(8), 670–684.

Chapter 8

Internet Use in Physician Practice and Patient Interaction

Ronald E. Rice
University of California, Santa Barbara

James E. Katz
Rutgers University

The Internet can be part of a technological bridge that can help both patients and physicians better manage health care processes and information (Rice & Katz, 2000) because more than half of Internet users in the United States seek health care information online. (While growth in such use is increasing worldwide, certainly there are wide disparities across and within nations and regions.) Although there has been good delineation of the types of activities for which health information seekers and physicians use the Internet, the interface of these two areas—how health information seekers and physicians bring information from the Internet to bear on one another—is less clear. Thus, this chapter looks at these relationships in greater detail, basing the analysis on a Robert Wood Johnson Foundation–sponsored survey of the topic. Much of the data from this study has already been reported by Murray, Lo, Pollack, Donelan, Catania, et al. (2003a), although neither in this framework or using these analyses.

Murray et al. (2003a) found that 85% of a national random sample of physicians report experiencing patients bringing Internet information to an office visit. If physicians felt that the quality of information the patient brings was accurate and relevant, they judged it to be beneficial. Inaccurate or irrelevant information was judged to harm health outcomes and the physician–patient relationship. The most consistent predictor of a perceived deterioration in the physician–patient relationship, the quality of health care, or in the health outcome, was physicians' feeling that patients were challenging their authority. A substantial minority of physicians (38%) believed that the patient bringing in information made the visit less time efficient, particularly if the patient wanted something inappropriate. Physicians also said that they, in part, agreed to clinically inappropriate requests of their patients based on the information from the Internet that the patients bring to them. This acquiescence may be due to fear of damaging the physician–patient relationship or because of the negative effect on time efficiency of not doing so (Murray et al., 2003a).

Our interest here is to analyze the data further, in the context of other reported research. This review is organized by research concerning use of the Internet by (a) physicians and (b) patients, and outcomes relevant to (c) physicians and (d) patients.

PHYSICIAN USE OF THE INTERNET

Physician E-Mail and Internet Searching

Physician use of the Internet is widespread; even as early as 2001, 90% of U.S. primary-care physicians and 55% of German ones had used the Internet (Risk & Dzenowagis, 2001). A 2001 Harris Interactive poll found that 59% of all U.S. physicians used the Internet daily (Harris Interactive, 2001a). Daily use varied by activity, led by searches for medical literature (42%), followed by seeking drug information (29%), patient education materials (20%), clinical trials information (19%), and continuing medical education (CME) courses (10%; Miller, Hillman, & Given, 2004). For e-mail, more than one third communicated with colleagues and more than half of those communications had to do with patient symptoms or treatment (Miller et al., 2004). A year later, 90% of doctors reported using the Internet to research clinical information, 74% to read medical journal articles, 63% to communicate with colleagues, 58% to complete continuing medical education (CME), 30% to access electronic medical records, and 25% to communicate with patients (Harris Interactive, 2003). An American Medical Association survey in late 2001 involving nearly 1,000 physicians found that 78% surfed the web, two thirds accessed the web daily, and 30% had a Web site (primarily to advertise their practice, or provide patient education; Greenspan, 2002).

Carney, Poor, Schifferdecker, Gephart, Brooks, and Nierenberg (2004) found that community-based clinical teachers and preceptors 60 years or older were four times more likely to use the Internet to assist in students' and residents' education, and at least twice as likely to use full-text Medline articles for patient care decisions than those under 60. Similarly, Houston, Sands, Nash, and Ford (2003) identified the average age of physicians who use the Internet daily for work as 49 years. So contrary to one's initial expectations, it may not be necessarily the case that the younger doctors are using the Internet most, at least in the United States. However, results from other studies disagree with this conclusion. Angelo and Citkowitz (2001) found that physicians under 55 years of age are more likely to participate in online physician discussion groups, although this is quite an old study in Internet terms because the data were collected in 1998. Miller et al. (2004) also found age inversely correlated with Internet reliance and use in practice (but with very small differences). And Potts and Wyatt (2002) found that more recently qualified doctors are more likely to see Internet information as reliable.

Non-U.S. surveys report physician age is correlated with Internet use. In Canada, younger physicians and specialists, not general practitioners, are more likely to be online; about 62% of those under age 44 report Internet access at work, compared to only 55% of those aged 55 to 64, and 42% of those 65-and-older (Martin, 2003). New Zealand family practitioners report similar results (Cullen, 2002). Regarding age, then, there is some evidence to reject the common assumption that younger doctors are more likely to use the Internet, but definitions of "older age" vary among sources. As well, over time, age effects could recede due to growing training efforts, popularization of e-health activities, and enhanced ease of use. On the other hand, there is reason to think that as new applications are created, other age gaps will emerge.

Influence of Physician Practice Characteristics

In terms of physicians' practice profile as related to patient perceptions and Internet use, very little data is available. Miller et al. (2004) reported that the strongest associations with increasing Internet use were with physician membership in group practice and the size of the practice. Some possible relationships can possibly be interpolated into some patient survey data. For instance, although there is no mention of how this health seeking is used in physician consultations, a Pew survey found that 66% of low-income California Internet users report that the Internet has improved the health information and services they receive (Fox, 2003). In contrast, 76% of higher income California Internet users report improved health services. But California may be an exception because the percentage of lower income Internet users who look for health information is equal to the percentage of higher income (84%)—this result is very atypical. Fox (2003) also introduced the intervening factor of health, as lower income Californians report being in much worse health than upper income Californians (27% of lower income respondents report excellent health vs. 48% for the higher income respondents, and 19% report a disability or chronic condition vs. 6%). So, it could be hypothesized that the poorer the practice profile, the more in need of health services the patients are, and thus the more the physician should be obtaining clinical information whether or not that information is gathered via the Internet.

Baker, Wagner, Singer, and Bundorf (2003) did not find a statistically significant relationship between living in a metropolitan area and Internet health seeking by patients. However, one study at the University of Iowa children's hospital (D'Alessandro, Kreiter, & Peterson, 2004) found that overall computer resources are used by only 17% of pediatricians to answer questions, whereas 28.6% use people resources and 44% use paper resources such as journals and textbooks. These non–urban doctors refer to paper resources more than twice as often as the Internet.

Kalsman and Acosta (2000) found that rural providers use the Internet with the same frequency as urban providers (85% of rural health providers had Internet access), and e-mail was the most frequently used Internet service (75% of respondents reported using the Internet either daily or one to four times a week). In a study of rural physicians in Australia, 84% had Internet access and 45.8% had videoconferencing access (White, Sheedy, & Lawrence, 2002). Of those with Internet access, 7.9% accessed it frequently for clinical purposes and 58.7% used it occasionally; pathology services and clinical information sheets were the higher uses reported (more than 50%). The authors concluded that rural physicians have embraced Internet technologies to a higher extent than their urban peers. This conclusion is supported by Jones and Lambros (2003), who saw at least equal Internet use and access among rural and urban physicians in Australia.

However, the findings of Angelo and Citkowitz (2001) may challenge these claims. In their study of physician online discussion groups, they concluded that urban physicians are more likely to take part. Nonetheless, as noted previously, their study was based on data collected in 1998. Moreover, it is not known to what extent various promotional efforts may be unique to the Australian context, especially given its particular geographic and infrastructural characteristics. Yet, overall it seems that rural providers are at least *as* versed in electronic communication as their urban colleagues.

Physician Referral of Patients to Web Sites

There is little information in the literature concerning physicians referring their patients to *specific* Web sites, although one source notes that a little more than half of physicians *occasionally* encourage Internet searches (Hollander & Lanier, 2001). A New Zealand study reports slightly higher results as 56% of responding physicians (67% of Internet users and 45%

of non-users) recommend the Internet to their patients (although it is unclear how often; Cullen, 2002). Still, what is more interesting is the discrepancy between the low physician referral rate of specific Web sites and the high patient demand for specific referrals. All Internet users in a study of postsurgery patients felt that Internet sites developed by their own health care provider would provide greater benefit than general Internet use (Murero, D'Ancona, & Karamanoukian, 2001). Likewise, Salo, Perez, Lavery, Malankar, Borenstein, and Bernstein (2004) noted that 59% of hospital patients who use the Internet would like to have web links provided by their physician.

The benefits of physician referrals of specific Web sites are demonstrated by D'Alessandro et al. (2004). This survey had physicians write "information prescriptions" (IPs) for patients, or listings of approved and evaluated Web sites that provide specific, evidence-based information that patients can use to help manage their health problems. The intervention group used the Internet more for general and child health information, and 31% of the intervention parents used the IPs. Compared to the 69% who did not use the IPs, these patients were more likely to use the Internet for health information, to say they would use the IP again, and to recommend the IP to family or friends. Hence the literature bolsters the idea that patient demand for web-savvy doctors well exceeds the levels at which they are encountering them.

E-Mailing and Discussing Internet Information With Patients

Nearly 90% of New Zealand physicians report that at least some patients bring Internet information to their visits, though 93% of those physicians reported that fewer than 10% of their patients did so (Cullen, 2002). Five percent of American Society of Clinical Oncologists were mailed a survey about Internet health information use and evaluation, with nearly 50% responding (Helft, Hlubocky, & Daugherty, 2003). They estimated that about 30% of their patients used the Internet for cancer information, and discussing such information added about 10 minutes to each patient encounter. The oncologists indicated that this information could make patients more hopeful and knowledgeable, but also more confused and anxious, and they reported both positive and negative effects of Internet use by their patients. Only 9% of the physicians felt threatened when patients brought Internet information to discuss. A defensive reaction from physicians to patients who bring Internet information to the visit can degrade the trust and communication between the physician and the patient. Rather, physicians should be more open to acting as a facilitator for patients' seeking and acquiring online medical information (Jacob, 2002).

The British Medical Association is still hesitant about physicians' using e-mail to provide services to patients, largely due to the lack of a personal contact that helps provide diagnosis clues, providing service to patients outside a doctor's licensing location, and the lack of confidentiality. However, the American Medical Association is more supportive, providing guidelines that say e-mail "can aid the health care delivery process by allowing written follow-up instructions, test results and dissemination of educational materials for patients, as well as a means for patients to easily reach their physician on routine health matters" ("UK Doctors Still 'Out of Office' to Patients Online," 2003).

But physicians themselves may be a barrier to online health care information access by patients. One study found that 43% of physicians do not think patients are knowledgeable enough to understand much of what is in Medline (Hollander & Lanier, 2001). Aside from qualms about patient knowledge, physicians' negative attitude may also stem from overall physician dissatisfaction with the quality of web-based information (Hollander & Lanier, 2001; Murray et al., 2003a; Potts & Wyatt, 2002). Indeed, although 75% of physicians believe electronic journals will make information easier to find, 26% also believe that electronic publication will lead to lower quality publications in medical literature (Wright, Tseng, & Kolodner, 2001). Concerning nonacademic Internet sources, Potts and Wyatt (2002) found that 48% of web-using physicians reported information to be "sometimes reliable," whereas only 20% believed it to be "usually reliable," and 29% saw it as "usually unreliable." This generally negative view is echoed by a small-scale survey that found 79% of physicians caution their patients against health content on the Internet (Hollander & Lanier, 2001).

PATIENT USE OF THE INTERNET

Characteristics of Patients Who E-Mail Their Physicians or Seek Online Health Information

Socioeconomic and health variables clearly are associated with people's access of online health care information. Online health information seekers are significantly more likely to be younger and have higher incomes and education. For instance, Cotton and Gupta (2004) found that the mean age of seekers versus nonseekers was 40 versus 52 years, and that 48% of seekers report having at least a bachelor's degree versus 18% for nonseekers. Even as use of the Internet for health information seeking has expanded, disparities along socioeconomic lines continue, and, thus, this may constitute yet another area in which a "digital divide" operates (Rice & Katz, 2003).

Patients' Perceptions of Reliability, Credibility and Usability of Online Health Information

Physicians seem to have some justification to be concerned about the reliability of online health information. Most patients who used the Internet rated the quality of that information as roughly the same as other information sources (including physicians as an information source). In an interesting juxtaposition, Diaz, Griffith, Ng, Reinert, Friedmann, and Moulton (2002) found that 60% of health seekers consider the quality of the information they found online as the same or better than that they obtain from their provider. Moreover, 62% rated the Internet quality as "excellent" or "very good," 32% "good," only 6% "fair," and none "poor." Fifty-nine percent of those using online health information did not discuss this information with their doctor. But those who did discuss this information with their doctors rated the quality of information higher. In another study, health seekers equivalently rated the quality of Internet information as good (70%) or excellent (25%), and the quality of other resources as good (66%) or excellent (28%; Peterson & Fretz, 2003). Further, Harris Interactive (2002a) reported that 82% of online health seekers consider the information is of good quality, 93% consider it is trustworthy, and 85% consider it is easy to understand. Patients decidedly rate the quality of Internet information as much higher than do physicians, and a significant 38% of Internet health seekers judge the information on their own without consulting a doctor (Harris Interactive, 2002b).

There is an additional irony of patient Internet use, which may trouble physicians. Although Internet users report overall high satisfaction with the Internet as a health resource (Williams, Nicholas, Huntington, & McLean, 2002), they also bemoan the search process as complex and unsuccessful (Gordon, Capell, & Madhok, 2002; Salo et al., 2004). Only one study by Harris Interactive (2002a) finds Americans believing that Internet health information is easy to find (72% of online health seekers). Rather, in a study of Internet health information searching involving postsurgery patients, 83% had difficulties completely understanding the information, and a third felt the retrieved information was overwhelming (Murero et al., 2001). The most common problems mentioned were: no new information, information too general, confusing interface/organization, and too much information to process (Williams et al., 2002). Yet, as Murero et al. (2001) further pointed out, 94% felt the information helped them cope with stress and anxiety about the surgery. Likewise, in

MEDLINEplus searches, the mean patient satisfaction rating was 6.1 on a scale of 1 to 10 and only 55% reported success (29% were unsuccessful); yet 74% of patients overwhelmingly indicated they would use the search engine again (Zeng, Kogan, Plovnick, Crowell, Lacroix, & Greenes, 2004). Similarly, of respondents in the Williams et al. (2002) experiment, only 30% said they found the information they were looking for (33% said maybe), 37% still said they would use the information. Again, in a U.K. study of rheumatology patients using the Internet, 83% found Internet information useful, whereas only 54% found any information not previously known (Gordon et al., 2002). So, several surveys conclude that the percentage of patients reporting they would use the retrieved information was higher than the percentage of patients reporting success in information retrieval.

Patients' Discussing Online Information With Physicians

Most Internet health seekers act independently (a mere 3% say they look up information only when told to do so by their doctor). Yet, there are contradictory reports as to how their Internet activity affects doctor–patient communication (Harris Interactive, 2002b). To begin, contrary to negative predictions, few health seekers are approaching their physicians specifically because of information they found on the Internet. Only 14% made an appointment to see their doctor as a direct result of Internet information (Harris Interactive, 2002a). Additionally, only one in five health seekers mentions information to their doctor at all (Tu & Hargraves, 2003). Diaz et al. (2002) put this in the negative, saying 59% *do not* discuss this information with their doctor. Tu and Hargraves (2003) further found that of those individuals who sought health information (Internet or otherwise) *and* saw their doctors, only 24% mentioned the information during a visit. The patient's tendency to mention information to their physicians was associated with the level of the patient's education, the number of chronic conditions, gender, race, and age. Overall, less than 40% of health seekers seem to bring up Internet information in doctors visits. Note that these reports are from the patient's viewpoint. Murray et al.'s (2003b) companion study surveyed a nationally representative sample of 3,209 patients. Nearly a third had looked for online health information in the past year, and 8% had taken that information to their physician. Nearly three quarters of those who did wanted the physician's opinion about the information. If the patients perceived that their physician had adequate communication skills, and did not appear to be challenged by the information, the patients felt that the effect was positive.

PHYSICIAN OUTCOMES

Providing Service

Many surveys report that physician Internet use significantly affects patient care decisions. Harris Interactive (2003) found that of doctors who regularly visit at least one health-related Web site, 96% report that it has had some impact on knowledge of new treatments (35% major impact, 61% minor impact), 76% note that it has had an impact on patient interaction (12% major impact, 64% minor impact) and 70% report that it has had at least a minor impact on the types of diagnoses made. Internet information brought in by patients sometimes influences treatment plans for 45.4% of physicians (Hollander & Lanier, 2001).

Similarly, the increased efficiency in physician time and operations with e-mail communication to patients is reflected in numerous articles and surveys (Mechanic, 2001). Kittler, Wald, Volk, Pizziferri, Jagannath, et al. (2004) found that in 63% of cases such communication did not increase the overall clinic workload, and generally it improved workflow and made it easier for patients to contact the practice. Half of those surveyed reported receiving between one to five e-mail requests per day for medication requests and refills, as well as for appointment requests, referral requests, and general electronic messaging. Likewise, Couchman, Forjuoh, and Rascoe (2001) demonstrated that patients would like e-mail for prescription refills, non-urgent consultations, and receiving test results. Furthermore, Sittig (2003) showed the desire of patients to go beyond administrative requests in their e-mail, as 75% of patient e-mail to physicians included requests for medication or treatment information or actions, or specific diseases or symptoms.

Physicians are generally neutral about their patients' overall experiences with Internet health material; 1% rated patients' experiences as excellent, 28% good, 62% neutral, and 9% poor (Potts & Wyatt, 2002). Yet 40% of physicians in that study reported that their patients received actual physical benefits from Internet use, whereas only 8% reported any harmful effects. Specifically, 27% did not report any benefits for their patients whereas 51% reported two or more benefits. Fifty percent did not report any problems for their patients whereas 29% reported two or more problems.

Discussions With Patients

Despite physicians' concern over web quality, and lack of confidence in their patients' ability to accurately judge and use such information, and reluctance to "prescribe" Internet searches, the literature overwhelmingly describes the favorable impact of patient-found Internet information on doctor–patient communication (Hollander & Lanier, 2001; Kittler et al., 2004; Murray et al., 2003a). Hollander and Lanier (2001) found that 69% of physicians believe that patients who secure information independently communicate better with health care providers, and 40% note that they are more compliant. In another study, 30% of online health seekers report that health information from the Internet had a major impact on discussions with their doctor (Harris Interactive, 2002a). In an Australian survey, 60% of patients said that Internet information led to more discussions with physicians, whereas only 1% reported it led to less; 34% felt that Internet information improved their relationship with their physician, and only 3% felt it worsened their relationship (Brotherton, Clarke, & Quine, 2002).

Not all studies report physician discussion about or use of patient-provided online information, however. In one survey, 51.5% of health professionals say they do not have the time to answer Internet-generated patient questions (Hollander & Lanier, 2001). And Cullen (2002) found that although 70% of New Zealand physicians say they take the information into account, only 38% of physician Internet users and 32% of non-Internet users indicated that they would actually read the information and discuss it at the patient's next visit.

There may be a slight discrepancy between the smaller figures of Internet information brought to visits (Tu & Hargraves, 2003) and the larger figures of the positive impact of Internet information in visits (Harris Interactive, 2002a, 2002b). But, this is not surprising, as physicians tend to underestimate the amount of Internet health seeking done by their patients. For example, in a U.K. survey, physicians report that only 1% to 2% of their patients had used the Internet for health information in the last month (Potts & Wyatt, 2002). What is, perhaps, likely is that patients are engaging in Internet health seeking and self-education without specifically stating such to their physicians.

PATIENT OUTCOMES

Use of Online Health Information

In 2001, a third of American health seekers said that Internet health information had a major impact on how they understood their health problems (Harris Interactive, 2002b). Among those without listed chronic conditions, 67% said that use of the Internet improved their understanding of health care issues (Baker et al., 2003). And one Australian study of oncology patients found that Internet information allowed 46%

of the respondents to better cope with their illness, versus only 1% saying it hurt their ability to cope (Brotherton et al., 2002). Online communication between physicians and patients demonstrates additional positive benefits for patient care. It seems to enhance health care in nearly three out of four; 63% of doctors who communicate online with patients note a minor impact on delivering better care, and an additional 10% note a major impact (Harris Interactive, 2003). Likewise, 48% of staff members in surveyed clinics (using a patient–physician e-mail program) believed that it improved the quality of care for the patient (Kittler et al., 2004). Seen from the doctors' point of view, online communication is having a sizable impact on patient satisfaction; 67% of doctors who see an impact consider it to be minor impact, and 19% see it as major (Harris Interactive, 2003).

A study by the Boston Consulting Group found that those who used the web for health-related purposes more frequently were two to three times more likely to take action that affected their own diagnosis and treatment, such as asking their physicians more detailed questions, suggesting a diagnosis to their physicians, and requesting specific treatments (Pastore, 2001). A survey of more than 12,000 online consumers by Gomez Advisors (Pastore, 2000a) reported that 77% had searched for online health information, and that desired features of health sites included being able to e-mail their own doctor, obtain lab results online, and manage health insurance eligibility and reimbursements.

Fostering Physician–Patient Discussion in General and About Web Sites

Americans are optimistic about the effect of Internet on the doctor–patient relationship: 40% think it will improve it whereas only 5% think it harms it (Harris Interactive, 2002a). Relationships between health practitioners and patients appear to be improved by e-mail communication, by increasing rapport and keeping communication lines open (Bysinger, 1997; Patt, Houstan, Jenckes, Sands, & Ford, 2003). Liederman and Morefield (2003) surveyed the staff and patients of a primary care clinic in California, who had a patient–practitioner web-messaging system made available to them. Of the patients who used the system and replied to the survey, 75% felt it improved access to their health care provider and 85% were satisfied with the system. However, this satisfaction was significantly associated with promptness of reply, with 83% patients expecting a reply to their e-mail within 48 hours. Health care providers were also generally satisfied with the system and preferred it to the telephone for non-urgent queries, although face-to-face contact was preferred for medical examinations and urgent illness.

If doctors are not confident in patients' ability to accurately use the Internet to look up health information, then talking over the information with the patients (to correct any misunderstandings) should result in increased approval for patient Internet health seeking as it affects their health care. This view is echoed from the patient's perspective. Diaz et al. (2002) discovered that respondents who shared Internet information with their providers rated its quality higher than those who did not (although this finding might also be a function of the quality of the information in the first place). From the physician's perspective, as well, 93% say they want their patients to discuss Internet information with them, and 62% even say it is a good idea for the physicians to explore the Internet in order to familiarize themselves with the information patients find (Hollander & Lanier, 2001). Interaction between physicians and their patients about Internet health sites is associated with greater site credibility. According to a LaurusHealth.com survey (Pastore, 2000b), the most credible health Web sites are those recommended by users' physicians (67%) or a local hospital (56%), whereas the least credible are those sponsored by a company that sells products or surveys on that site (9%); even those recommended by friends were not very credible (32%).

Effects on Physician–Patient Relationship

Concerns about Internet health information leading patients to challenge physicians appear to have little foundation. The research literature overwhelmingly indicates that the increase in patient health-seeking behavior does not necessarily lead to patients desiring to replace or challenge their physician. Neither does it appear that Internet health information will replace reliance on physicians. Only 11% of health seekers use the Internet instead of speaking with their physician (Diaz et al., 2002). Nearly a third (31%) of U.K. rheumatology patients using the Internet report that Internet information searches are easier than asking questions of their physician (Gordon et al., 2002). Yet generally speaking, Internet information does not appear to decrease doctor's visits. A survey of nearly 5,000 households in early 2002 (Baker et al., 2003) found that about 40% of those with Internet access had sought online health information, and 6% used e-mail to contact a physician or health care professional. Very few reported any effect on measurable health care use, physician visits, or telephone contacts with physicians, though about a third indicated that their use affected a decision about health or their health care, and 5% reported ordering prescriptions or pharmaceutical products online. However, the Boston Consulting Group found that those who used the web for health-related purposes more frequently, were two to three times more likely to take action that affected their own diagnosis and treatment (Pastore, 2001). This proactive behavior includes asking their physicians more detailed questions, suggesting a diagnosis to their physicians, and requesting specific treatments.

Clearly, patients still rely on their physicians to a large degree (Brotherton et al., 2002). 60% of independent health seekers only rely on Internet information when their doctors tell them to (Harris Interactive, 2002b). Likewise, of American adults who discussed Internet information with their doctor, only 14% asked the doctor for prescription medication and only 9% started an alternative treatment (Harris Interactive, 2002a). In another survey, 41% of Internet health seekers use the Internet only as a second opinion (Diaz et al., 2002). Although Sciamanna, Clark, Diaz, and Newton (2003) discovered that non-Internet users consider the Internet as a substitute for insufficient doctor communication, when they do have access, participants found the Internet less useful than expected and treated it more as a second opinion/source. Patients would much rather discuss Internet information with their doctors than use it to replace them, and those patients who do discuss information with their doctors are more positive about its quality and health benefits.

METHODOLOGY

A random sample of 2,000 physicians providing at least 20 hours a week of direct patient care, stratified by medical specialty, was selected from the Medical Marketing Service, Inc.'s national list of physicians, derived from the American Medical Association's database of more than 650,000 physicians.

The survey (Murray et al., 2003a) was developed through literature reviews, focus-group discussions, and pilot administration. It included three parts. The first asked general questions about views toward online health information as well as direct-to-consumer advertising (DTCA). The second section included either specific questions about the last time a patient brought Internet health information to an appointment, or specific questions about the last time a patient brought in DTCA information. The third section asked demographic, patient, practice and workload questions, which were later extended with specialty, year of graduation, region, office or hospital based, and training. Each version of the survey was sent to a random half of the sample.

The questionnaire was mailed in the United States in November of 2000, with a $35 check as incentive, followed up with three mailed reminders and a telephone call. Of the original 2,000 physicians sent the survey, 38 were ineligible because they were deceased, retired, or no longer in practice; and 1,050 physicians completed the questionnaire (response rate 53%). This study reports on the 515 physicians who had received the survey version with Internet questions in the second section. As the sample very closely reflected the characteristics of the physicians in the Medical Marketing Service database, data were not weighted for the present study. For more detail, see Harris Interactive (2001b) and Murray et al. (2003a).

ANALYSIS FRAMEWORK

Some of the measures reported by Murray et al. (2003a) are reconceptualized and in some cases recomputed for parsimony and improved reliability. The measures address individual characteristics, Internet use and perceptions, and outcomes, for physicians and patients. Physician and patient characteristics can be used to explain physician and patient Internet use, and those in turn can be used to explain physician and patient outcomes. Table 8.1 provides the descriptive statistics for the variables and scales used in the analyses, organized by the six concepts. Table 8.2 summarizes the final multiple regressions for usage and outcomes, also organized by the six concepts.

RESULTS

Descriptive Results

Physician E-Health Outlook and Practice Characteristics. Respondents were slightly positive about the recent increase in health information available to the public, felt that health-related information available to the public from ads, articles, Web sites and family/friends is somewhat accurate, slightly agreed that a range of negative effects are associated with health-related information on the Internet, and sometimes encourage their patients to look for information about their own medical conditions or treatments.

Concerning their practice, about half earned at least $250,000 per year, three quarters engage in joint decision making with their patients, nearly all work out of their office, and three quarters were male. The physicians saw, on average, 84 patients per week (spending 30 minutes with each), and devoted about 12 hours per week to other tasks relating to patient care and 5.9 hours on practice finances. Almost a quarter of

TABLE 8.1
Descriptive Statistics for Measures and Scales (With Reliabilities) Used in Analyses

Physician Characteristics	Min	Max	Mean	S.D.	N
increase health inf good/bad? 1vgood 5vbad	1	5	2.30	.91	1041
accuracy ads arts webs friends/family? 1VA 4NotAtAll; α = .55	1	4	2.44	.39	1047
mean 9 items health info effects 1SA 4SD high = worse; α = .68	1	4	2.24	.42	1029
encourage patients look for inf? 1often 4never	1	4	1.96	.82	1047
age	28	90	49.23	11.05	998
role play in Pt's decisions? (Pt and family together 11.6%; Together 73.3%)	Physician 15.1%				1040
% Pts talked internet? (61–80% 2.3%; 41–60% 7.6%)	81–100% .2%	21–40% 30.8%	1–20% 59.1%		861
1999 income med practice (-$150K 31.1%; -$200K 20.4%)	< $100K 18.7%	-$250K 13.2%	> $250K 16.7%		957
office or hospital based? (Hospital 10.8%)	Office 89.2%				1050
gender (Female 10.8%)	Male 78.4%				1036

Patient Characteristics	Min	Max	Mean	S.D.	N
enough time spend w/patients? 1often 4never	1	4	1.65	.72	1044
how many patients see typical wk?	1	300	83.75	46.42	1018
min./patient typical week	3	300	30.62	23.69	1001
hours per week with Patients?	1	148	33.48	15.84	1016
hours/week related to other tasks related to care?	0	90	12.16	9.72	985
hours per week on finances?	0	55	5.90	5.69	954
mean medicaid minority < $20K; α = .75	0	100	23.37	18.83	994

(Continued)

TABLE 8.1
(Continued)

Physician Internet Use	Min	Max	Mean	S.D.	N
use Internet for practice? 1Y 2N	1	2	1.39	.49	1043
use Internet for clinical information? 1Often 4Never	1	4	3.12	1.1	636
communicate with patients by e-mail? 1Often 4Never	1	4	3.45	.84	637
refer patients to Web sites? 1Often 4Never	1	4	2.88	.86	866
Patient Internet Use					
how relevant to patient was inf? 1Vrel 4NotRel	1	4	2.02	.65	408
accuracy of inf patient talked about? 1VAcc 4NotAcc	1	4	2.20	.59	407
reliability of inf on net? 1VConc 4NotConc	1	4	1.83	.67	865
patients assess inf reliable? 1Exc 5Poor	1	5	4.15	.76	866
patient brings printed material? 1Y 2N	1	2	1.51	.50	393
% Pts talked internet? 81-100% .2% 61-80% 2.3%	21-40% 30.8%	41-60% 7.6%	1-20% 59.1%		861

Physician Outcomes	Min	Max	Mean	S.D.	N
do what the patient wanted? 1Y 2Part 3N	1	3	1.92	.39	409
mean relation timeeff quality health (high = worse); α = .74 1help 2nodiff 3hurt	1	3	1.92	.39	409
Patient Outcomes					
mean 4 items 1HelpLot 3NoDiff 5HurtLot; α = .77	1	5	2.31	.50	867
mean challenge, not appropriate 1Y 2N; α = .55	1	2	1.76	.35	409

Note. "α =" is Cronbach's alpha.

TABLE 8.2

Summary Results From Multiple Regressions Explaining Physician and Patient Usage, and Physician and Patient Outcomes

Explaining Physician Usage		Explaining Physician Outcomes	
1. Use for purposes related to practice		*11. Most recent occasion patient talked about info saw on Internet they thought relevant to their own health—did what patient wanted?*	
Encourage patients look for info	.16 ***	Use to e-mail patients	.12 *
Evaluation of public health info	.11 ***	Accuracy online info patient talked about	.31 ***
Adj R^2 = .04, F = 21.3 ***, N = 877.		Adj R^2 = .11, F = 17.5 ***, N = 262	
2. Use to obtain clinical information		*12. As result of patient bringing this info, mean of: relationship changed; time efficiency; quality of care; health outcomes*	
Evaluation of public health info	.10 **	Use to e-mail patients	.16 **
Enough time to spend w/ patients	.10 *	Often refer patients specific Web sites or other online resources for health-related info	.13 *
Adj R^2 = .02, F = 5.3 *, N = 627		Accuracy online info patient talked about	.18 **
		Relevance info to disease or condition	.22 ***
		Concerned reliability of online health info your patients access	-.16 **
		Adj R^2 = .23, F = 16.9 ***, N = 268	
3. Use to e-mail patients			
Hours/week on practice finances	-.16 ***		
Accuracy public health-related info	.11 **		
Encourage patients look for info	.11 **		
Effects of public health-related info	.09 *		
Adj R^2 = .06, F = 10.8 ***, N = 585			
4. Often refer patients specific Web sites or other online resources for health-related info			
Encourage patients look for info	.42 ***		
Patient type	.09 **		
Effects of public health-related info	.08 *		
Adj R^2 = .20, F = 63.9 ***, N = 743			

(Continued)

TABLE 8.2
(Continued)

Explaining Patient Usage		Explaining Patient Outcomes	
5. % patients talked with physician Internet info		*13. Mean of how your patients' access to online health information hurt: comm with physician, confident they are making own health decisions, take care of their own health, understand their health*	
Encourage patients look for info	.24 ***	Use to e-mail patients	.14 **
Number patients seen/week	.08 *	Often refer patients specific Web sites or other online resources for health-related info	.15 **
Adj R² = .06, F = 22.8 ***, N = 683		Accuracy online info patient talked about	.18 **
		How good patients assessing health Web site	.20 ***
		Relevance info to disease or condition	.17 **
		Adj R² = .24, F = 18.0 ***, N = 286	
6. Relevance info to disease or condition		*14. Mean feeling patient was challenging physician authority, wanted physician to do something was not appropriate*	
Effects of public health-related info	.26 ***	Accuracy online info patient talked about	-.24 ***
Accuracy public health-related info	.19 ***	How good patients assessing Web site	-.14 **
Hours/week related to care	-.12 *	Relevance info to disease or condition	-.12 *
Adj R² = .16, F = 20.7 ***, N = 310		Adj R² = .15, F = 23.2 ***, N = 405	
7. Accuracy of online info patient talked about			
Effects of public health-related info	.31 ***		
Evaluation of public health info	.16 **		
Accuracy public health-related info	.15 **		
Adj R² = .24, F = 33.6 ***, N = 311			

8. *Concerned reliability of online health info your patients access*

Effects of public health-related info	-.25 ***
Evaluation of public health info	-.14 ***
Gender	.07 *
Encourage patients look for info	.08 *
Adj R^2 = .11, F = 21.7 ***, M = 686	

9. *How good patients assessing health Web site*

Effects of public health-related info	.20 ***
Accuracy public health-related info	.22 ***
Encourage patients look for info	.09 **
Enough time to spend w/patients	.08 *
Evaluation of public health info	.08 *
Adj R^2 = .17, F = 28.8 ***, N = 688	

10. *Brought printed material*

Practice income	-.14 **
Hours/week on practice finances	-.15 **
Adj R^2 = .04, F = 7.0 ***, N = 299	

Note. Both physician and patient measures are from the physician's perspective. All results are final summary regressions using two blocks of explanatory variables, with variables entered stepwise within blocks. For usage, the blocks are Physician Characteristics and Patient Characteristics. For outcomes, the blocks are Physician Usage and Patient Usage. Values are standarized beta coefficients. None of the variables in each dependent set was intercorrelated more than r = .3, except *Accuracy of online info patient talked about* was correlated with *Relevance info to disease or condition* r = .45 *** and with *How good patients assessing health Web site* r = .33 ***. No simple dimensional or reliable scales were derivable from the six patient use variables, so each use variable was run in a separate regression. However, there is some shared variance across some of the dependent variables, so significance levels are somewhat overestimated.

their patients were on Medicaid, members of minority groups, or had incomes less than $20,000.

Physicians' Use of the Internet.   Concerning physicians' use of the Internet, 61% had used the Internet for some aspect of their practice, rarely to obtain clinical information, rarely to communicate by e-mail with their patients, and hardly ever referred their patients to specific Web sites or other online resources for health-related information.

Patients' Use of the Internet.   Eighty-four percent of the physicians reported that, in the prior 12 months, their patients had talked to them in person about information they thought was relevant to their own health that they had seen on the Internet. However, this does not represent large percentages of patients; nearly 60% indicated that 20% or less of their patients had done so, about a third indicated that between 21% and 40% had done so, and less than 10% indicated that more than 40% of their patients had done so. The physicians felt that the information was somewhat relevant, but the accuracy of the information that the patient talked about was less than somewhat accurate. They were fairly concerned about the reliability of the online health information that their patients accessed, especially as they felt that their patients were not good at assessing the reliability of online health information. About half of the time, patients brought some printed information from the Internet with them.

Physician Outcomes: How Did the Physicians Feel This Affected Their Own Practice?   In general, the physicians did, in part but not completely, what the patient had requested. They felt that bringing the information to the visit neither helped nor hurt (using the mean of relationship with patient, time-efficiency of visit, quality of care, ultimate health outcomes).

Patient Outcomes: And How Did They Feel This Affected Their Patients?   Overall (considering how well they communicate with the physician, how confident they are in making their own health decisions, how well they take care of their own health, and how much they understand their health conditions and treatments), they felt that their patients' access to online health information helped a little. Three quarters of the physicians did not feel that the patients were challenging their authority or wanting them to do something inappropriate by bringing health information from the Internet to the visit.

Summary Multiple Regression Results

Influences on Physicians' Use of the Internet. Table 8.2 shows that (1) physicians were more likely to use the Internet for practice-related purposes if they also encouraged their patients to look for online information about their own medical conditions or treatments, and if they more positively evaluated the recent increase in Internet health information available to the public. In particular, they (2) used the Internet to obtain clinical information if they had a more positive evaluation of public health information (ads, articles, Web sites, friends/family), and had enough time to spend with their patients; and (3) used it to communicate by e-mail with their patients if they spent less time on their practice finances, more positively evaluated public health information, encouraged their patients to look for information, and more positively assessed the effects of Internet health-related information. They were also more likely to (4) refer their patients to specific Web sites or other online health information if they generally encouraged their patients to seek out more medical information, had wealthier patients, and more positively assessed the effects of Internet health information.

Influences on Patients' Use of the Internet. Physicians (5) reported that a greater percent of their patients talked with them about Internet information if they encouraged them to look for medical information in general, and if they saw fewer patients per week. Physicians were then asked several assessments of this information they talked about. They were (6) more likely to assess this information as relevant to the patient's disease or condition if they had more positive assessments of the effects of Internet health information, felt that public health information was more accurate, and spent fewer hours per week on patient-related care. The information was (7) seen as more accurate if the physician had more positive assessments of the effects of Internet health information, more positively evaluated the recent increase in public health information, and felt public health information was more accurate. They were (8) more concerned about the reliability of the online health information that their patients accessed if they had more positive assessments of the effects of Internet health information, more positively evaluated the recent increase in public health information, were male, and encouraged patients to look for medical information. They were (9) more likely to feel their patients were good at assessing health Web sites if they had more positive assessments of the effects of Internet health information, felt public health information was more accurate, encouraged their patients to look for medical information, had enough time to spend with their patients, and had more positive evaluations of general public health information. Finally (10), their patients were more likely to bring printed material from the Internet to their visit if the physician's practice income was lower, and the physician spent less time on practice finances.

Influences on Physician Outcomes: How Did the Physicians Feel This Affected Their Own Practice?
Physicians were (11) more likely to do what the patient wanted in the most recent occasion when a patient talked about information they saw on the Internet if they also used e-mail more frequently to communicate with their patients, and had more positive evaluations of the accuracy of the online information the patient talked about. They were (12) more likely to feel that, as a result of their patient bringing this information, improvements in their relationships with the patient, their time efficiency, the quality of care, and the patient's health outcomes, all improved, if they used e-mail more frequently to communicate with their patients, referred their patients more frequently to specific Web sites or other online resources for health information, felt the online information the patient talked about was more accurate and was more relevant to their disease or condition, and were more concerned about the reliability of the online health information their patients accessed.

Influences on Patient Outcomes: And How Did They Feel This Affected Their Patients?
Physicians were (13) more likely to feel that patients' access to online health information helped their communication with the physician, and improved their confidence in making their own health decisions, taking care of their own health, and understanding their health, if the physicians used e-mail more frequently to communicate with patients, more frequently referred patients to health Web sites or online resources, and felt the accuracy of the online information was better, their patients were better able to assess the health Web sites, and the information was relevant to the patients' disease or condition. They were (14) more likely to feel that patients were not challenging physician authority, or wanting the physician to do something that was not appropriate, if they felt that the accuracy of the online information was better, their patients were better able to assess the health Web sites, and the information was relevant to the patients' disease or condition.

Figure 8.1 summarizes these relationships, showing both the unique and common influences across physician and patient Internet use and outcomes. The strongest influences on usage overall are physicians' perceptions of the evaluation, accuracy, and effects of publicly available health information and encouraging their patients to look for their own medical and health information. The strongest influences on outcomes

Influences on Physician Internet Use (from 4% to 20% variance explained)	Use Outcomes →	Influences on Physician Outcomes (from 11% to 23% variance explained)

Physician Characteristics
• Evaluation of public health info
• Accuracy public health-related info
• Effects of public health-related info
• Encourage patients look for info
    Patient Characteristics
• Hours/week on practice finances
• Patient type
• Enough time to spend w/patients
		Physician Use
		• Use to email patients
		• Often refer patients specific websites or other online resources for health-related info
		    Patient Use
		• Accuracy online info patient talked about
		• Relevance info to disease or condition
		• Concerned about reliability of online health info your patients access

Influences on Patient Internet Use (from 4% to 24% variance explained)	Use Outcomes →	Influences on Patient Outcomes (from 15% to 24% variance explained)

Physician Characteristics
• Evaluation of public health info
• Accuracy public health-related info
• Effects of public health-related info
• Encourage patients look for info
• Gender
    Patient Characteristics
• Enough time to spend w/patients
• Number patients seen/week
• Hours/week on practice finances
• Hours/week related to care
• Practice income
		Physician Use
		• Use to email patients
		• Often refer patients specific websites or other online resources for health-related info
		    Patient Use
		• Accuracy online info patient talked about
		• How good patients assessing health website
		• Relevance info to disease or condition

FIG. 8.1.   Summary of influences of physician and patient characteristics on physician and patient use, and of physician and patient use on physician and patient outcomes.

overall are physicians' use of e-mail to communicate with their patients, their evaluations of the accuracy and relevance of the online health information their patients talk about, and how good their patients are at assessing health Web sites.

CONCLUSION

Analysis of survey responses lends further evidence of the positive side of the Internet in terms of information and self-empowerment. At the same time, they reveal little evidence of negative effects in precisely one of those areas that had elicited concern, namely how it would affect the quality of physician delivery of health care.

Views of the Internet among physicians tend to cohere around a dimension of sentiment towards digital resources. Those who like the Internet and e-mail, for instance, also are more positive about their patients' use of them. This is not unexpected, perhaps, but needs highlighting to remind the reader of the limitations of an area-by-area or service-by-service approach to the analysis of the diffusion of new services.

Although many of the physician-based conclusions reached from our analysis of the Robert Wood Johnson survey data support prior research findings, there are conflicts in need of further study. More investigation needs to be done about exactly *how* patients represent Internet health information in doctors' visits, the effect of time constraints on referring patients to health sites and discussing Internet information during appointments, and the somewhat ironic relationship between physicians' reporting somewhat positive benefits from their patients' using Internet information and their skepticism about the accuracy, relevance, and reliability of their patients' Internet information.

Another result worthy of further investigation is the surprising inverse relationship between positive views of Internet health care information accuracy and the number of hours per week devoted to patient care. One possible explanation is that those physicians who have positive views of Internet information accuracy are engaging in wishful thinking in that they would want their patients to be more positive in their outlook. It may also suggest that anticipatory efficiencies exist in terms of exploiting the Internet as a better source of information for patient health care.

The most significant questions about physician views of patient use of Internet information can only be answered by comparative research. A study that combined both patients' and physicians' behaviors and attitudes in controlled situations would allow a combined and comparative analysis of doctors' views on patient Internet health seeking with patients' views on their own health seeking.

Although physicians remain skeptical of the merits of Internet health information, it appears that the Internet does indeed have the ability to contribute positively to the patient–physician relationship. This remains an underdeveloped resource, however, as barriers of communication and constraints of time remain. Technological and service innovations could help create an environment that would enhance patients' ability to care for their health, and physicians' ability to play a more effective role in the process. This might be accomplished, for example, by creating a virtual space for discussion and mutual decision making. Some of the financial pressures on the health care system in the United States, where most patients pay at least part of their health bills and some pay all, might be alleviated while also empowering both physicians and patients.

At the same time, it is intriguing to put health care communication in perspective with the way in which increasing bandwidth and computing power has been applied to animate and enrich home entertainment, mobile gaming, and portable music. Many consumers are able to effectively create their own rich and highly personalized environments, and tailor them precisely to their own situation. By contrast, it would seem that barriers to enhanced and personally tailored health care information for patients stem from financial, legal, and organizational issues, rather than from computer architecture and richness of communication. The research discussed in this chapter highlights the perceptual and content gap between highly trained experts (physicians) and lay people (patients) who use a vast information resource to address health care needs. Understanding the gap and how to close it could be an important service to increasing health care efficiency and effectiveness.

REFERENCES

Angelo, S., & Citkowitz, E. (2001). An electronic survey of physicians using online clinical discussion groups: A brief report. *Connecticut Medicine, 65*(3), 135–139.

Baker, L., Wagner, T., Singer, S., & Bundorf, M. (2003). Use of the Internet and e-mail for health care information: Results from a national survey. *Journal of the American Medical Association, 289*(18), 2400–2406.

Brotherton, J., Clarke, S., & Quine, S. (2002). Use of the Internet by oncology patients: Its effect on the doctor–patient relationship. *Medical Journal of Australia, 177*(7), 395.

Bysinger, B. (1997). Using the Internet to support provider–patient collaboration. *Health Management Technology, 18*(1), 44–45.

Carney, P., Poor, D., Schifferdecker, K., Gephart, D., Brooks, W., & Nierenberg, D. (2004). Computer use among community-based primary care physician preceptors. *Academic Medicine 79*(6), 580–590.

Cotton, S., & Gupta, S. (2004). Characteristics of online and offline health information seekers and factors that discriminate between them. *Social Science & Medicine, 59,* 1795–1806.

Couchman, G., Forjuoh, S., & Rascoe, T. (2001). E-mail communications in family practice: What do patients expect? *Journal of Family Practice, 59*(5), 414–418.

Cullen, R. (2002). In search of evidence: Family practitioners' use of the Internet for clinical information. *Journal of the Medical Library Association, 90*(4), 370–379.

D'Alessandro, D., Kreiter, C., Kinzer, S., & Peterson, M. (2004). A randomized controlled trial of an information prescription for pediatric patient education on the Internet. *Archives of Pediatrics and Adolescent Medicine, 158*(9), 857–862.

D'Alessandro, D., Kreiter, C., & Peterson, M. (2004). An evaluation of information-seeking behaviors of general pediatricians. *Pediatrics, 113*(1 Pt. 1), 64–69.

Diaz, J., Griffith, R., Ng, J., Reinert, S., Friedmann, P., & Moulton, A. (2002). Patients' use of the Internet for medical information. *Journal of General Internal Medicine, 17*(3), 180–185.

Fox, S. (2003). Wired for health: How Californians compare to the rest of the nation. *Pew Internet & American Life Project.* Retrieved October 5, 2004, from http://www .pewinternet.org/pdfs/PIP_CA_Health_Report.pdf

Gordon, M., Capell, H., & Madhok, R. (2002). The use of the Internet as a resource for health information among patients attending a rheumatology clinic. *Rheumatology, 41*(12), 1402–1405.

Greenspan, R. (2002). Physicians' net usage up. *CyberAtlas.* Retrieved December 6, 2003, from http://www.cyberatlas.internet.com/markets/healthcare/print/0,,10101_ 1430741,00.html

Harris Interactive. (2001a). New data show Internet, website and email usage by physicians all increasing. *Health Care News, 1*(8), 1–3.

Harris Interactive. (2001b). *The impact of the Internet and advertising on patients and physicians: Methodology report for survey of physicians.* New York: Harris Interactive.

Harris Interactive. (2002a). 4-country survey finds most "cyberchondriacs" believe online health care information is trustworthy, easy to find and understand. *Health Care News, 2*(12), 1–3.

Harris Interactive. (2002b). Four-nation survey shows widespread but different levels of Internet use for health purposes. *Health Care News, 2*(11), 1–4.

Harris Interactive. (2003). eHealth's influence continues to grow as usage of the Internet by physicians and patients increases. *Health Care News, 3*(6), 1–7.

Helft, P. R., Hlubocky, F., & Daugherty, C. K. (2003). American oncologists' views of internet use by cancer patients: A mail survey of American Society of Clinical Oncology members. *Journal of Clinical Oncology, Mar 1, 21*(5), 942–947.

Hollander, S., & Lanier, D. (2001). The physician–patient relationship in an electronic environment: A regional snapshot. *Bulletin of the Medical Library Association, 89*(4), 397–399.

Houston, T., Sands, D., Nash, B., & Ford, D. (2003). Experiences of physicians who frequently use e-mail with patients. *Health Communication, 15*(4), 515–525.

Jacob, J. (2002). Consumer access to health care information: Its effect on the physician–patient relationship. *Alaska Medicine, 44*(4), 75–82.

Jones, C., & Lambros, M. (2003). Use of the Internet for patient care: A nationwide survey of Australian anesthetists. *Anesthesia and Intensive Care, 31*(3), 290–293.

Kalsman, M., & Acosta, D. (2000). Use of the Internet as a medical resource by rural physicians. *The Journal of the American Board of Family Practice, 13*(5), 349–352.

Katz, J. E., Rice, R. E., & Acord, S. (2004). E-health networks and social transformations: Expectations of centralization, experiences of decentralization. In M. Castells (Ed.), *The network society: A cross-cultural perspective* (pp. 293–318). London: Edward Elgar.

Kittler, A., Wald, J., Volk, L., Pizziferri, L., Jagannath, Y., Harris, C., Lippincott, M., Yu, T., Hobbs, J., & Bates, D. (2004). The role of primary care non-physician clinic staff in e-mail communication with patients. *International Journal of Medical Informatics, 73,* 333–340.

Liederman, E., & Morefield, C. (2003). Web messaging: A new tool for patient–physician communication. *Journal of the American Medical Information Association, 10,* 260–270.

Martin, S. (2003). MDs' office Internet use hits 57%. *The Canadian Medical Association Journal, 168*(4), 475.

Mechanic, D. (2001). How should hamsters run? Some observations about sufficient patient time in primary care. *British Medical Journal, 323*(7307), 266–268.

Miller, R., Hillman, J., & Given, R. (2004). Physician use of IT: Results from the Deloitte Research Survey. *Journal of Healthcare Information Management, 18*(1), 72–80. Retrieved September 25, 2004, from http://www.216.239.41.104/search?q=cache:HZRlGVoc_ 90J:www.himss.org/content/files/jhim/18-1/contribution_physician.pdf +Deloitte+ Research/Fulcrum+Analytics&hl=en

Moyer, C. A., Stern, D. T., Dobias, K., Cox, D., & Katz, S. (2002). Bridging the electronic divide: Patient and provider perspectives on e-mail communication in primary care. *American Journal of Management Care*, 8(5), 427–433.

Murero, M., D'Ancona, G., & Karamanoukian, H. (2001). Use of the Internet by patients before and after cardiac surgery: Telephone survey. *Journal of Medical Internet Research*, 3(3), e27.

Murray, E., Lo, B., Pollack, L., Donelan, K., Catania, J., Lee, K., Zapert, K., & Turner, R. (2003a). The impact of health information on the Internet on health care and the physician–patient relationship: National U.S. Survey among 1,050 U.S. physicians. *Journal of Medical Internet Research*, 5(3), e17. Retrieved September 24, 2004, from http://www.jmir.org/2003/3/e17

Murray, E., Lo, B., Pollack, L., Donelan, K., Catania, J., White, M., Zapert, K., & Turner, R. (2003b). The impact of health information on the internet on the physician–patient relationship: Patient perceptions. *Archives of Internal Medicine*, 163(14), 1727–1734.

Pastore, M. (2000a). The mess known as online healthcare. *CyberAtlas*. Retrieved December 6, 2003, from http://www.cyberatlas.internet.com/markets/healthcare/print/0,,10101_1496801,00.html

Pastore, M. (2000b). Consumers choose health sites with doctors' input. *CyberAtlas*. Retrieved December 6, 2003, from http://www.cyberatlas.internet.com/markets/healthcare/print/0,,5931_335121,00.html

Pastore, M. (2001). Online health consumers more proactive about healthcare. *CyberAtlas*. Retrieved December 6, 2003, from http://www.cyberatlas.internet.com/markets/healthcare/print/0,,10101_755471,00.html

Patt, M., Houstan, T., Jenckes, M., Sands, D., & Ford, D. (2003). Doctors who are using e-mail with their patients: A qualitative exploration. *Journal of Medical Internet Research*, 5(2), e9.

Peterson, M., & Fretz, P. (2003). Patient use of the Internet for information in a lung cancer clinic. *Chest*, 123(2), 452–457.

Potts, H., & Wyatt, J. (2002). Survey of doctors' experience of patients using the Internet. *Journal of Medical Internet Research*, 4(1), e5.

Rice, R. E., & Katz, J. E. (Eds.). (2000). *Internet and health communication: Experience and expectations*. Thousand Oaks, CA: Sage.

Rice, R. E., & Katz, J. E. (2003). Comparing Internet and mobile phone usage: Digital divides of usage, adoption and dropouts. *Telecommunications Policy*, 27(8–9), 597–623.

Risk, A., & Dzenowagis, J. (2001). Review of Internet health information quality initiatives. *Journal of Medical Internet Research*, 3(4), e28. Retrieved September 24, 2004, from http://www.jmir.org/2001/4/e28

Salo, D., Perez, C., Lavery, R., Malankar, A., Borenstein, M., & Bernstein, S. (2004). Patient education and the Internet: Do patients want us to provide them with medical Web sites to learn more about their medical problems? *The Journal of Emergency Medicine*, 26(3), 293–300.

Sciamanna, C., Clark, M., Diaz, J., & Newton, S. (2003). Filling the gaps in physician communication: The role of the Internet among primary care patients. *International Journal of Medical Informatics*, 72, 1–8.

Sittig, D. (2003). Results of a content analysis of electronic messages (e-mail) sent between patients and their physicians. *BMC Medical Informatics Decision Making*, 3(1), 11.

Tu, H., & Hargraves, J. (2003). Seeking health care information: Most consumers still on the sidelines. *Center for Studying Health System Change*, 1–4. Retrieved September 24, 2004, from http://www.hschange.org/CONTENT/537/

UK doctors still "out of office" to patients online. (2003). Retrieved September 25, 2003, from http://www.e-health-media.com/news/item.cfm?ID=531

White, C., Sheedy, V., & Lawrence, N. (2002). Patterns of computer usage among medical practitioners in rural and remote Queensland. *The Australian Journal of Rural Health, 10*(3), 137–146.

Williams, P., Nicholas, D., Huntington, P., & McLean, F. (2002). Surfing for health: User evaluation of a health information website. Part two: Fieldwork. *Health Information & Libraries Journal, 19*(4), 214–225.

Wright, S., Tseng, W., & Kolodner, K. (2001). Physician opinion about electronic publications. *The American Journal of Medicine, 110*(5), 373–377.

Zeng, Q., Kogan, S., Plovnick, R., Crowell, J., Lacroix, E.-M., & Greenes, R. (2004). Positive attitudes and failed queries: An exploration of the conundrums of consumer health information retrieval. *International Journal of Medical Informatics, 73*, 45–55.

Chapter 9

Delivering the Goods: Midwives' Use of the Internet

Sarah Stewart

Otago Polytechnic, New Zealand

MIDWIFERY AND THE INTERNET

Midwives provide maternity care for women and their families. In the New Zealand (NZ) context, a midwife is responsible for the provision of care to a woman from conception until 6 weeks after the baby is born. Midwifery care relies heavily on personal one-to-one communication and physically "being there." Some would argue that e-health is "dangerous nonsense" (Coddington, 2000) and there is no place for computers and the Internet in the midwifery practice environment; after all, being a midwife means "being with woman" not "being with computer." However, both health consumers and midwives are increasingly accessing health information and resources via the Internet, which is bound to have implications for midwifery practice, and how midwives utilize the Internet. This chapter discusses the results of a web-based survey that questioned NZ midwives about their use of Internet resources. The study sought to find out what resources midwives used and wanted to be developed, and the barriers to use of the Internet. The study also aimed to discover how consumers' use of the Internet affected midwifery practice and how midwives felt about it.

Background

In New Zealand, maternity care is provided by the Lead Maternity Carer (LMC), from conception to 6 weeks after the baby is born. The government funds the LMC; therefore maternity care is free to the woman.

177

More than 70% of women have midwives as their LMC, the remaining providers being general practitioners and obstetricians (New Zealand Ministry of Health, 2003). The midwife is responsible for providing information to the woman and preparing her for life as a mother, and is accountable for the clinical decisions she makes. Midwives may prescribe medications that are pertinent to childbirth, order diagnostic tests such as blood tests and ultrasound scans, and refer to obstetricians or pediatricians when problems are detected (Calvert, 1998). The majority of these midwives are self-employed, claiming fees for service directly from the government. Hospital core services, including secondary maternity care for women with complex health needs, are provided by employed midwives who work on rostered shifts. Hospital midwives run the antenatal clinics and inpatient wards, as well as delivery suites.

The NZ midwife has a strong philosophy of working in partnership with each woman and providing continuity of care. However, the partnership model that is the foundation of NZ midwifery practice emphasizes that the woman has the right to control her own pregnancy and birthing experience, which involves informed choice and consent (Guilliland & Pairman, 1995).

Potential of the Internet for Midwives

The potential of the Internet for midwives ranges from being a source of evidence-based information that can be integrated into midwifery practice, to networking and collaboration with other midwives both nationally and internationally, as well as a source and tool for research (Petersson, Forsgreen, Sjodin, Kublickas, & Westgren, 2003; Sinclair, 1997). E-mail discussion groups and online bulletin boards have been successful tools for facilitating professional communication and collaboration (Brooks, Rospopa, & Scott, 2004), and have the potential to be particularly valuable for the large number of midwives in New Zealand who are self-employed or working in independent practices. There are a vast number of e-mail discussion groups for midwives, including the New Zealand Midwives Group (http://www.health.groups.yahoo.com/group/nzmidwives), which is a closed group specifically designed for the support of NZ midwives, and the open international discussion group for people interested in midwifery research (http://www.jiscmail.ac.uk/lists/MIDWIFERY-RESEARCH.html).

This type of communication has the potential to be especially valuable for those midwives who are geographically or professionally isolated from colleagues because it facilitates support, education, and camaraderie (Stensland Kurokawa, 1996). Brooks et al. (2004) evaluated an online discussion forum that was set up in a British National Health Trust, United

Kingdom (UK) over a period of 2 years, with the aim of giving midwives the opportunity to discuss health care policy. Participants felt the forum allowed them to make a very real contribution to decision making, as opposed to the traditional methods of communication, especially as it did away with the traditional hierarchical barriers of face-to-face communication. The forum allowed participation at any time of the day or night, and fostered a sense of belonging to a community. Changes in practice and resolution of issues were the end result of many discussions (Brooks et al., 2004).

There is a dearth of research into how midwives use the Internet in practice and few midwives use the Internet as a research tool for surveying and collecting data. Loy (2001) carried out the first national survey of midwives, both practitioners and students, in the United Kingdom (n = 141). Loy (2001) found that 55% of respondents had access to the Internet at work, and 95% had home access. The midwives who had the greatest access were midwifery lecturers and students, who had 100% access through the university at which they worked or studied. Hospital midwives had 55% work access, although more than 20% of these midwives found it inconvenient or difficult to use. Respondents were using the Internet frequently, with 45% using it two to three times per week. The vast majority of midwives accessed the Internet to find out an explicit piece of information or to keep current with news and research. Although midwives were very positive about the idea of e-mail discussion lists in that they were seen to facilitate the dissemination of information as well as provide stimulating discussion, only 30% of respondents had used them. Respondents were familiar with online databases, with more than 75% having used an online database, and nearly 50% had taken advantage of the electronic version of the *British Medical Journal* or *Lancet*.

Other disciplines have carried out Internet research that is relevant to midwifery practice. For example, Beck (2004) described women's experiences of posttraumatic stress disorder (PTSD) following childbirth. E-mail was used to collect data from 36 of the 38 participants, who were based in New Zealand, the United States, Australia and the United Kingdom—the other two women posted their stories by traditional mail. Mothers who suffered PTSD described four themes: experience of flashbacks and nightmares; feelings that they were a shadow of their former selves; the need to know the details of their traumatic births; and the feelings of anger/rage, anxiety/panic attacks, and depression that permeated their everyday lives.

Clinical Applications

Internet technology is developing in a way that can provide practical clinical support for midwives, such as home monitoring of the fetal heart rate in utero (Di Lieto, Catalano, Pontillo, Pollio, De Falco, Lannotti, &

Schiraldi, 2001) or home monitoring of babies once they have been born (Gray, Safran, Davis, Pomilio-Weitzner, Stewart, Zaccagnini, & Pursley, 2000). This is an attractive option for women and midwives, especially in rural communities in New Zealand. Laboratory results can be sent via the Internet to the midwife, allowing her to make clinical decisions at a much greater speed than when receiving results by conventional post. Applications of Internet technology such as these would keep women at home with their families, and reduce traveling and time costs, which are a constant tension particularly for rural midwives (Hendry, 2003; Patterson, 2001). Furthermore, the Internet has the capability for keeping maternity records on an Internet-based program, which would make them accessible from wherever the midwife and woman were located. These measures could facilitate data consultations at any time or place, allow patient access their personal records, facilitate ease of electronic claiming, and transfer of data into national databases. As yet, there have been few examples of these applications being utilized in midwifery practice. However, the Midwifery Provider Organisation, which is affiliated with the New Zealand College of Midwives (NZCOM), has devised a practice management system for self-employed midwives that includes data collection software, an interface that allows midwives to claim electronically, and access to an online pharmacology resource (http://www.midwife.org.nz/index.cfm/services).

Communicating the Midwifery Business

Personal midwifery Web sites provide an avenue for advertising and generating information for women and their families, as well as communicating with colleagues. There is a growing number of personal Web sites belonging to NZ midwives, as well as several sites where a midwife can advertise her services, such as the NZCOM "Search for a Midwife" (http://www.midwife.org.nz/index.cfm/search) and "Everybody" (http://www.everybody.co.nz/midwife_search.html). However, it appears that the majority of midwives rely on word-of-mouth recommendation or listings in the telephone yellow pages to gain clientele, although there is currently no data to support that supposition.

Searching for Online Evidence-Based Information

One of the rapidly growing concepts in health care is that of evidence-based practice (EBP). Midwives constantly have to make decisions together with women, yet it can be time-consuming and expensive to keep track of the latest research evidence, especially if midwives subscribe to more than one relevant journal (Estabrooks, O'Leary, Ricker, & Humphrey, 2003). The Internet provides easy and convenient access to sources of evidence-based practice such as the "Cochrane Pregnancy and Childbirth Database" (http://www.nelh.nhs.uk/cochrane.asp) and evidence-based guidelines including "Caesarean Section" (http://www.nice .org.uk) and "Care of Women with Breech Presentation or Previous Caesarean Section" (http://www.nzgg.org.nz). There is conflicting evidence about the uptake of resources such as these by health practitioners, including general practitioners (GPs), nurses and other health care personnel (Westbrook, Gosling, & Cohera, 2004). Kerse, Arroll, Lloyd, Young, and Ward (2001) surveyed 456 GPs about their use of the Internet; half of the GPs knew about the Cochrane database, but only 15% made use of it.

Similarly to GPs, midwives are autonomous practitioners and there is evidence that they access evidence resources on the Internet. Petersson et al. (2003) evaluated the use of an Internet-based database about infectious diseases (INFPREG) that was available in all antenatal clinics in Sweden, as well as medical departments such as obstetric and pediatrics. Of the Swedish midwives ($n = 404$) who participated in the evaluative survey in 2002, 88% had access to the Internet, with 66% reporting that they used it for finding medical information. Fifty-eight percent midwives had visited INFPREG, with 81% implementing information found on the database into practice, and with 26% midwives informing patients about INFPREG. Resources such as bibliographic databases are valuable tools for midwifery practice with the potential power to improve midwifery standards of care by ensuring that midwives are kept up to date with recent developments in clinical practice (Kinniburgh, 2001).

The Internet allows consumers to have the same access to information as midwives, increasing consumer empowerment and involvement in decision making (Harding, 2000). This, in turn, is an added incentive for midwives to provide evidence-based information, as consumers are increasingly likely to challenge them because of what they find on the Internet (Murray, Lo, Pollack, Donelan, Catania, et al., 2003).

INTERNET AND MIDWIFERY EDUCATION

Statutory requirements around professional development for NZ midwives mean they have to show evidence of ongoing education (Midwifery Council of New Zealand, 2004). Historically, midwives who have mostly worked as hospital employees have accessed their ongoing education in the form of in-service programs offered by their employer. Nowadays, hospital and self-employed midwives are expected to look further afield for professional development opportunities. The increasing national and international move toward online delivery of undergraduate and postgraduate midwifery education is likely to appeal to midwives in New Zealand, especially those who live some distances from education providers (Avery, Ringdahl, Juve, & Plumbo, 2003). The extra cost of flights and accommodations are all factors that the rural midwife has to carefully consider before she embarks on a postgraduate program of study. Time away from her practice may mean the midwife loses revenue from missing a birth. Online education allows the midwife to stay at home and organize her study around the commitments of her practice.

The Internet lends itself well to certain aspects of undergraduate midwifery education. The growing trend to flexible delivery as a means to attract more students will inevitably result in a proliferation of online undergraduate courses (Camacho Carr & Farley, 2003). Certainly some courses will lend themselves very well to online delivery, such as those that contain core knowledge and critical thinking. Decision making can be facilitated in computer-stimulated scenarios, but there will always be a need for the acquisition and assessment of psychomotor clinical skills to be carried out in a face-to-face setting (Camacho Carr & Farley, 2003). Nevertheless, there is room for creative use of online resources even in the clinical setting. One example is the use of a web-based computerized data collection tool developed by the University of Michigan School of Nursing, as described by Walker and Pohl (2003). Midwifery students record each of their clinical encounters in the electronic log. Lecturers are then able to tailor the students' clinical experience according to their learning needs as revealed in the log.

Health Consumers

The Internet has the potential to provide services that have far-reaching effects for health consumers. Consumers have been quick to recognize the potential for sharing advice, opinions, and personal experience, as well as searching for health information. The Pew Internet and American Life Project (2003) telephone survey of 2,038 adults in America in 2002 found that 85% of women with Internet access had researched health information online, compared to 75% of men. Most health information seekers (73%) felt that the Internet improved information and services they received, and some participants believed their relationships with doctors were affected, although not necessarily for the better.

Pregnancy and childbirth rates highly as a topic for exploration on the Internet (Bernhardt & Felter, 2004). Pregnant women can obtain advice or opinions about any number of birthing issues such as vaginal birth following Caesarean section (http://www.childbirth.org). Parents are using the Internet to share their birth stories with the world (http://

www.thelaboroflove.com/birthstories/index.shtml), and support each other on e-mail discussion lists, bulletin boards, and chat groups (http://www.midwiferytoday.com/forums). Bernhardt and Felter (2004) used focus groups to explore how 20 mothers used the Internet to find information. Most of the women sought information during their pregnancy and continued to use the Internet to diagnose or treat conditions once the baby was born, or obtain advice about child development and parenting. Quality was an issue and the women preferred information that was provided either by health professionals or other parents.

Audio and video capabilities of the Internet add another dimension to the maternity experience for women and the midwife by facilitating synchronous communication. Women even "broadcast" the births of their babies over the Internet (http://www.time.com/time/community/transcripts/chattr061798.html), which may be an alarming prospect for the attending midwife depending on her desire for publicity.

EFFECT OF THE INTERNET ON RELATIONSHIPS BETWEEN CONSUMERS AND MIDWIVES

The potential for consumers to become more knowledgeable than the "all-knowing" health professional because of their access to information on the Internet has caused concern about the effects that has on the relationship between the health professional and "patient" (Jeannot, Scherer, Pittet, Burnard, & Vader, 2003; see also Rice & Katz, chap. 8, this volume). However, in their qualitative study about the role of the Internet in patient–practitioner relationships, Hart, Henwood, and Wyatt (2004) argued that patients have high levels of trust in health practitioners and only a few patients challenged medical authority. Cotten and Gupta (2004) established in personal interviews with 385 patients that, although people use online and offline sources of health information, the majority of participants (80%) sought information from doctors and nurses. Indeed, practitioners' concern about the Internet may be tied up with their own lack of Internet competencies (Hart et al., 2004). Loy (2001) established in his survey of U.K. midwives that 65% of respondents were aware of an increase in the use of the Internet by women in their care, and nearly 50% of midwives had been asked to discuss information presented to them by their clients. The midwives were extremely positive about women using the Internet for finding information, and welcomed any move that would increase the partnership between women and midwives. Having said that, few midwives used the Internet to supply women with information (Loy, 2001).

Barriers to Use of the Internet

The main barriers to use of the Internet appear to be a lack of skills and training as well as time. Sinclair (2001) carried out a survey of 1,082 registered midwives in Northern Ireland, which had a 41% response rate. Only 2% of respondents felt they had a high level of skills for searching Web sites for evidence-based information compared to 65% who rated themselves as having "very low" or no skills. Forty-five percent of respondents had received formal computer training. In the survey carried out by Loy (2001), 24% of respondents cited lack of training a barrier to Internet use, and lack of time was cited by 34% of respondents.

Critiquing Midwifery Information Found on the Internet

Health professionals and consumers may access information that is of poor quality. When reading material in journals or books, there is a good chance that it has undergone some sort of editorial or peer review. However, anyone can publish information on the Internet and for some Web sites, there is no form of quality control. Semere, Karamanoukian, Levitt, Edwards, Murero, et al. (2003) surveyed 150 parents of outpatients at the Pediatric Surgery Clinic in the Children's Hospital of Buffalo. Nearly three quarters of the parents (73%) accessed the Internet for health information. Nearly all the parents (98%) felt the information found was comprehensive and helpful; however 31% of parents visited sites that they did not remember. The authors found it worrying that people would make decisions based on the information they found (52%), yet a high number were unaware of where they obtained the information. The call for evidence-based information that is presented in a manner that is easily accessible, consistent, and reliable is echoed by Spink, Yang, Jansen, Nykanen, Lorence, et al. (2004) who established in their study of medical and health queries to web search engines that many queries related to pregnancy or health of the baby. They analyzed thousands of queries to search engines (www.Excite.com, AlltheWeb.com and www .AskJeeves .com) and found that many people did not fully understand how a web search engine worked, ascribing it human capabilities that went beyond the search engines' abilities. Users become emotional and frustrated with search engines that did not respond to their own personal needs and concerns. Christopher, Hardwick, and MacKensie (2003) analyzed information in Web sites that contained information about miscarriage. They discovered a number of Web sites that did not give even the most basic information. Of 19 Web sites, merely eight sites had the author's name; nine sites mentioned diagnosis of miscarriage by ultrasound scanning, blood or urine testing; only three sites stated all three management options as included in the U.K. Royal College of Obstetrics and Gynaecology evidence-based guidelines.

AIM OF THIS STUDY

The aim of the study carried out in 2002 was to find out about NZ midwives and their use of Internet resources. How did midwives use the Internet and what resources did midwives want to be developed? Did midwives use the Internet solely for searching for information, or did they exploit it more fully for communication and collaboration, as well as practice development and support? Has consumers' use of the Internet had an effect on their practice and how did midwives feel about it? What were the barriers to midwives' use of the Internet?

METHODS

This study was informed by the research carried out by Loy (2001). Permission was obtained from Loy to use his questionnaire as a framework. The questions were revised and reformatted to improve the quality of data received and suit the NZ context. Ethical approval was obtained from the Victoria University of Wellington Ethics Committee. The final questionnaire was pretested by six midwives and two Internet scholars, and consisted of 72 questions, which consisted of 63 structured questions and nine open-ended questions and took between 10 and 15 minutes to complete. The questionnaire was divided into eight sections. Section I asked general questions about use of the Internet, which aimed to gain the respondents' interest in the survey. In Sections II, III, and IV, respondents were asked about use of the Internet at work, home, and institution of study. Section V solicited information about use of the Internet by consumers; Section VI enquired about use of e-mail discussion lists/groups; Section VII elicited information about Internet resources. Demographic data was gathered in the last section of the questionnaire. The survey was posted for 1 month on a Web site that had been developed for that particular purpose. The Web site was made up of three pages, which contained information about the survey. Once completed, questionnaire data was e-mailed to the author in an anonymous, numerical form.

The study was restricted to a convenience sample of registered midwives in New Zealand. Midwives were recruited by using an e-mail "snowballing" technique. The researcher e-mailed all the midwives whose e-mail address was already known, or could be found on the

Internet. The e-mail contained details on the study, how to access the Web site, and invited midwives to complete the web-based survey. The midwives were also asked if they could pass on the survey by e-mail to other colleagues to recruit other participants. Ninety-three midwives were invited to complete the survey via e-mail and to pass on the survey information to colleagues. A total of 54 midwives completed the questionnaire.

RESULTS

Location and Frequency of Internet Use

All but one respondent had access to the Internet at home, and that person used the Internet at work. Out of 51 respondents who answered the question, 30 (58.8%) had access to the Internet at work. However, respondents were most likely to use the Internet "mainly at home" as shown in Table 9.1. Internet usage was high. Out of 51, 46 (85.2%) respondents accessed the Internet at least once a week. Respondents (n = 30, 55.6%) were more likely to describe their use of the Internet as an equal combination of personal, work and study.

Searching for Midwifery Information

The main reason for using the Internet was satisfying personal information needs (54.3%), followed by keeping up to date (37.7%) and satisfying information needs for women in the midwives' care (30.3%). Lack of time (38.9%) and insufficient training (18.5%) were the main barriers to use of the Internet. Thirteen (43.4%) of the 30 respondents who answered had been offered training in use of the Internet at work; seven (43.8%) of 16 respondents had been offered training at the institution where they study. Midwives are beginning to incorporate information found on the Internet into their practice (n = 27 of 33; 81.2%).

TABLE 9.1
Location of Internet Use

Location	Percentage
Mainly at home	77.7%
Mainly at work	11.1
An equal combination of home and university/polytechnic	5.6
An equal combination of work and home	3.7
Missing	1.9
Total (n = 54 respondents)	100%

Respondents were asked to give examples of the information found on the Internet in three open-ended questions. Content analysis was used to categorize the information into four groups: clinical practice ($n = 127$) such as water birth, breastfeeding, and breech birth; professional issues ($n = 45$) including information about jobs abroad and purchasing a water birthing pool; information for women ($n = 4$), for example, pregnancy calendar; teaching and learning ($n = 7$), for instance, trends in education. Respondents ($n = 33$; 61.2%) were most likely to think that the information found on the Internet was on average of good quality. Almost half the respondents felt they were able to say reasonably well whether information found on the Internet was reliable or not ($n = 23$; 42.7%).

Use of the Internet by Consumers

Thirty-eight out of 49 respondents (70.4%) were aware of an increase in use of the Internet by women in their care and talked to them about information they found on the Internet. Respondents felt that consumers accessing information on the Internet had an impact on midwifery practice ($n = 32$; 59.25%) with half of the respondents who answered this question feeling positive about it ($n = 23$; 42.49%). Ten (18.5%) of 48 respondents had procured a client through the Internet. Respondents were asked if they delivered midwifery care via the Internet. Of the 44 (81.48%) who answered, eight (18%) utilized the Internet mostly to give advice (6/8; 75%) and other midwifery care (3/8; 37.5%). Six out of the eight respondents (75%) corresponded with women in their care, and four out of the eight (50%) corresponded with casual acquaintances who approached them because they were known to be midwives.

Internet Resources Available to Midwives

Just over half ($n = 28/54$; 54.9%) the respondents had experience with e-mail lists. Respondents felt that e-mail discussion lists were a good means of tracking information ($n = 21/28$; 75%), an invaluable way of keeping up to date ($n = 14/28$; 50%), and great way of networking ($n = 11/28$; 39.3%). Disadvantages included too many messages being posted or not enough ($n = 7/28$; 25%), discussion had no relevance ($n = 7/28$; 25%), and the list was a lazy way of doing research ($n = 8/28$; 28.6%). Of the respondents who answered ($n = 20/54$), eight (28.57%) expressed that they changed their midwifery practice as a result of e-mail discussion.

The most commonly used resources by midwives in the sample were bibliographic databases ($n = 41$; 75.9%), professional bodies such as NZCOM ($n = 40$; 74%), electronic journals ($n = 39$; 72.2%), midwifery

TABLE 9.2
Desired Resources for the Future

---

2 Responses Each:

• Drug information
• Online mentoring system

---

1 Response Each:

• Access from work
• British Journal of Midwifery
• Develop my Web site to be more comprehensive on breech birth
• Free Cochrane database access
• Hospital midwives can access information from other hospitals in New Zealand
• Interactive clinical scenarios
• Midwifery management of aspects of care network
• Network for rural/remote midwives
• New midwifery developments
• NZCOM newsletters—local and national
• NZ midwifery educator's forum
• Online educational sessions that can be used for portfolio for rural midwives
• Order equipment from New Zealand
• Specific midwifery search engine
• Topic focused with medical/midwifery/sociological/psychological publications
• Up-to-date midwifery textbook

---

resources shop ($n = 37; 68.51\%$), and reports or research papers ($n = 36; 66.7\%$). As well as those Internet resources, respondents felt it would be useful in the future to be able to access resources such as conference and course details ($n = 44; 81.4\%$), newsletters/updates ($n = 41; 75.9\%$) and online tutorials ($n = 41; 75.9\%$). Nearly all the respondents had used on-line databases ($n = 48; 90.6\%$). Respondents were most likely to use Cochrane ($n = 43; 81.2\%$), Medline ($n = 42; 79.25\%$) and CINAHL ($n = 36; 66.6\%$). The majority of respondents found data bases easy to use ($n = 40; 80\%$). Eight (15.1%) out of 53 respondents who answered the question had their own Web site. Respondents were asked in an open-ended question to specify what other resources they would like made available in the future (Table 9.2).

Demographics

The average age of respondents was 40–44 years ($n = 18; 33.3\%$). Thirty-six of 54 respondents were in full-time employment ($n = 36; 66.7\%$). Thirty-three of 54 respondents (61%) were currently enrolled in

TABLE 9.3
Employment

Characteristics	Respondents (Multiple Characteristics Allowed)
Self-employed LMC	24
Midwifery lecturer	16
Hospital midwife	15
Midwifery manager	5
Employed LMC	4
Research midwife	3
Midwifery adviser	1
Expert witness	1
Rural midwife	10
Urban midwife	8
Total (n = 54 respondents)	87

a class, or had undertaken a course of study in the last 3 years. Respondents defined themselves as having multiple midwifery roles and practice in more than one geographical area (Table 9.3).

Limitations

The survey only attracted 54 respondents, probably because of the method of recruiting midwives to the survey. The sample was made up of midwives who used the Internet, but did not include midwives who did not use the Internet. The Internet will become increasingly effective as a tool for research as more midwives become familiar with it. In the meantime, it is recommended that the Internet be included as part of a mixed-methods research approach, for example, used in conjunction with paper questionnaire and/or interview (Dillman, 2000). The major flaw of this study was the initial definition of midwives and their employment. Respondents were able to select more than one role, such as lecturers who also defined themselves as self-employed LMCs. Thus, respondents did not differentiate themselves into a single given group, which together with the small sample size made it impossible to carry out detailed analysis. In future research midwives should be only "allowed" to choose one main category of employment. One would then be able to answer more complex questions about midwifery role and use of the Internet. The small numbers also meant it was impossible to clearly differentiate between how rural midwives used the Internet compared to urban midwives.

DISCUSSION

In the current study, the sample of midwives clearly embraced the Internet, for an equal combination of work, study, and personal reasons. Those midwives were proficient in the use of the Internet with only 10 (18.5%) feeling they had been insufficiently trained. The Internet played an active role in the midwives' practice, for example helping them to keep up to date ($n = 20$; 37.7%) and enabling them to share information with women in their care ($n = 16$; 30.3%). This study suggests that those midwives were keen to use Internet resources such as bibliographic databases and electronic journals.

However, there are areas that require further exploration. Half ($n = 23$; 42.7%) of the respondents were able to critique information found on the Internet reasonably well (Table 9.4). But what about those midwives who could not critique information very well ($n = 7/54$; 13%) or those who were not sure ($n = 13/54$; 24.1%), given that they incorporate information found on the Internet into their practice ($n = 27/33$; 81.8%)? What are the implications for the profession if midwives are acting on inaccurate information found on the Internet, or are analyzing the information inappropriately? Consideration needs to be given to resources/training to help midwives who are not able to assess quality of information found on the Internet.

There was a high level of uptake of Internet resources such as bibliographic databases and professional bodies. Respondents also planned to access a wide range of resources in the future including conference and course details, newsletters/updates, and online tutorials. Nonetheless, there was no demand for more clinical applications of Internet technology such as access to clients' data or remote interactive consultations. This may be because midwives do not see a need for such technology, or because there is no immediate possibility of it being available in New Zealand.

A future survey could investigate the potential for midwives to exploit to a much greater extent the Internet for advertising and marketing of

TABLE 9.4
Ability to Critique Information

Ability to Critique Information	Percentage
Very well	9.2%
Reasonably well	42.7
Not sure	24.1
Not very well	13.0
Missing	11.0
Total ($n = 54$ respondents)	100%

their services, how much knowledge midwives have about these potential functions, and whether they are seen to be desirable resources. Advertising may be seen by midwives as an admission that one's own personal reputation is not adequate to build and maintain a practice, or an emphasis on the business rather than the caring side of practice (Rothchild, 2002). Nevertheless, as the Internet becomes more ubiquitous in New Zealand (Statistics New Zealand, 2005), parents may use it to critically evaluate the midwife's services, qualifications and outcomes before engaging her as their midwife (Rothchild, 2002).

Most respondents (38/49; 70.4%) were aware of an increase in use of Internet by their patients, and had talked to them about information found on the Internet. This result shows that in this sample online information is affecting midwives' practice, and potentially their clients as well. Although there were respondents who were positive about the impact ($n = 23$; 44.7%), there were also midwives who were unsure or concerned about the impact on midwifery practice ($n = 24$; 41.3%). This reflects the concerns of other health professionals (Jeannot et al., 2003) and further research is required to identify exactly what midwives' concerns may be. A small number of respondents (8/44; 18%) used the Internet to deliver midwifery care including advice ($n = 6/8$; 75%). However, the potential for midwives to be sued for these activities are as high as with other health professionals (Liederman & Morefield, 2003). Guidelines for New Zealand doctors' use of the Internet have been produced by the Medical Council of NZ (2001). They acknowledge that the Internet and e-mail play an increasing part in medical practice but emphasize the risks of providing medical advice by electronic means. Although the number of midwives using the Internet to deliver midwifery care is small, nonetheless this study shows there is a need for similar guidelines to be issued for NZ midwives.

CONCLUSION

There is no doubt that the Internet is an innovation whose influence is growing steadily in our everyday lives, and that it has a role to play in the provision of evidence-based practice in midwifery care. This study of a small sample of NZ midwives shows that they regularly use the Internet for searching information, which they utilize in their professional practice and pass on to midwifery clients. There are a number of midwives who are unable to adequately assess what information is reliable, which suggests that resources and training should be provided to aid these midwives, especially as they utilize that information in practice. Midwives were very interested in resources such as bibliographic databases, online journals, and tutorials to be made available on the Internet. Midwives have noted an increase in the use of the Internet by the women they care for. As the Internet grows in popularity, midwives need to keep up with the latest advances in Internet technology in order to meet consumer and professional demands. At the same time, guidelines for use of the Internet in practice need to be developed so that midwives can be confident that the quality of the care they give women is not compromised.

REFERENCES

Albisser, A., Albisser, J., & Parker, L. (2003). Patient confidentiality, data security, and provider liabilities in diabetes management. *Diabetes Technology and Therapeutics*, 5(4), 631–640.

Anderson, J., Rainey, M., & Eysenbach, G. (2003). The impact of cyberhealthcare on the physician–patient relationship. *Journal of Medical Systems*, 27(1), 67–84.

Avery, M., Ringdahl, D., Juve, C., & Plumbo, P. (2003). The transition to web-based education: Enhancing access to graduate education for women's health providers. *Journal of Midwifery and Women's Health*, 48(6), 418–425.

Beck, C. (2004). Post-traumatic stress disorder due to childbirth. *Nursing Research*, 53(4), 216–224.

Bernhardt, J., & Felter, E. (2004). Online paediatric information seeking among mothers of young children: Results from a qualitative study using focus groups. *Journal of Medical Internet Research*, 6(1), e7. Retrieved from http://www.jmir.org/2004/1/e7/

Brooks, F., Rospopa, C., & Scott, P. (2004). Midwifery on the net: New communication technology. *British Journal of Midwifery*, 12(2), 107–110.

Calvert, I. (1998). *Birth in focus*. Palmerston North, New Zealand: Dunmore Press.

Camacho Carr, K., & Farley, C. (2003). Redesigning courses for the World Wide Web. *Journal of Midwifery and Women's Health*, 48(6), 407–417.

Christopher, J., Hardwick, R., & MacKensie, F. (2003). Information contained in miscarriage-related websites and the predictive value of website scoring systems. *European Journal of Obstetrics & Gynaecology and Reproductive Biology*, 106, 60–63.

Coddington, D. (2000). Dot.com.docs. *North and South*, 173, 62–67.

Cotten, S., & Gupta, S. (2004). Characteristics of online and offline health information seekers and factors that discriminate between them. *Social Science and Medicine*, 59(9), 1795–1806.

Di Lieto, A., Catalano, D., Pontillo, M., Pollio, F., De Falco, M., Lannotti, F., & Schiraldi, P. (2001). Telecardiotocography in prenatal telemedicine. *Journal of Telemedicine and Telecare*, 7, 119–120.

Dillman, D. (2000). *Mail and Internet surveys: The tailored design method*. New York: Wiley.

Estabrooks, C., O'Leary, K., Ricker, K., & Humphrey, C. (2003). The Internet and access to evidence: How are nurses positioned? *Journal of Advanced Nursing*, 42(1), 73–81.

Freed, D. (2003). Patient–physician e-mail: Passions or fashion? *The Health Care Manager*, 22(3), 265–274.

Gray, J., Safran, C., Davis, R., Pomilio-Weitzner, G., Stewart, J., Zaccagnini, L., & Pursley, D. (2000). Baby CareLink: Using the Internet and telemedicine to improve care for high-risk infants. *Pediatrics*, 106(6), 1318–1324.

Guilliland, K., & Pairman, S. (1995). *The midwifery partnership: A model for practice.* Wellington, NZ: Department of Nursing and Midwifery, Victoria University of Wellington, New Zealand.

Harding, C. (2000). Making choices in childbirth. In L. Page (Ed.), *The new midwifery: Science and sensitivity in practice* (pp. 71–85). Edinburgh, Scotland: Churchill Livingstone.

Hart, A., Henwood, F., & Wyatt, S. (2004). The role of the Internet in patient–practitioner relationships: Findings from a qualitative research study. *Journal of Medical Internet Research*, 6(3), e36. Retrieved from http://www.jmir.org/2004/3/e36/

Hendry, C. (2003). The organisation of maternity services in rural localities within the South Island of New Zealand. *New Zealand College of Midwives' Journal*, 28, 20–24.

Jeannot, J., Scherer, F., Pittet, V., Burnard, B., & Vader, J. (2003). Use of the World Wide e12. Retrieved Web to implement clinical practice guidelines. *Journal of Medical Internet Research*, 5(2), from http://www.jmir.org/2003/2/e12/

Kerse, N., Arroll, B., Lloyd, T., Young, J., & Ward, J. (2001). Evidence databases, the Internet and general practitioners: The New Zealand story. *New Zealand Medical Journal*, 114(1127), 89–91.

Kinniburgh, J. (2001). Using the Internet to support evidence-based practice. *Journal of Community Nursing*, 15(8), 4, 6, 8.

Liederman, E., & Morefield, C. (2003). Web messaging: A new tool for patient–physician communication. *Journal of the American Medical Information Association*, 10, 260–270.

Loy, J. (2001). Midwives and their use of the Internet. *MIDIRS Midwifery Digest*, 11(1), 25–27.

Medical Council of New Zealand. (2001). *Guidelines for doctors using the Internet*. Retrieved November, 6, 2004, from http://www.mcnz.org.nz/portals/1/Guidance/Internet%20guidelines-revised2001.pdf

Midwifery Council of New Zealand. (2004). *Recertification programme: Competence-based practising for midwives. A discussion document*. Retrieved December 17, 2004, from http://www.midwiferycouncil.org.nz

Murray, E., Lo, B., Pollack, L., Donelan, K., Catania, J., Lee, K., Zapart, K., & Turner, R. (2003). The impact of health information on the Internet on health care and the physician–patient relationship: National U.S. survey among 1,050 U.S. physicians. *Journal of Medical Internet Research*, 5(3), e17. Retrieved from http://www.jmir.org/2003/3/e17/

New Zealand Ministry of Health. (2003). *Report on maternity: Maternal and newborn information 2002* (Vol. 2004): New Zealand: Author.

Patt, M., Houstan, T., Jenckes, M., Sands, D., & Ford, D. (2003). Doctors who are using e-mail with their patients: A qualitative exploration. *Journal of Medical Internet Research*, 5(2), e9. Retrieved from http://www.jmir.org/2003/2/e9/

Patterson, J. (2001). Rural midwifery: Challenges of the last decade and where to from here? *Midwifery News*, 20, 1–6.

Petersson, K., Forsgreen, M., Sjodin, M., Kublickas, M., & Westgren, M. (2003). Evaluation of an Internet-based database on infectious disorders during pregnancy: INFPREG. *Acta Obstetricia et Gynecologica Scandinavica*, 82, 116–119.

The Pew Internet and American Life Project. (2003). *Internet health resources: Health searches and email have become more commonplace, but there is room for improvement in searches and overall Internet access*. Retrieved December 17, 2004, from http://www.pewinternet.org/pdfs/PIP_Health_Report_July_2003.pdf

Reynolds, S. (2003). Making sense of information technology. *British Journal of Midwifery*, 11(3), 178–183.

Rothchild, M. (2002). Marketing your practice on the Internet. *Otolaryngologic Clinics of North America*, 25, 1149–1161.

Semere, W., Karamanoukian, H., Levitt, M., Edwards, T., Murero, M., D'Ancona, G., Donias, H., & Glick, P. (2003). A pediatric surgery study: Parent usage of the Internet for medical information. *Journal of Pediatric Surgery*, 38(4), 560–564.

Sinclair, M. (1997). Midwives, midwifery and the Internet. *Modern Midwife*, 7(9), 11–14.

Sinclair, M. (2001). Information technology skills of midwives in Northern Ireland. *The Practising Midwife*, 4(1), 23–28.

Spink, A., Yang, Y., Jansen, J., Nykanen, P., Lorence, D., Ozmutlu, S., & Ozmutlu, H. C. (2004). A study of medical and health queries to web search engines. *Health Information and Libraries Journal*, 21, 44–51.

Statistics New Zealand. (2005). *Household access to the Internet*. Retrieved February 12, 2005, from http://www.stats.govt.nz/products-and-services/Articles/hhold-access .inet.htm

Stensland Kurokawa, J. (1996). Rural midwifery and electronic communications. *Journal of Nurse-Midwifery*, 41(3), 263–264.

Walker, D., & Pohl, J. (2003). Web-based data collection in midwifery clinical education. *Journal of Midwifery and Women's Health*, 48(6), 437–443.

Westbrook, J., Gosling, A., & Cohera, E. (2004). Do clinicians use online evidence to support patient care? *Journal of American Medical Informatics Association*, 11(2), 113–120.

Chapter 10

The Mysterious Maze of the World Wide Web: How Can We Guide Consumers to High-Quality Health Information on the Internet?

Joshua J. Seidman
Center for Information Therapy, Washington, DC

Consumers are turning to the Internet in growing numbers for answers to their health care questions. As of 2002, 73 million Americans reported that they went to the web for health information (Pew Internet and American Life Project, 2002). At the same time, a number of studies have suggested that much of the health information available on the Internet is, to varying degrees, incomplete, inaccurate, oversimplified, and/or misleading (Craigie, Loader, Burrows, & Muncer, 2002; Culver, Uerr, & Frurnkin, 1997; Hatfield, May, & Markoff, 1999; Impicciatore, Pandolfini, Casella, & Bonati, 1997; Kunst, Groot, Latthe, Latthe, & Khan, 2002; Meric, Bernstam, & Mirza, 2002; Pandolfini & Bonati, 2002; Purcell, Wilson, & Delamothe, 2002; Rice, 2001; Risk, 2002; Thompson, 1999; Wilson, 2002; Zeng, Kogan, Plovnick, Crowell, Lacroix, & Greenes, 2004).

For example, a RAND study conducted in the fall of 2000 that assessed the quality of health care Web sites found that they were generally incomplete (Berland, Elliott, Morales, Algazy, Kravitz, et al., 2001). Of 10 English-language sites for each condition, only 36% had more than minimal coverage and complete accuracy for childhood asthma; 37% for obesity; 44% for depression; and 63% for breast cancer. Without an adequate medical background, consumers who rely on the web for health information may seize on misleading, incorrect, or oversimplified information that can be potentially harmful to them.

Although some organizations have begun to develop tools that would help consumers navigate the health care information on the web, there is not yet any widely accepted method for evaluating the quality of health and medical information on the Internet. Moreover, the existing tools generally do not attempt to look directly at the information that is provided on health care conditions and assess its accuracy and comprehensiveness. Instead, they evaluate the quality of health care Web sites through proxy measures of information quality that include how the Web site was developed and is operated (i.e., "structural" measures such as whether the Web site discloses the names of its authors, explains the process used to develop its content, and appropriately dates its content) and characteristics of the site's sponsor (e.g., whether it is sponsored by a for-profit company). However, no research has addressed whether these proxy measures actually provide useful guidance to consumers about the accuracy and comprehensiveness of the information they are gathering from the web.

In an effort to investigate further the quality of health care information on the web, as well as to evaluate the existing tools available to help consumers navigate health care information on the web, this study analyses 90 diabetes Web sites using a new evaluation tool. There was little connection between the quality of information on diabetes Web sites and the structural indicators that consumers are advised to use to select reliable health information Web sites. In light of these findings, this chapter suggests a series of strategies and policy recommendations for improving Web site accreditation efforts and providing more effective guidance to consumers.

CONSUMER STRATEGIES FOR NAVIGATING HEALTH INFORMATION ON THE WEB

In general, consumers show relatively little skepticism about the quality of health information on the web. The Pew Internet & American Life Project (2002) found that 72% of the 73 million Americans who have gone online for health information say you can believe all or most of the health information online. At the same time, consumers will occasionally reject the information provided on the web—close to 75% in the Pew study had done so at some point. When they do, it is for the following reasons:

- The site is "too commercial and seemed more concerned with selling products than providing accurate information" (47%).
- They couldn't determine the source of the information (42%).
- They couldn't determine when the site was last updated (37%).

The popular press reinforces the notion that sponsorship characteristics can help consumers find reliable Web sites. Despite a lack of evidence supporting this theory, advice articles in magazines such as *Money* (Lee, 2000) generally tell laypeople that they should look for sites that have no commercial interests, are run by government agencies, and/or are affiliated with respected academic institutions.

One of the country's independent health care organization accrediting bodies, known as URAC (formerly the Utilization Review Accreditation Commission), launched the first attempt at third-party Web site accreditation in 2001. URAC's voluntary, consumer Web site accreditation system relies on a set of ethical and quality standards that address several issues including privacy protection, security, and the process used for developing content. URAC derived its standards primarily from the principles developed by Health Internet Ethics (Hi-Ethics), another not-for-profit organization created in the late 1990s primarily by health content vendors to establish standards for ethical provision of Internet health information to consumers. As of January 2005, URAC's Web site listed 49 sites as accredited or "in process," although only 26 of these had accreditation dates that were current (i.e., the accreditation was "valid through" a date that had already past).

URAC's effort represents an important step forward, but they also have substantial limitations in guiding consumers to credible health information. URAC's quality standards are primarily designed to assess structural issues in Web site design and management and do not assess the specific quality or credibility of the information provided on the Web site. URAC accreditation is analogous in some ways to licensure of physicians; it is an important minimum threshold, but not all licensed physicians provide high-quality care.

PROPOSED MODEL FOR EVALUATING
THE QUALITY OF INTERNET HEALTH INFORMATION

Structural and Performance Criteria

In order for a tool to be systematic and objective, it needs to rely on elements that are valid and measurable. A set of criteria (presented in Table 10.1) to include in a health information Web site quality evaluation tool was developed through the lens of a quality-of-care conceptual framework, in which measurement can be thought of in the context of Donabedian's (1980) structure–process–outcomes measure paradigm and other efforts in building performance measures (Seidman, Steinwachs, & Rubin, 2003a). Both existing research available and tools that have been

TABLE 10.1

Proposed Measurable Criteria for Credibility Score for Diabetes Sites

Category	Measurement	How Measured
I. Explanation of methods	a. Content generation explanation b. Identification and disclosure	a. Site has explanation of process for generating its health content b. Author(s) listed and affiliations, credentials, and contact information provided
II. Validity of methods	a. Referenced material b. Peer review	a. Assertions supported by referenced material b. Material on site has gone through peer review
III. Currency of information	a. Updating process b. Content dating c. Timely update	a. Site has explanation of process for updating its health content b. Each web page indicates date of last update c. Page updated within last 6 months
IV. Comprehensiveness of information	a. Screening b. Glycemia tests c. Nutrition d. Exercise e. Acute episodes f. Secondary diabetes g. Foot care h. Dyslipidemia i. Smoking cessation j. Nephropathy k. Retinopathy l. Immunization m. Insulin administration n. Oral medications o. Glucose monitoring p. Care of children q. Gestational diabetes r. DCCT implications s. UKPDS implications t. Insulin/glucose explanation	Each of these aspects (primarily drawn from the clinical practice recommendations of the American Diabetes Association) is addressed and discussed on the Web site

u. Prevention
v. Psychological aspects
w. Neuropathy
x. Obesity

V. Accuracy of information

a. Type 1 versus Type 2
b. Secondary causes
c. Diagnostic tests
d. HbA1c test
e. Albumin tests
f. Cholesterol tests
g. Warning signs
h. Hypoglycemia prevention
i. Oral medications
j. Rezulin

a. Explain Type 1 (lack of insulin) and Type 2 (insulin doesn't work effectively)
b. Explain main secondary causes: drugs (pentamidine, corticosteroids, thiazides, niacin), pancreatic disease (chronic pancreatitis, hemochromatosis, cystic fibrosis, pancreatic surgery), endocrine disorders (Cushing's disease, acromegaly, pheochromocytoma, thyrotoxicosis), genetic syndromes (lipodystrophies, myotonic dystrophy, ataxia telangiectasia), insulin-receptor syndromes
c. Explain diabetic threshold for fasting blood glucose test (> 125 mg/dl) and oral glucose tolerance test (> 199 mg/dl)
d. Explain risk associated with HbA1c levels > 8%: impact on risk of CAD, kidney disease, and retinopathy.
e. Explain macroalbuminuria test (goal: negative) and microalbuminuria test (goal: < 30 mg/g creatinine)
f. Explain HDL/LDL difference and LDL target level (< 100 mg/dl)
g. Explain warning signs of acute diabetic episodes (fainting, seizures, state of serious confusion)
h. Explain what brings on hypoglycemia (not eating enough/on time, exercise without food/insulin adjustment, weight loss, too much insulin/oral medications)
i. Explanation of all five classes of oral medications (sulfonylureas, meglitinides, biguanides, glitazones, alpha glucosidase inhibitors)
j. Explain liver problems associated with the glitazone Rezulin and why pulled back from market

Note. Categories I, II, and III comprise the structural criteria, and Categories IV and V comprise the criteria for performance measures of information quality.

developed by health services researchers, physicians, Web experts and medical librarians were used to identify candidate criteria (for an extensive analysis of general health Web site features, see Rice, Peterson, & Christine, 2001).

Although the set of criteria does not represent the entire universe of important aspects of health information, it does provide a reasonably good cross-section of structural criteria and performance measures that can be assessed objectively. *Structural measures* address the underlying systems and infrastructure, whereas *performance measures* assess the extent to which health care providers have done the right things. Structural characteristics include those in Categories I, II, and III of Table 10.1: explanation of methods, validity of methods, and currency of information. Performance measures of information quality include comprehensiveness (IV) and accuracy (V) in that they address how well the Web site performed in creating accurate and comprehensive (or high-quality) information against a set of criteria that were created based upon review of evidence-based practice guidelines and expert opinion.

There are undoubtedly other aspects of health information quality and communication that affect quality of care. Certainly, user needs and expectations should be considered when evaluating information quality. Moreover, high-quality information by itself will not produce high-quality care, but it generally is a prerequisite for it. In order to create valid and widely applicable measures of comprehensiveness and accuracy, such an evaluation tool would use a generic, "gold" standard; but none exists for overall health information. Therefore, the model focuses on one specific disease—diabetes—for which a reasonable standard exists, the American Diabetes Association's (ADA's) Clinical Practice Recommendations (2000). Diabetes was used because the evidence base is stronger than in many other clinical areas due to specific, exceptional clinical trials (e.g., the Diabetes Control and Complications Trial in 1993; the United Kingdom Prospective Diabetes Study in 1998; and The Diabetes Prevention Program in 1999). As a result, it was possible to use evidence-based guidelines and performance measurement experts to develop a reasonable comprehensive standard for the content and scope of information on diabetes that should be included in a Web site on the disease (Seidman et al., 2003b).

Development of the Measures

The Diabetes Quality Improvement Project (DQIP) performance measurement experience provides a useful model for developing and applying diabetes Web site information quality performance measures, particularly with respect to content validity, a combination of face validity (or expert validity) and sampling validity. Initially 20 criteria to evaluate comprehensiveness and 10 criteria that relate to accuracy were extracted from the ADA's largely evidence-based practice guidelines. The comprehensiveness criteria reflected the breadth of content covered in the ADA guidelines, an important aspect of sampling validity. The ADA determined the coverage of topics based on their expert panels' assessment of the clinical evidence. These 30 measures then were included with the seven structural characteristics (content generation explanation, identification and disclosure, referenced material, peer review, updating process, content dating, and timely update; see Table 10.1) that were extracted from the existing tools and suggested evaluation criteria in the literature. Each item in the tool was operationalized to explicitly indicate what constituted a positive score.

The next stage of measure development involved a review of measures by relevant experts for the purpose of strengthening the instrument's face validity. Feedback was obtained from three experts in diabetes performance measurement, all of whom served on the DQIP technical expert panel (Barbara Fleming, MD, PhD; Sheldon Greenfield, MD; and Richard Kahn, PhD). Comments focused primarily on the comprehensiveness and accuracy sections, and can be grouped into two categories. First, the experts believed that the set of comprehensiveness criteria was inadequate if it was to ensure that all major areas of diabetes care were addressed. Specifically, they suggested inclusion of four additional criteria in the comprehensiveness set (prevention, psychological aspects, neuropathy, and obesity), further strengthening the content validity of the tool, which now included 34 items. The experts were satisfied that the set of accuracy items were representative of the broader comprehensiveness set.

Second, one of the experts raised concerns about the feasibility of measuring accuracy based upon the measures' proposed definitions. That concern was addressed in three ways. First, the technical definitions for the accuracy measures were revised and clarified. Second, a reviewer training session was added to improve the likelihood that the tool would be used according to objective criteria. Finally, actual reliability assessment testing of the proposed measures was conducted (as described later), just as it had been done prior to the approval of DQIP's performance measures.

In the reviewer training session, each measure and technical definition was explained to an external reviewer, a physician and master's degree candidate at the Johns Hopkins School of Public Health. A small sample of diabetes sites was assessed with the evaluation tool to demonstrate its application. Those initial reviews raised seven specific questions, four of which related to accuracy criteria. These items were clarified. Then Table 10.2 was provided to the reviewer during their respective independent re-

TABLE 10.2
Issues Identified in Initial Sample
of Diabetes Sites During Reviewer Training

Issue	What to Do About It
Many sites merely aggregate miscellaneous information	Can still judge site by overall performance
Extent to which sites cover both childhood and adult diabetes	Sites specifically stating their focus on Type 1 diabetes are excluded; all others are included
Some structural criteria may be hard to assess, partially because some pages document structural issues well and other pages within the site may not	Judge based on whether the anchor site (main home page) documents structural characteristics, etc.
Accuracy/Secondary Causes (V.b.) measure: Some sites may address some, but not all, of the causes	Score positive if they include at least four of the five causes
Accuracy/Albumin Tests (V.e.) measure: Some sites may use "proteinuria" instead of "macroalbuminuria"	Either "proteinuria" or "macroalbuminuria" is fine
Accuracy/Hypoglycemia (V.h.) measure: Some sites may address some, but not all, of the prevention methods	Score positive if they include at least three of the four prevention methods
Accuracy/Oral Medications (V.i.) measure: Some sites may refer to acarbose rather than the broader drug class name of alpha glucosidase inhibitors	Score positive if either term is used

views. Each item in the evaluation tool had a specific definition, and the scoring was binary (yes or no). This tool is designed to be applied by those with some public health background, but not necessarily with clinical experience; future assessment of the tool should examine the minimum skills required for reviewers.

Sampling Strategy

To identify the sample of Web sites, a specific search term ("diabetes") was entered into the Direct Hit search engine (http://www.directhit.com/; DirectHit is now subsumed by Teoma, but DirectHit.com is still functional), which claims that it tracks the most "popular" sites by search term. Any sites coming from a duplicate parent were eliminated, as they were covered in the review of the parent site (e.g., "www.diabetes.com" would include any pages that include "www.diabetes.com/xxx"). We also developed a standardized set of eligibility criteria. Sites were excluded for four reasons. First, sites addressing only Type 1 diabetes or "juvenile diabetes" were excluded because some of the comprehensiveness criteria would not apply to Type 1. Second, a site in which there was a clear explanation that it was not designed for consumers would not be appropriate for an evaluation of consumer health Web sites. Third, sites that only included "news" and were not designed to offer general diabetes content were not evaluated. Finally, sites were excluded if the Web site address led to a "dead" link.

Analysis Method

The analyses used Spearman rank correlations to measure the strength of association between structural variables (the seven criteria from I, II, and III of Table 10.1) and Web site quality as judged by comprehensiveness and accuracy (the 34 criteria from IV and V of Table 10.1). Two-sample t tests assessed the relationship between sponsorship characteristics and the accuracy and comprehensiveness of health information. Sponsorship categories were: for-profit versus not-for-profit, government versus private, academic versus nonacademic, and those that accept advertising versus those that do not. Finally, these sponsorship categories were jointly included in a multiple linear regression to assess unique influence of sponsorship on the quality of health information Web sites.

Reliability of the Tool

Perhaps the most important assessment of the tool itself involved an assessment of *instrument reliability*, the extent to which the research instrument produces reproducible results. One way to test instrument reliability in this instance is an interobserver test. Therefore, having trained another reviewer to use the tool, the author and the reviewer evaluated a sample of the same 30 Web sites using the 34 accuracy and comprehensiveness items.

The kappa statistic is the most common approach to measuring *interrater reliability* to assess how much agreement existed between reviewers relative to expected agreement by chance on each criterion. However, statisticians have identified multiple problems with kappa in these types of circumstances. Feinstein and Cicchetti (1990) argued that two paradoxes affect the meaningfulness and appropriateness of kappa. Like epidemiological measures of positive and negative predictive value, the kappa value is influenced substantially by "prevalence" so that rare events are likely to have low kappas even when agreement is high. In addition, a lack of balance in the kappa 2×2 table also produces idiosyncrasies in the reporting of reliability using kappa. Finally, because the reliability of the overall index—rather than the individual items—is of central concern here, a better measure of a continuous variable makes sense as well. Therefore, the most useful measure of reliability is Lin's (1989) concordance correlation coefficient, which attempts to measure how close the two raters' judgments fall along a 45-degree line from the origin (or a slope of exactly 1.00). For comparison, results from a similar measure of reliability, Bland and Altman's (1986) limits of agreement, and Pearson's r, are also provided.

Lin's concordance correlation coefficient produced a rho of .76 with a standard error of .08. The Pearson's r was similar, at .77. Bland and Altman's (1986) 95% limits of agreement were −.197 to .232, with a difference average of .017 and a standard deviation of .109. This set of values suggests moderate to high agreement between raters on the performance index.

THE QUALITY OF DIABETES INFORMATION ON THE WEB

Structural Criteria and Performance/Web Site Quality

The tool included seven structural criteria; structure was measured by the percent of the seven criteria each Web site demonstrated. For the seven structural criteria, scores ranged from 0% to 100%, with a mean of 31% and a median of 29%.

The performance of diabetes information on the Internet was varied, with a fairly normal distribution. The tool included 34 accuracy and comprehensiveness criteria; the quality was measured by the percentage of times a given site provided appropriate information according to each of the criteria. Quality scores ranged from 14% to 97% among the sample of 90 Web sites evaluated, with a median of 55% and a mean of 56%; one quarter of sites were below 41%, and one quarter were above 70%.

In other words, on a quarter of the Web sites that have information on diabetes, a consumer would get inaccurate or incomplete information on 60% of the criteria. For example, a consumer might have gone to one Web site sponsored by an academic institution that did not provide accurate information about the warning signs of an acute diabetic episode.

Given the potentially dangerous consequences of such poor information and the reasonably high chance of getting it, there's great benefit in determining the characteristics associated with high-quality Web sites. Such proxies for information quality could provide a valuable and simple strategy for steering consumers to credible information.

What Do Structural Measures Tell You About Web Site Quality?

The structural measures, similar to those developed by URAC, do offer some limited indication of diabetes Web site accuracy and comprehensiveness. There was a statistically significant but modest correlation between the sum of the performance measure and the sum of the structural measure. The Spearman rank correlation coefficient was .42 for the combined performance measure (.45 for comprehensiveness and .28 for accuracy, separately, all statistically significant at $p < .01$). Although there seems to be some small utility in considering structural measures of Web sites when assessing the quality of information that they provide, these measures alone are not sufficient to consistently guide consumers to high-quality Web sites.

What Do Sponsorship Characteristics Tell You About Web Site Quality?

Contrary to the advice often proffered by the popular press, sponsorship characteristics are a poor predictor of Web site quality in terms of the accuracy and comprehensiveness of health information. Pairwise comparisons using two-sample t tests revealed no statistically significant differences in terms of the impact of different sponsorship characteristics on Web site quality. Not-for-profit sites (55 of the 90 sites), government-sponsored sites (12) and—somewhat surprisingly—nonacademic sites (78) and sites that accept advertising (32) performed slightly better than those that did not accept advertising (58), although none of these differences was statistically significant (see Table 10.3).

What Makes Web Site Information High Quality?

The limited relationship between proxy measures of quality (first, structural, and second, sponsorship) and the accuracy and comprehensiveness of diabetes information on the Internet suggests there is a compelling need to develop other methods for guiding consumers. This research demonstrates that one cannot simply use proxy measures or follow the advice common in the popular press to "just look for sites with certain characteristics."

Qualitative Analysis of Performance Factors

The study also included a qualitative review of the findings to see if there was anything else that easily and readily explained variation in the quality of diabetes Web sites. Unfortunately, this review suggested that there

TABLE 10.3
t Tests to Evaluate the Impact of Four Sponsorship Categories—
Profit Status, Private/Government Sponsorship, Advertising,
and Academic Affiliation—on Web Site Quality

Sponsorship Category	Overall	Outcome Composite	Comprehensiveness	Accuracy
For-profit	47%	53%	56%	43%
Not-for-profit	53%	57%	61%	45%
Significance of difference	n.s.	n.s.	n.s.	n.s.
Private	50%	55%	59%	43%
Government	56%	58%	61%	53%
Significance of difference	n.s.	n.s.	n.s.	n.s.
Advertising	52%	57%	59%	47%
No Advertising	50%	55%	60%	43%
Significance of difference	n.s.	n.s.	n.s.	n.s.
Academic	48%	50%	53%	37%
Nonacademic	51%	56%	60%	46%
Significance of difference	n.s.	n.s.	n.s.	n.s.

are no ready alternatives to the proxy measures currently in use. Three of the top four performing sites provided information exclusively on diabetes, but the highest-quality site and seven of the top 10 sites provided information on a broader array of health conditions.

The qualitative analysis suggested that some of the high-quality sites performed well because they simply took a more serious approach than others in developing information that would be helpful to consumers. For example, one site trains all of its medical writers in evidence-based medicine methodologies, uses trained medical librarians to conduct literature searches, has generalist physicians involved with the structuring of content, and has specialist physicians review all of the content when it is originally prepared as well as when it is updated. However, it would be difficult to objectively measure and verify whether a site uses these kinds of processes when developing its content.

POLICY IMPLICATIONS

This research indicates that the likelihood that consumers will find accurate and comprehensive diabetes content varies dramatically depending on what Web sites they view. It also suggests that it may be necessary to evaluate the content provided on each individual health Web site if we want to provide meaningful guidance to consumers about where they can obtain accurate and comprehensive information.

An Alternative Model

Although existing independent review bodies, such as URAC, provide useful information about some of the key proxy measures that might help lead people to higher quality Web sites, our research suggests that structural measures do not correlate highly with performance in the realm of health information quality. Rather than completely replacing existing Web site accreditation efforts, the URAC structural measures should be supplemented by evaluations of information accuracy and comprehensiveness using tools such as the one developed for diabetes Web sites. Performance measures aimed at evaluating condition-specific content would be complemented by information that addresses a Web site's adherence to generic but important principles such as privacy concerns, ethics, and other structural characteristics (for a discussion of such approaches, see Wilson, 2002).

If URAC moves in the direction of adding a review of information content, one of the major challenges will be to develop a practical and feasible strategy for extending the reach of a content-based tool that only offers information about one condition (diabetes) to a much broader array of health conditions. What mechanisms might exist to create comparable tools for a breadth of conditions? One could convene interested parties to train them in the process of developing a content-based tool and then have individual organizations dedicated to specific health conditions take responsibility for development and maintenance of a tool for their area. For example, the American Heart Association and American College of Cardiology might take responsibility for accreditation of Web sites with information about heart disease. Alternatively, the federal government might be able to play a key role; for example, the National Heart, Lung, and Blood Institute could oversee cardiovascular content. Given the enormous array of health conditions for which information is available on the web, it would be important to establish priorities. Content-based accreditation efforts might begin with the conditions associated with the Centers for Disease Control and Prevention's list of most common reasons for mortality or the Institute of Medicine's recently published list of the 15 top priority health care areas for national quality improvement (Adams & Corrigan, 2003).

In many ways, the recommendation that it may be beneficial to add a review of actual content to Web site accreditation efforts is not surprising given the experience of other initiatives aimed at helping consumers assess the quality of health plans. For example, efforts to evaluate the quality of care provided by health plans undertaken by organizations such as the National Committee for Quality Assurance (NCQA)—an independent not-for-profit organization that has been providing information about the quality of health plans since 1990—often began considering only structural measures. However, in 1999, NCQA began to base 25% of a health plan's overall accreditation score on a set of clinical performance measures (known as HEDIS, the Health Plan Employer Data and Information Set) and member satisfaction measures (based on the consumer survey CAHPS, the national Consumer Assessment of Health Plans Study). Applying the same principles to Web site accreditation, performance measurement could begin primarily with a system similar to the diabetes tool presented here, but could ultimately incorporate a CAHPS corollary by adding a user satisfaction survey component that would assess user perceptions of Web sites' usefulness, understandability, and other important issues.

Would It Make a Difference?

Given that such an approach will involve considerable effort, it is worth exploring the question: Would comparative Web site performance measurement make a difference in terms of improving the quality of Internet health information and, would external evaluation and assessment lead to more informed use by searchers and thus improved health care? If one looks to the quality-of-care measurement experience, there is some reason to think that report cards and publishing of comparative performance data do have an impact, although it may arise in a different way than might be expected. Whereas some had hoped that consumers and purchasers would use comparative performance data to select providers and health plans or that clinicians would use that data to make referrals, most evidence thus far suggests that has only occurred in limited ways (Schneider & Epstein, 1996).

What comparative performance measurement and its public reporting have done, however, is to stimulate behavior change on the part of the organizations being profiled. This has happened at both the provider level, such as with the reporting of bypass surgery rates in New York state (Hannan, Kilburn, Racz, Shields, & Chassin, 1994), and at the health plan level, with reporting of HEDIS data, as described in the NCQA State of Managed Care Quality Report (2004). Given the corollaries in the development of performance measurement systems, public reporting of Web site information quality could have a similar impact.

Approaches to Quality Oversight

Creating a performance measurement-based system of consumer health Web site evaluation leaves many options available for how that information can be used. In a regulatory approach, Web sites would have to meet certain levels of accuracy and comprehensiveness in order to be allowed to deliver medical information to consumers. Some might argue that such limitations constitute an infringement on free speech in that the Internet is simply one vehicle for offering viewpoints and opinions that are constitutionally protected in the United States. An opposing perspective could equate delivery of health information over the Internet to the delivery of that same information interpersonally during a clinical encounter. That is, a clinician requires state licensure to be able to deliver certain types of information to patients and can be sued for malpractice for delivering inaccurate health information to a patient. Some would argue that some Web sites purport to communicate comparable information without bearing the same responsibility.

In truth, such strict regulation of health Internet content seems unlikely and probably unconstitutional, but the findings from this research demonstrate that an objective mechanism of oversight is needed; several options for how that might be conducted are offered here. Such oversight could emanate from the private sector or some public–private partnership. Private and public sector entities may reimburse for information dissemination at some point in the future, in which case they would be able to mandate quality assurance for content delivered. Under such a system, either the government could fill that role itself or could deem existing or new private sector organizations appropriate for measuring and accrediting Web sites. It is true, however, that these approaches raise questions of feasibility, as Web sites can change overnight, and it's very laborious to code each and every site. For example, Risk (2002) argued that none of the current procedures (as summarized by Wilson, 2002) work because (a) they create burdens on providers and users, especially to maintain the programs, (b) there is inadequate provision of user education programs, (c) cost of developing and maintaining quality assessment programs is significant, and (d) they are not useful for the developing world. He suggests that quality assurance systems need to be transparent in two ways: Web sites that do not conform are filtered out, and users can apply their own quality criteria.

FUTURE RESEARCH DIRECTIONS

Three categories of future related research would be helpful. First, with respect to the need for research on Web site evaluation tools for other conditions, one of the critical factors is dealing with the varying evidence base across diseases. Whereas treatment for diabetes has a relatively strong evidence base (and treatments for some conditions like cardiovascular disease probably are even stronger in that respect), other conditions have much more limited or rapidly changing evidence on which a Web site can base its information. This has implications for criteria selection in terms of both what should be covered on a Web site (comprehensiveness) and precisely what the site should say (accuracy).

Second, more research on how consumers use web information would be valuable. Specifically, how do they search for information, what influences their use of the information that they find, and how does that information affect how they make health care decisions for themselves and their families? Although high-quality information is a prerequisite for fostering positive consumer health behavior, it is not a sufficient requirement for stimulating behavior change on the part of consumers.

Third, the research regarding how to integrate this tool with URAC's existing accreditation effort probably could benefit from the experience NCQA has had with integrating performance measurement into an accreditation system based on structural measures. Specific issues to address include:

- How to weight the relative portions of each system in an overall score,
- What the timeline should be for system integration,
- What conditions should be addressed initially, and how the specific conditions should evolve over time, and
- What private and public sector organizations should be involved in a multicondition evaluation system.

CONCLUSION

Wide variation exists in the accuracy and comprehensiveness of online diabetes information, and there is no existing mechanism for consumers to get detailed, objective information about Web site quality. This research also demonstrates that proxies such as sponsorship characteristics and structural, descriptive issues are of limited use in helping consumers search for Internet health information. Objective review of performance in producing health information quality, expressed in terms of accuracy and comprehensiveness of information, can offer consumers a tangible and useful tool in navigating the online health universe.

REFERENCES

Adams, K., & Corrigan, J. M. (Eds.). (2003). *Priority areas for national action: Transforming health care quality.* Washington, DC: National Academies Press.

American Diabetes Association. (2000). Clinical practice recommendations. *Diabetes Care, 23*(Suppl. 1).

Berland, G., Elliott, M., Morales, L., Algazy, J., Kravitz, R., Broder, M., Kanouse, D., Munoz, J., Puyol, J., Lara, M., Watkins, K., Yang, H., & McGlynn, E. (2001). Health information on the Internet: Accessibility, quality, and readability in English and Spanish. *Journal of the American Medical Association, 285*(20), 2612–2621.

Bland, J. M., & Altman, D. G. (1986, February 8). Statistical methods for assessing agreement between two methods of clinical measurement. *The Lancet, 1*(8476), 307–310.

Craigie, M., Loader, B., Burrows, R., & Muncer, S. (2002). Reliability of health information on the Internet: An examination of experts' ratings. *Journal of Medical Internet Research, 4*(1), e2.

Culver, J. D., Uerr, F., & Frurnkin, H. (1997). Medical information in the Internet. A study of an electronic bulletin board. *Journal of General Internal Medicine, 12,* 466–470.

The Diabetes Prevention Program Study Group. (1999). The Diabetes Prevention Program: Design and methods for a clinical trial in the prevention of Type 2 diabetes. *Diabetes Care, 22,* 623–634.

Donabedian, A. (1980). *Explorations in quality assessment and monitoring: Vol. 1. The definition of quality and approaches to its assessment.* Ann Arbor, MI: Health Administration Press.

Feinstein, A. R., & Cicchetti, D. V. (1990). High agreement but low kappa: I. The problems of two paradoxes. *Journal of Clinical Epidemiology, 4,* 543–549.

Hannan, E. L., Kilburn, H., Jr., Racz, M., Shields, E., & Chassin, M. (1994). Improving the outcomes of coronary artery bypass surgery in New York State. *Journal of the American Medical Association, 271,* 761–766.

Hatfield, C. L., May, S. K., & Markoff, J. S. (1999). Quality of consumer drug information provided by four Web sites. *American Journal of Health-System Pharmacy, 56,* 2308–2311.

Impicciatore, P., Pandolfini, C., Casella, N., & Bonati, M. (1997). Reliability of health information for the public on the World Wide Web: Systematic survey of advice on managing fever in children at home. *BMJ, 314,* 1875–1881.

Kunst, H., Groot, D., Latthe, P., Latthe, M., & Khan, K. (2002). Accuracy of information on apparently credible websites: Survey of five common health topics. *BMJ, 324*(9), 581–582.

Lee, J. (2000). The Internet can save your life. *Money,* March, 119–125.

Lin, LI-K. (1989). A concordance correlation coefficient to evaluate reproducibility. *Biometrics, 45,* 255–268.

Meric, F., Bernstam, E. V., & Mirza, N. Q. (2002). Breast cancer on the World Wide Web: Cross-sectional survey of quality of information and popularity of Websites. *BMJ, 324,* 577–581.

National Committee for Quality Assurance. (2004). *The state of health care quality: 2004.* Retrieved December 2, 2005, from http://www.ncqa.org/communications/SOMC/SOHC2004.pdf

Pandolfini, C., & Bonati, M. (2002). Follow-up of quality of public-oriented health information on the World Wide Web: Systematic re-evaluation. *BMJ, 324,* 582–583.

Pew Internet & American Life Project. (2002). *Vital decisions: How Internet users decide what information to trust when they or their loved ones are sick.* Retrieved May 22, 2002, from http://www.pewinternet.org/

Purcell, G. P., Wilson, P., & Delamothe, T. (2002). The quality of health information on the Internet. As for any other medium it varies widely; regulation is not the answer. *BMJ, 324,* 557–558.

Rice, R. E. (2001). The Internet and health communication: A framework of experiences. In R. E. Rice & J. E. Katz (Eds.), *The Internet and health communication: Expectations and experiences* (pp. 5–46). Thousand Oaks, CA: Sage.

Rice, R. E., Peterson, M., & Christine, R. (2001). A comparative features analysis of publicly accessible commercial and government health database Web sites. In R. E. Rice & J. E. Katz (Eds.), *The Internet and health communication: Expectations and experiences* (pp. 213–231). Thousand Oaks, CA: Sage.

Risk, A. (2002). Commentary: On the way to quality. *BMJ, 324*(9), 601–602.

Schneider, E. C., & Epstein, A. M. (1996). Influence of cardiac-surgery performance reports on referral practices and access to care. *New England Journal of Medicine, 335*, 251–256.

Seidman, J. J., Steinwachs, D., & Rubin, H. R. (2003a). Design and testing of a tool for evaluating the quality of diabetes consumer-information Web sites. *Journal of Medical Internet Research, 5*(4), e29. Retrieved December 2, 2005, from http://www.jmir.org/2003/4/e29

Seidman, J. J., Steinwachs, D., & Rubin, H. R. (2003b). Conceptual framework for a new tool for evaluating the quality of diabetes consumer-information Web sites. *Journal of Medical Internet Research, 5*(4), e30. Retrieved December 2, 2005, from http://www.jmir.org/2003/4/e30

Shrout, P. E., & Fleiss, J. L. (1979). Intraclass correlations: Uses in assessing rater reliability. *PsychiatricBulletin, 86*, 420–428.

Thompson, S. (1999). The Internet and its potential influence on suicide. *Psychiatric Bulletin, 23*(8), 449–451.

UKPDS Group. (1998). Intensive blood-glucose control with sulphonylureas or insulin compared with conventional treatment and risk of complications in patients with type 2 diabetes (UKPDS 33). UK Prospective Diabetes Study (UKPDS) Group. *Lancet, 352*, 837–853.

URAC. (2001). *Health Web site standards, draft. Feb 25 2001.* Retrieved October 3, 2003, from http://www.Webapps.urac.org/Websiteaccreditation/Portal/Business/Docs/Web%20site%20stds%20v1-0.doc

URAC. (2005). *URAC's health Web site check-up service and accreditation program.* Retrieved January 7, 2005, from http://www.urac.org/prog_accred_HWS_verify.asp?navid=accreditation&pagename=prog_accred_HWS

Wilson, P. (2002). How to find the good and avoid the bad or ugly: A short guide to tools for rating quality of health information on the Internet. *British Medical Journal, 324*(7337), 598–602.

Zeng, Q., Kogan, S., Plovnick, R., Crowell, J., Lacroix, E.-M., & Greenes, R. (2004). Positive attitudes and failed queries: An exploration of the conundrums of consumer health information retrieval. *International Journal of Medical Informatics, 73*, 45–55.

IV

SUPPORT GROUPS
AND COMMUNITIES

Chapter 11

Online Communities for Mutual Help: Fears, Fiction, and Facts

Gerald Kral

Zentrum Rodaun, Wien, Austria

HEALTH ISSUES AND THE INTERNET

During the last decade, the Internet has become an increasingly important mass-communication media touching on all areas of life and providing information concerning health issues. Here the Internet plays two roles: it is a medium of information, and a medium of communication for groups as well as for individuals. The possible effects on individuals obtaining health-related information from the Internet and joining health-related online groups are controversial. Eysenbach and Köhler (2004) classified 4.5% out of 2,985 search expressions, randomly selected from a sample of 298,512 query strings taken from the Metaspy Exposed Web site, as health related. It is estimated that more than 100,000 health-related Web sites exist in the United States (Morahan-Martin, 2004). On a typical day at the end of 2004, 7 million adult Americans went online to get health or medical information and 93 million have used the Internet for health or medical purposes (Pew Internet & American Life Project, 2005). Online, it is possible to attain information about almost every kind of disease, even about those that are extremely rare.

This possibility can create three different kinds of problems:

- initially, the quality, reliability, readability and accessibility of the information from the Internet has a wide variability (Berland, Elliott, Morales, Algazy, Kravitz, et al., 2001);

- patients have more—qualified or unqualified—information about diseases;
- at this time, there is not enough evidence about the impact of this amount of information on the patients (Murero, D' Ancona, & Karamanoukian, 2001)

ONLINE COMMUNITIES

The Internet does not only provide information, it also offers various possibilities for direct communication between individuals concerned with health issues (Katz & Rice, 2002). They could be patients, family, or friends or health professionals. They can profit from the large number of specific forums, newsgroups, and virtual self-help-groups found on the Internet.

During the last decade, there has been some research about the concept of "community." Hillary (1963) concluded that this term is used in a wide variability of meanings. Other authors state that "community" often is used in relation to certain places and typical kinds of processes and structures (Weis, 1982). One review of the physical and online community literature identified four primary conceptualizations: traditional, social network, pseudo-community, and imagined community (Katz, Rice, Acord, Dasgupta, & David, 2004). Authors such as Rheingold (1993) and Suler (1999) have shown that many of the important characteristics for communities can be transferred onto the "online world." Suler (1999) stated that cyberspace is a kind of "psychological space," where spatial metaphors such as "worlds," "domains," or "rooms" are common in articulating online activities. In the literature both of the terms *online community* and *virtual community* are used for groups of people meeting each other online on virtual places. This chapter uses these terms as synonyms.

People join online health communities because they may be suffering from an illness, maybe have major emotional problems, could be worried about their health, etc. (Rice & Katz, 2001). They could join to find emotional support, or to meet other people who share their interests, fears or experiences and therefore can understand them. They meet in a kind of virtual shelter where they think they can be together with likeminded others, and not be subjected to scientific studies. For a long time, virtual communities, especially in health contexts, have been a kind of *terra incognita*. This has lead to major misunderstandings about their nature and major underestimations about the importance and support they can have for their members (Becker, El-Faddagh, & Schmidt, 2004). Knowledge and empirical evidence about virtual self-help-groups can possibly help and encourage people to go online and find support (Eysenbach, Powell, Englesakis, Rizo, & Stern, 2004). It could also aid health professionals to allow their patients join online communities for self-help without worrying about the outcome. For this reason, research about online-self-help groups seems to be legitimate, if it is carried out under conditions following ethical guidelines.

Ethical Issues Concerning Studies About Online Communities

King (1994, 1996) provided one of the first systematic approaches to ethical issues related to online communities, which stresses the importance of the protection of the individual posting and the anonymity of the person who posted it in an online community. Another author concerned about ethical issues is Suler (2000). His suggestions for guidelines for ethical research are similar to those by King (1996), but beyond this he postulates the informed consent from the subjects and responsible authorities. Flicker, Haans, and Skinner (2004) formulated guidelines of ethical conduct, where the informed consent of the subjects, too, as well as description of the aims of the study to the subjects, potential harms, and competing commercial interests are key points. Finally, the ethics committee of the Association of Internet Researchers A(o)IR has edited recommendations about the ethics of Internet research in 2002 (Ess & the AoIR Ethics Working Committee, 2002). In this document, all the considerations cited above are summarized, so that it is an important, well-elaborated and valid guideline to use in planning one's studies. For the publishing of health-related Web sites, the Health on the Net Foundation (HON) has elaborated some principles, concerned with the quality of the available information, confidentiality of data, privacy, advertising and funding policy.

ONLINE SELF-HELP GROUPS IN THE HEALTH CONTEXT

Literature concerning online groups for mutual help was initially published in the middle of the 1990s, although some studies could already be found in the middle of the 1980s (Winzelberg, 1997). These groups usually have the format of newsgroups (or bulletin board systems or message boards), mailing lists, chats or MUDs (Multiuser Dungeons/Domains) (Döring, 2000). The most important and most widely spread formats are the newsgroups or www-forums. They utilize asynchronous communication: postings can be read and it is possible to follow discussion threads.

The advantages of virtual self-help groups are evident: The ability to transcend geographical and temporal constraints is much better for virtual support groups. There is less risk in disclosure of health information and there is greater access to diverse sources of health information than in face-to-face support groups. Due to reduced social status cues, more heterogeneous supportive relationships are possible. And writing about health problems and formulating disclosure of personal concerns has a therapeutic value by itself (Wright & Bell, 2003).

It is an open question whether there are disadvantages in using health information and electronic support groups on the Internet. There exist theoretical as well as empirical approaches and efforts to explain the efficacy mechanisms and processes of communication in "virtual self-help groups."

Walther (1996) developed the concept of "hyperpersonal interaction" in computer mediated communication (CMC) in order to explain the phenomenon that such contacts frequently and very quickly reach a high level of intensity and intimacy. He assumed that in CMC, the "reduction" of social indicators can lead to a concentration on what is essential, that is, on the message the sender wants to pass on. In the reactions to these messages again the essential aspects are reinforced and emphasized: "(CMC is hyperpersonal) when users experience commonality, are self-aware, physically separated, and communicate via a limited-cues channel, they selectively self-present and edit; to construct and reciprocate representations of their partners and relations without the interference of environmental reality. Perhaps more so when this communication is asynchronous and/or when the CMC link is the only link there is" (Walther, 1996, p. 33).

Research about health-related online groups (Dublin, Simon, & Orem, 1997; King & Moreggi, 1998; Lasker, Sogolow, & Sharim, 2005; Madara & White, 1997; Salem, Bogar, & Reid, 1997; Turner, Grube, & Meyers, 2001) has identified some characteristics of these communities. Online groups have higher levels of expressed emotional support and self-disclosure, less formal structure and group process than face-to-face self-help-groups (Salem et al., 1997); the therapeutic value of virtual groups is assessed as very high by their members (Madara & White, 1997); and the main reason for participating in health-related online groups is the wish to share personal experiences with others (Dublin, Simon, & Orem, 1997). There are positive correlations between the perceived amount and the depth of the support, and the amount of time that participants spend in reading the contributions (Turner et al., 2001). Lasker, Sogolow and Sharim (2005) observed that the messages exchanged on a biomedical mailing list contained "very frequent expressions of emotional support."

Online Self-Help Groups for Eating Disorders

One of the early research studies about an online self-help group for eating disorders was done by Winzelberg (1997). He investigated all contributed postings within a period of 3 months; 306 messages in total were sent by 70 participants of which 97% were women. Winzelberg does not give any clues about gender classification as names people use to log in, as they are often based on "gender-swapping" (or "gender-switching"; Bruckman, 1993) or are "neutral" or fantasy nicknames, and cannot be easily classified. However, the percentage of women in this group seems plausible because of the well-known distribution of eating disorders within the gender groups. Thirty-six percent of the participants classified themselves as anorexic, 23% as bulimic. The largest group (31%) of postings were those referring to personal problems; 23% contained information in form of medical, psychological, and nutritious advice; 16% provided emotional support; and 15% referred to other kinds of requests like advice in love matters, problems with parents, or at school. An interesting aspect of this study seems the finding that 31% of the postings were sent between 11.00 p.m. and 7.00 a.m. These findings led Winzelberg to a generally positive assessment of the effect of the community. Still, he remained cautious because no other research was available for comparisons at that time: "In the meantime, caution should be exercised before recommending participation in ESG" (Winzelberg 1997, p. 405).

Walstrom (2000) did a qualitative microanalysis of threads of interaction in an online forum for eating disorders. She focused in particular on assessing the process of establishing a secure and supportive environment from which the users can benefit in a therapeutic way. In her conclusions, Walstrom argues that online self-help groups can be considered an ideal addition to face-to-face groups.

Grunwald and Busse (2002) analyzed 619 questions that were sent to an online counseling service for people suffering from eating disorders. Fifty-nine percent of respondents could be classified as belonging to the symptom area of bulimia; not quite 15% to anorexia; 11.5% referred to the Binge Eating Disorder; the rest could not be classified unambiguously. Eight percent of the mails could not be classified in relation to eating disorders. Three-quarters of the e-mails were by women and 17% by men; the other 9% of the e-mails could not be classified as belonging to a specific gender. Information about age was only given for not quite 38% of the users. The average age of this group was calculated to be 21 years. The authors concluded that "a remarkably high number of questions came from very young women. This group of users often expresses that until that moment they had not been able or willing to confide in anybody to ask such questions. These e-mails must be considered as an initial contact of persons with a beginning or recent eating disorder" (online).

These research studies generally point at virtual self-help groups as having a relatively high value for participants, male and female; mutual exchange is very important and quite personal issues are shared. As far as the data of the users of eating disorder Web sites could be gathered, they seem to be compatible with clinical experiences.

STUDYING AN ONLINE SELF-HELP GROUP FOR EATING DISORDERS

Method

For this research (Kral, Presslich, & Nedoschill, 2003) a questionnaire with 25 items was developed that, after a trial period of about 1 month (May–June, 2001), was set up on the web page of the largest German-language forum for persons with eating disorders called "hungrig-online" (in English: "hungry-online"). "Hungrig-online" is a moderated Web site (http://www.hungrig-online.com), which means that there are persons who observe the exchange of messages and intervene if necessary. On the homepage of the "hungrig-online" forums, a link was established pointing directly to the questionnaire.

In the described period of time we received a total of 605 completed questionnaires, only six of which had to be excluded because of not plausible or largely incomplete data (less than 50% of the questions were answered). The following data therefore are based on 599 evaluated questionnaires. After the first week we had already obtained almost 59% of all responses. And, because it was possible to maintain the questionnaire on the Web site over a long period of time, those users who also visited the Web site between longer intervals could be reached.

Results

Characteristics of the Respondents.   The users reportedly visited "hungrig-online" several times a week (30.1%); 22% visited the Web site several times a day; 17% once a day; 15.4% once a week; and only 13.5% less than weekly (2% did not answer this question). The peak of the distribution of age lies in the age group between 20 and 25 years (about 29% of the subjects); about 75% were between 16 and 30 years old; 95.2% were females and 4.8% were males. As for the question about their present employment, 37.1% reported to be still going to school; 24.5% were working; 23.2% were attending university; 6.8% were serving an apprenticeship; 4.5% reported to be unemployed; 2.8% were in other professional training or education; and 1.0% did not answer this question.

Eating-Disorder-Specific Data.   In our sample, 90.5% reported suffering from an eating disorder: Forty-six percent reported bulimia, 30% reported anorexia, 12% indicated some other kind of eating disorder, 8% said they have no eating disorder, 3% reported binge eating, and 1% provided no response. Relating the kind of eating disorder with the gender shows that out of the 29 men who answered this question, 15 reported suffering from an eating disorder (six with anorexia, four bulimia, two binge eating, and three others).

Table 11.1 shows the duration of the eating disorder and the percentage of subjects who are or have been in psychotherapeutic treatment. Interestingly, 53.5% of our sample has been suffering from their eating disorder for more than 3 years, and of those, 63.9% are not in treatment at present. These numbers are lower than the ones collected by Madara and White (1997; quoted by King & Moreggi, 1998), who found not quite 50% to be in individual therapy and almost 60% to be in group therapy.

Table 11.2 illustrates the results of the question about the therapy-motivating effect of "hungrig-online." This question showed that there

TABLE 11.1
Duration of Eating Disorder and Treatment

	Disorder Since				
In Treatment	up to 1 year	up to 2 years	up to 3 years	> 3 years	Total
At present	3.0%	6.6%	5.0%	19.4%	33.9%
In the past	1.5	1.7	2.8	14.2	20.1
Never	12.4	7.2	6.3	20.1	45.9
Total	16.8%	15.5%	14.0%	53.7%	100.0%

TABLE 11.2
Increase of Therapy Motivation

	Kind of Eating Disorder	
Increasing Therapy Motivation	Anorexia	Bulimia
Yes	22.6%	30.5%
Maybe	33.3	39.5
No	44.0	30.1
N	168	259

was a correlation with the eating disorder category: women who stated they were suffering from anorexia tended towards having a lower therapy motivation for using "hungrig-online." These results are congruent with clinical experiences with regard to the psychological strain and the therapy motivation of clients with eating disorders. For this question, there were no significant correlations involving the period of time over which they had been suffering from the eating disorder.

Our data can be summarized as follows: Amongst the respondents (and, as can be assumed, also among the users of "hungrig-online," male or female) we find almost only persons who are suffering from eating disorders (here it needs to be emphasized that this understanding was based on a personal, and not on a medical, diagnosis), that in 50% of the cases have lasted for more than 3 years, and of which nearly 50% were never treated. These data imply that institutions like "hungrig-online" are of great significance if we want to reach groups of persons suffering from eating disorders, which otherwise would not be discovered and therefore could not be addressed.

The "Hungrig-Online" Forums. The usually high-visiting frequency in "hungrig-online" implies that many reactions to incoming postings—depending on the time of the day—are posted rather quickly. It often happens that after an initial posting, a few minutes later others post their reactions and dozens within the next hour. The content of these postings shows that there is a very frank exchange between the participants, and that often problems are disclosed, even though nobody knows the "real life" of the author of the posting.

Table 11.3 provides the reasons why the participants visit the forum and write such contributions. The result that 80.6% report to visit the "hungrig-online" forums in order to meet other people with similar problems or a similar fate is more unambiguous than in the research done by Dublin et al. (1997) where 63% of the visitors of an online self-

TABLE 11.3
Expectations From Visiting the Forum

What Do You Expect from Visiting the [Eating Disorder] Forum?	
To get to know people with similar problems	80.6%
Valuable information and advice	12.4
Simply felt lonely	3.8
Hope to find people who support me, because together it is easier	0.7
Tips to lose weight	1.2
Information about counsellors or therapists	0.0
No answer	1.3
N	599

TABLE 11.4
Contact Outside of the Forums

Direct Contact?	Often	Sometimes	Seldom	Never	No Answer	N
By e-mail	5.2%	24.0	23.0	43.7	4.0	599
Personally	1.5%	5.3	6.8	84.1	2.2	599

help group declared the reason for their visit to be their wish to share their experiences with others; 12.4% were looking for information and advice; tips for losing weight were not much looked for (1.2%); and none reported looking for possibilities for therapy.

Data concerning types of communication, provided in Table 11.4, show that contacts mainly take place virtually, and personal encounters in real life have hardly any importance. An interesting fact seems to be that only 10% of the respondents explicitly feel that they get better advice from the moderators than from the other participants; about half of them do not experience any difference between the moderators and the participants; a bit less than 12% specifically give credit to participants they have known in the forum for quite some time. These data imply that the "hungrig-online" group is a virtual community with a relatively high degree of mutual trust and rather intensive contacts.

Of those forum participants who had already introduced discussion threads by themselves ($n = 381$), about 70% report to have experienced the responses as "giving them hope," for about 20% they were neutral, about 8% experience the reactions as rather depressing.

Interestingly enough a simple classification of the postings gives a somewhat different impression: With regard to their content, 67% of the evaluated postings were classified by us as neutral, about 15% as positive, and about 18% as negative.

Discussion

Where it concerns the perception of the forum participants in our sample, we see a shift towards positive experiencing of the responses to their postings. It seems as if the fact that there is some resonance itself already has a positive connotation. In our sample, where problems of self-value and fighting for acknowledgment play a major role, this seems natural. Salem et al. (1997, quoted by King & Moreggi, 1998) in their research findings concerning an online group for persons suffering from depression found much more frequently support, acceptance, and positive feelings than contradiction and negative expression of feelings.

In contrast to early studies that were very careful about stating any positive effects of online self-help-groups (e.g., Winzelberg, 1997), due to further research the positive effects and potency for emotional support of these communities seem to be evident. The "hungrig-online" is predominantly visited by people who rate themselves as suffering from an eating disorder (approximately 92%) and who are female (95%); so it is a forum that addresses the target group exactly. The fact that 46% of the visitors never had psychotherapeutic treatment seems worrying on the one hand, but on the other hand, it again underlines the value of this virtual place.

The fact that almost nobody is looking for tips on how to lose weight seems surprising as well as gratifying and could be an argument against fears concerning such types of online self-help groups. Less optimistic is the relatively weak reported effect for starting psychotherapeutic treatment. This could be a useful hint for providers and moderators of online-self-help groups to perhaps take more advantage of the potential of these groups. But another result suggests that they have to be careful: Only 10% feel that they get their best advice from the forum moderators, which again shows the predominant "peer-to-peer" characteristics of the studied forum. On the other hand therapists, too, seem to have their reservations: only 1% out of our sample knew about the forum from a therapist.

What is perhaps most impressive in the results of the "hungrig-online" study is the frequency and intensity of the communication among the users and the large amount of emotional support they can get from each other. The comparison of the ratings of the postings with the perceived support shows this quite convincingly. These findings seem to support the linking of "weak-tie network theories" with online self-help groups (Wright & Bell, 2003) as well as the concept of "hyperpersonal interaction" (Walther, 1996).

ONLINE SELF-HELP GROUPS
FOR SUICIDAL PEOPLE

In 2000, a young Austrian girl traveled to Norway to meet a young Norwegian man whom she had met in an Internet forum; they then committed suicide by jumping off the cliffs. This led to the first "Internet suicide" in history. Immediately after, a discussion arose in the media about the destructive nature and danger of the Internet, especially for adolescents. The media reported a lot of unproven statements and generalizations about this tragic but singular case. Fiedler and Lindner (2001) analyzed these statements:

- Causes of suicides ("Suicidal thoughts are generated in individuals by the Internet," "Adolescents who are initially not suicidal are driven into suicidal thoughts by group dynamics and identification processes in suicide forums");
- Effects of "infection" and the "snowball effect" ("Communication about methods to commit suicide increases the probability to commit suicide," "Suicides will become epidemic because of suicide forums");
- Content of suicide forums ("Discussions about effective suicide methods and trading with deadly drugs or weapons dominate the communication," "Mutual help means assistance for dying together"); and
- Motivations to visit suicide forums ("Dating for dying together," "Get information and tips about effective suicide methods").

There are some publications, but very few evidence-based studies about suicide forums online communities. As Fiedler and Lindner (2001, 2002) stated, many of the reports about Internet and suicide are based on wrong assumptions, generalizations of single incidents, and unproven statements. The authors conclude that suicide forums do not generate, only portray, suicidal tendencies that online users already have. Other authors (e.g., Bronisch, 2002; Prass, 2000) have described suicide forums as dangerous. Most of the publications that illustrate skeptical opinions in reference to suicide forums are based on a single case study (e.g., Becker, Mayer, Nagenborg, El-Faddagh, & Schmidt, 2004) describing two female adolescents who made parasuicidal attempts. At the present (late 2005) only few empirical studies have been done to clarify the nature of the effects of participating in online suicidal forums. In an online questionnaire Winkel, Groen, Waldmann, and Petermann (2003) found that suicide forums presented a number of positive aspects for their users, and they found no evidence that could support concerns.

STUDYING AN ONLINE SUICIDE FORUM

At the moment there are approximately 30 German-speaking suicide forums on the Internet. In order to obtain some empirical evidence and contribute to understanding of what is really happening in these virtual communities, including what they mean to those who visit them, we analyzed the biggest German-language suicide forum, "selbstmordforum.de" (Eichenberg & Kral, 2003).

Method

We created a questionnaire of 29 questions about biographical data, users' habits concerning their visits to the suicide forum, their motivation for visiting, their postings and their answers to posts from other users, the kind of communication, and the suicidal thoughts those users have. Before starting with the main study we performed a pilot test by presenting the questionnaire in another suicide forum. For the main study the questionnaire was online for 4 weeks in March and April, 2003. The sample consisted of 164 subjects who responded to all of the 29 questions.

Results

Characteristics of Respondents.   Our sample seems rather young (more than half of our respondents are between 16 and 20 years old, nearly 80% are under 25), and exactly 50% were females, 50% males. Nearly 60% of our sample attend school or are university students, and 7.8% are apprentices. Three-quarters were single, 20.2% were married or lived in a steady relationship; the rest were separated or were widow(er)s. These results seem to be in good accordance with the distribution of age.

Data Concerning Suicidal Thoughts.   Table 11.5 shows at what point in time their thinking of suicide started. There are possibly two subgroups: approximately 28% had suicidal thoughts for the first time between 1 and 3 years ago, whereas approximately 34% had such thoughts more than 5 years ago, which is quite a long time. Only 12% of our subjects never had any suicidal thoughts.

TABLE 11.5
Duration of Suicidal Thoughts

The First Time I Thought of Committing Suicide Was . . .	Percentage
less than 1 month ago	3.0%
1–3 months ago	1.8
3–6 months ago	4.7
6–12 months ago	4.7
1–2 years ago	15.4
2–3 years ago	13.0
3–4 years ago	4.1
4–5 years ago	7.1
more than 5 years ago	34.3
I never thought of suicide	11.8
N	164

Table 11.6 shows that there is a decrease in intensity of any suicidal thoughts during the respondents' participation in the suicide forum: Thirty-one percent say that this decrease is due to their attendance at the forum; 61% of respondents say there is no causal relationship with the decrease and joining the forum, and only 8% have the feeling that joining the forum reinforced their suicidal thoughts. Subjects rate the amount of their suicidal thoughts after attending the forum as lower than before.

Another interesting result is that only 40% of the sample had received medical or psychotherapeutic treatment because of their suicidal thoughts, whereas 60% had not. On the other hand, only 22% say that attending the forum has reinforced their motivation to look for professional help, whereas 78% say that this is not the case. So we have 88% of people with, in most cases, a high amount of suicidal thoughts in the studied suicide forum, 60% of whom never had been treated properly. Fifty-four percent of our sample had made at least one suicide attempt in their life (26% of them once, 21% twice or three times), 46% have not made any.

The Suicide Forum.   One of our questions aimed at the motivation for attending the forum. Our statements were rated with 1 for very low agreement and 5 for very high agreement. They are ranked according to the mean value of the answers. The most important motivation to attend the forum is "to meet people with similar problems and thoughts," followed by the motivation "to speak about any problems that have lead to my suicidal thoughts," "to find people I can talk to in an acute suicidal crisis," "to help others," "curiosity," "to overcome a crisis together with other people who have similar problems and thoughts, because it is easier if you are not alone," and "to get rid of my suicidal thoughts." The motivation "to get tips for effective suicide methods" only ranks sixth. The motivation "to find somebody who commits suicide together with me" is ranked

TABLE 11.6
Intensity of Suicidal Thoughts

Amount of Suicidal Thoughts	Before Attending the Suicide Forum	Now
0	1.3%	9.4%
1	7.4	16.1
2	3.4	15.4
3	14.1	20.8
4	20.1	8.7
5	26.8	15.4
6	26.8	14.1
Mean value	5.3	4.1

TABLE 11.7
Reactions to the Postings and Their Assessment by the Posters

Reaction to the Postings (range 1–5)	Response	This helps me . . .
I am receiving answers which make me feel understood	3.2	3.4
I receive comforting reactions	3.1	3.1
I am cheered up/distracted	2.8	3.0
I am receiving concrete advice how to overcome my problems	2.7	2.8
I do not receive any reactions	1.9	1.7
My wish to commit suicide is being reinforced	1.7	2.5

eighth, the next to last position, and the weakest motivation is "to obtain information about how to deal with people I know who have suicidal thoughts." Corresponding with these findings are the contents of the postings. Here, "I describe the problems which have led to my suicidal thoughts" is most frequent; followed by "I am responsive to other people's suicidal thoughts," "I try to solve other people's problems that have led to their suicidal thoughts," "I am trying to make people who have suicidal thoughts change their minds," and "I give expression to my suicidal thoughts." At the sixth ranking was "I simply communicate with other participants; the "suicide" issue is of no importance," then "I share my experiences how to overcome my suicidal thoughts," lastly, "I ask for help."

Table 11.7 shows the ranking of the reactions to the postings and the assessment of the reactions by the posters. The results displayed in this table again underline the importance of feeling understood and receiving comforting reactions in the forum. Being reinforced in suicidal tendencies is the least of all reactions.

Comparing our empirical findings with the initially quoted statements (Fiedler & Lindner, 2001), we can see that most of them are not confirmed by our data. There was no evidence that suicidal thoughts are generated in people by visiting the online group and no evidence for increased likelihood of committing suicide or dating for suicide or for mutual help for dying together.

FACTS, FICTION, AND FEARS: A COMPARISON

Data obtained from the two studied health-related online groups—that are very different concerning the topics they deal with and were collected at two different time periods—showed relatively similar results. Both of the studied online communities clarify the *fact* that participants are able to address their respective target group. In the "hungrig-online" sample, 92% were suffering from an eating disorder, and about 88% of the "selbstmordforum.de" sample said that they have suicidal thoughts. Participants of online forums not only reach their target groups, but there is a good deal of frank communication and mutual support among participants; this latter point seems to be the reason for the perceived helpfulness of these communities.

What, to a certain extent, turned out to be *fiction* is the idea that online communities like the two forums studied could be a powerful resource to motivate their visitors to seek professional help. Out of the "hungrig-online" sample, approximately 27% stated that visiting the forum strengthened their motivation to seek proper therapeutic treatment, and out of the "selbstmordforum.de" sample, approximately 22% said so. These numbers do not seem very high, but if the forum could help one out of 20% to 25% of persons to attend therapy, this is a positive outcome.

Data obtained from the studies about two different kinds of health-related online communities show very clearly that *fears* concerning such communities seem to be unnecessary. "Hungrig-online" is not a platform for dieting together, and "selbstmordforum.de" is not a place for dying together. So, there is no reason for trying to get people to avoid contact with online communities concerned with their specific interest. The data possibly suggest that most health professionals have some kind of fears about recommending that their patients or clients visit online communities. The reasons for this seem to be various, as just discussed. However, the problem is that patients may lack emotional support. And as mentioned before, writing about health problems and formulating disclosure of personal concerns can have a therapeutic value by itself. As shown in the "selbstmordforum.de" study, visiting the forum is likely to reduce suicidal thoughts. In both of the studies reported here, the subjects emphasized the great supportive character of joining the communities and communicating with others. Perhaps the most important finding is that comparing our empirical findings with Fiedler and Lindner's (2001) discussion of media statements about suicide forums not being empirically based, results show that most of the media statements are not confirmed by our empirical findings. There was no evidence that suicidal thoughts are generated in people by visiting the online group and no evidences for increased likelihood of committing suicide or dating for suicide or for mutual help for dying together. Due to the controversial nature of suicidal forums in the literature and the little number of studies available (Becker, El-Faddagh, & Schmidt, 2004), our findings are intended to contribute to the ongoing discussion; future empirical studies need to further clarify the nature of the phenomenon.

In both eating disorders and suicide study groups, where one could suppose activities that could be harmful for the visitors such as exchanging powerful tips for losing weight or effective suicide methods, there was no evidence that these points played a major role. So, the results we obtained seem helpful for understanding the important factors of how online groups for mutual help work and that they are a resource, not a risk, for people who visit them. This could also be helpful for health professionals in dealing with this topic. In particular, linking online and offline support could be considered as an optimal care for people with health concerns.

REFERENCES

Becker, K., El-Faddagh, M., & Schmidt, M. H. (2004). Cybersuizid oder Werther–Effekt online: Suizidchatrooms und –foren im Internet. *Kindheit und Entwicklung, 13*(1), 14–25.

Becker, K., Mayer, M., Nagenborg, M., El-Faddagh, M., & Schmidt, M. H. (2004). Parasuicide online: Can suicide websites trigger suicidal behavior in predisposed adolescents? *Nordic Journal of Psychiatry, 58*, 111–114.

Berland, G. K., Elliott, M. N., Morales, L. S., Algazy, J. I., Kravitz, R. L., Broder, M. S., Kanouse, D. E., Muñoz, J. A., Puyol, J. A., Lara, M., Watkins, K. E., Yang, H., & Mcglynn, E. A. (2001). Health information on the Internet: Accessibility, quality, and readability in English and Spanish. *Journal of the American Medical Association, 285*(20), 2612–2621.

Bronisch, T. (2002). Suizidforen im Internet. Eine Stellungnahme zu Georg Fiedler und Reinhard Lindner. *Suizidprophylaxe, 29*(3), 107–111.

Bruckman, A. (1993). *Gender-swapping on the Internet.* Paper presented at the Internet Society, San Francisco, CA. Retrieved May 28, 2005, from http://www.cc.gatech.edu/pub/people/asb/papers/gender-swapping.txt

Döring, N. (2000). Selbsthilfe, Beratung und Therapie im Internet. In B. Batinic (Hg.), *Internet für Psychologen* (pp. 509–548). Göttingen: Hogrefe.

Dublin, J., Simon, V., & Orem, J. (1998). Analysis of survey results. In J. Glackenbach (Ed.), *Psychology and the Internet: Intrapersonal, interpersonal and transpersonal implications* (pp. 77–109). San Diego: Academic Press. Retrieved May 28, 2005, from http://www.webpages.charter.net/stormking/Chapter5/index.html

Eichenberg, C., & Kral, G. (2003, July). *Suicide forums on the Internet.* Paper presented at the 8th annual European Federation of Psychology Associations Congress, Vienna, Austria.

Ess, C., & The AoIR Ethics Working Committee. (2002). *Ethical decision-making and Internet research: Recommendations from the AOIR ethics working committee.* Retrieved May 5, 2005, from http://www.aoir.org/reports/ethics.pdf

Eysenbach, G., & Köhler, C. (2004). Health-related searches on the Internet. *Journal of the American Medical Association, 291*(24), 2946.

Eysenbach, G., Powell, P., Englesakis, M., Rizo, C., & Stern, A. (2004). Health-related virtual communities and electronic support groups: Systematic review of the effects of online peer to peer interactions. *British Medical Journal, 328*, 1166–1170.

Fiedler, G., & Lindner, R. (2001). *Suizidforen im Internet.* Retrieved May 12, 2005, from http://www.uke.uni-hamburg.de/extern/tzs/online-text/suizidforen.pdf

Fiedler, G., & Lindner, R. (2002). Suizidforen im Internet. *Suizidprophylaxe, 29*(1), 26–31.

Flicker, S., Haans, D., & Skinner, H. (2004). Ethical dilemmas in research on Internet communities. *Qualitative Health Research, 14*(1), 124–134.

Grunwald, M., & Busse, J. C. (2002). Online-Beratung bei Essstörungen: Chancen für eine bessere Versorgung. *Deutsches Ärzteblatt 99*/18. Retrieved November 9, 2003, from http://www.aerzteblatt.de/v4/archiv/artikel.asp?id=31494

Hillary, G. (1963). Villages, cities and total institutions. *American Sociological Review, 28*, 779–791.

Katz, J. E., & Rice, R. E. (2002). *Social consequences of Internet use: Access, involvement and interaction.* Cambridge, MA: The MIT Press.

Katz, J. E., Rice, R. E., Acord, S., Dasgupta, K., & David, K. (2004). Personal mediated communication and the concept of community in theory and practice. In P. Kalbfleisch (Ed.), *Communication and community, communication yearbook 28* (pp. 315–371). Mahwah, NJ: Lawrence Erlbaum Associates.

King, S. A. (1994). Analysis of electronic support groups for recovering addicts. *Interpersonal Computing and Technology: An Electronic Journal for the 21st Century, 2*(3), 47–56. Article retrieved May 20, 2003, from http://www.helsinki.fi/science/optek/1994/n3/king.txt

King, S. A. (1996). Researching Internet communities: Proposed ethical guidelines for the reporting of the results. *The Information Society, 12*(2), 119–127.

King, S. A., & Moreggi, D. (1998). Internet therapy and self help groups—the pros and cons. In J. Glackenbach (Ed.), *Psychology and the Internet: Intrapersonal, interpersonal and transpersonal implications* (pp. 77–109). San Diego: Academic Press. Retrieved June 25, 2003, from http://webpages.charter.net/stormking/Chapter5/index.html

Kral, G., Presslich, C., & Nedoschill, J. (2003). Analyse und Evaluation von Selbsthilfe-Ressourcen im Internet (www) anhand eines Forums für Menschen mit Essstörungen. *Psychologie in Österreich, 13*(1), 48–54.

Lasker, J. N., Sogolow, E. D., & Sharim, R. R. (2005). The role of an online community for people with a rare disease: Content analysis of messages posted on a primary biliary cirrhosis mailinglist. *Journal of Medical Internet Research, 7*(1), e10. Retrieved May 28, 2005, from http://www.jmir.org/2005/1/e10/

Madara, E. J., & White, B. J. (1997). On-line mutual support: The experience of a self-help clearinghouse. *Information & Referral, 19*, 91–108. Retrieved May 17, 2005, from http://webpages.charter.net/stormking/Chapter5/index.html

Morahan-Martin, J. M. (2004). How Internet users find, evaluate, and use online health information: A cross-cultural review. *CyberPsychology & Behavior, 7*, 497–510.

Murero, M., D' Ancona, G., & Karamanoukian, H. (2001). Use of the Internet in patients before and after cardiac surgery: An interdisciplinary study. *Journal of Medical Internet Research, 3*(3), e27.

Pew Internet & American Life Project. (2005). *Internet: Mainstreaming the online life.* Retrieved May 20, 2005, from http://www.pewinternet.org/pdfs/Internet_Status_2005.pdf

Prass, S. (2000). Suizid-Foren im Internet—eine neue Kultgefahr? Retrieved May 31, 2005, from http://www.religio.de/dialog/300/22_16-19.htm

Rheingold, H. (1993). *The virtual community: Homesteading on the electronic frontier.* Reading, MA: Addison-Wesley.

Rice, R. E., & Katz, J. E. (Eds.). (2001). *The Internet and health communication.* Thousand Oaks, CA: Sage.

Salem, D. A., Bogar, G. A., & Reid, C. (1997). Mutual help goes on-line. *Journal of Community Psychology, 25*(2), 198–207.

Suler, J. (1999). *Cyberspace is a psychological space.* Retrieved May 25, 2005, from http://www.rider.edu/~suler/psycyber/psychspace.html

Suler, J. (2000). Ethics in cyberspace research. Retrieved March 1, 2005, from http://www.rider.edu/~suler/psycyber/ethics.html

Turner, J. W., Grube, J. A., & Meyers, J. (2001). Developing an optimal match within on-line communities: An exploration of cmc support communities and traditional support. *Journal of Communication, 51,* 231–251.

Walstrom, M. (2000). "You know, who's the thinnest?": Combating surveillance and creating safety in coping with eating disorders online. *CyberPsychology & Behavior, 3*(5), 761–783.

Walther, J. B. (1996). Computer-mediated communication: Impersonal, interpersonal, and hyperpersonal interaction. *Communication Research, 23*(1), 3–43.

Weis, R. (1982). *A dynamic view of questioning in an organization.* Unpublished doctoral dissertation, University of Washington.

Winkel, S., Groen, G., Waldmann, H-C., & Petermann, F. (2003). Suizidforen im Internet. Bedeutung einer virtuellen Lebenswelt aus Sicht der Nutzer. *Medien + Erziehung Merz. Zeitschrift für Medienpädagogik, 5,* 115–124.

Winzelberg, A. (1997). The analysis of an electronic support group for individuals with eating disorders. *Computers in Human Behavior, 13*(3), 393–407.

Wright, K. B., & Bell, S. B. (2003). Health-related support groups on the Internet: Linking empirical findings to social support and computer-mediated communication theory. *Journal of Health Psychology, 8*(1), 39–54.

Chapter 12

The Use of the Internet for Health Information and Social Support: A Content Analysis of Online Breast Cancer Discussion Groups

George A. Barnett
State University of New York, Buffalo

Jennie M. Hwang
State University of New York, Buffalo

THE INTERNET AND HEALTH, ESPECIALLY CANCER, INFORMATION AND SUPPORT

The Internet has become a popular medium for people seeking online health information and social/emotional support (Rice & Katz, 2001). Several different patient populations have found benefits from Internet-based resources. Those groups include persons with chronic debilitating illness (Dickerson, Flaig, & Kennedy, 2000; Johnson, Ravert, & Everton, 2001), dementia and Alzheimer's disease (Brennan, Moore, & Smyth, 1992; Smyth & Harris, 1993), eating disorders (Winzelberg, 1997), cancer (Chen & Siu, 2001; Wienberg, Schmale, Ulken, & Wessel, 1995, 1996), cardiothoracic disease (Murero, D' Ancona, & Karamanoukian, 2001) and postsurgical rehabilitation (Brennan, Moore, Bjornsdottir, Jones, Visovsky, et al., 2001). In addition, health care organizations have increasingly utilized Internet services for self-help and mutual aid groups for individuals with disabilities (Finn, 1999; Ritchie & Blank, 2003).

Numerous studies have shown that patients and their families and friends participate in online support groups to cope with disease (Fogel, Albert, Schnabel, Ditkoff, & Neugut, 2002; Hilton, 1993; Kral, chap. 11, this volume; Kristjanson & Ashcroft, 1994; Winzelberg, Classen, Alpers,

Roberts, Koopman, et al., 2003). Generally, the members of online support groups express very positive attitudes toward the usefulness of the web for seeking health information (Lieberman, Golant, Giese-Davis, Winzlenberg, Benjamin, et al., 2003; Marton, 2000). Computer-mediated forms of social interaction afford people the means for overcoming barriers to social support systems such as geographical isolation, physical debilitation, and fear of self-disclosure (Rice & Katz, 2001). Through the use of the Internet, patients can transform roles and change their involvement in their own health care to become competent social actors despite serious illness (Ziebland, 2004; Ziebland, Chapple, Dumelow, Evans, Prinjha, & Rozmovits, 2004).

Cancer patients, in particular, suffer a serious, often terminal illness, that also undermines their self-images as competent members of society. More than 1.2 million people worldwide will be diagnosed with breast cancer this year (World Health Organization, 2005). The disease is the second leading cause of death among the female population worldwide today, and the leading cause of mortality in adult women. Women with breast cancer have distinct needs for information throughout their breast cancer journeys (Boman, Andersson, & Bjorvell, 1997; Degner, Kristjanson, Bowman, Sloan, Carriere, et al., 1997; Fogel, Albert, Schnabel, Ditkoff, & Neugut, 2003). An overview of the Internet and information on breast cancer by Santoro (2003) indicated that many Internet breast cancer resources (i.e., medical journals, clinical trial registries, medical guideline databases) have appeared, allowing users to keep themselves up to date on medical progress. Moreover, breast cancer patients and their family members actively discuss and share personal experiences and professional issues in online support groups related to treatments (Braithwaite, Waldron, & Finn, 1999; Brennan, Moore, & Smyth, 1992), reduction in distress and pain (Michie, Rosebert, Heaversedge, Madden, & Parbhoo, 1997), support networks (Lamberg, 1997b; Wienberg, Schmale, Uken, & Wessel, 1996), aid coping (Fogel, 2004; Lieberman, 1992; Shaw, Wilson, & O'Brien, 1994), empowerment (Fogel et al., 2002; Sharf, 1997), and developing hyperpersonal communication (Scheerhorn, Warisse, & McNeilis, 1995; Sutter, 2001; Turner, Grube, & Meyers, 2001). In a review of computer-mediated communication support communities for cancer patients, Turner et al. (2001) wrote, "Individuals join social support online communities because they are seeking information, empowerment, encouragement, emotional support and empathy regarding their specific concern" (p. 235). Ziebland's (2004) analysis of the DIPEx Web site (www.dipex.org) also found that cancer patients have used the Internet to not only gather information and gain support from others, but also to make sense of the experience of cancer.

Computer-mediated support groups may have certain advantages over face-to-face groups, including allowances for anonymity, self-presentation concerns, and the idealized other. For example, patients may feel more comfortable discussing sensitive health-related issues without disclosing their identities to others online rather than in face-to-face communication. Computer-mediated communication also helps to idealize the receiver and to optimize the self-presentation of the sender (Walther, 1996). Because the acquisition of face-to-face social support for persons with health problems may be problematic due to limitations in time, mobility, or access, online support groups may be a particularly useful alternative. Participants can post messages 24 hours a day, 7 days a week or whenever they feel anxiety concerning their disease. Some researchers (e.g., Wellman & Gulia, 1999) suggest that the web has an additional advantage of allowing individuals to seek support from *weak ties*. Weak ties are contacts with those who exist outside the context of family and close friends and can be more objective than close personal relations (Granovetter, 1973). Fogel et al. (2003) found that minority individuals' use of the Internet for breast health issues offers them the perception that someone is talking with them about their health issues, and the Internet offers them tangible benefits including concrete advice about breast cancer.

Although online support holds promise as a new mode of communication for patients and providers, it raises issues regarding inaccurate and misleading information (Lewis & Behana, 2001; Rozmovits & Ziebland, 2004). For example, in Marton's study (2000), participants rated the quality of health information on health Web sites authored by organizations and practitioners quite highly, whereas the quality of health information on unmoderated newsgroups and Web sites developed by individuals was given a low rating. Lamberg (1997b) stated, "The problem with the Internet is not too little information but too much," and cautioned that "novices and savvy Internet users alike can have trouble distinguishing the wheat from the chaff" (p. 1423). Previous findings have noted that one cannot separate web design considerations from content, data should be collected directly from patients, and clinical management suggestions should be provided directly to them (Lewis & Behana, 2001; Marton, 2000). Health care professionals can also benefit by providing accurate information and quality assistance in online support groups (Finn, 1999; LaCoursiere, 2001; Wilson, 2002).

CONTENT ANALYSIS OF DISCUSSION GROUPS

Computer-mediated communication refers to methods of electronic communication such as e-mail, bulletin boards, chat rooms, and instant messaging. Members can exchange information on specific topics, such as diagnosis, treatment, and therapy for breast cancer, through public network-based discussion forums or private services such as subscription-based chat rooms or bulletin boards. Thus, within the context of computer-mediated social support, messages posted during discussions or on listserves may be content-analyzed to determine the topics about which patients and their significant others seek information (Till, 1995).

Prior research has begun to identify the content of messages posted on breast cancer support Web sites. Wienberg et al. (1996) found that breast cancer patients discussed their medical conditions, shared personal concerns, and offered support through a computer bulletin board. The postings of six women who had been diagnosed with breast cancer could be placed into 11 categories including personal and medical information about oneself, concern or liking of other members of the group, and positive aspects or feelings about one's own situation.

Sharf (1997) examined the content of the Breast Cancer List, an unmoderated discussion list supported by the Canadian government, open to researchers, physicians, patients, family, and friends, that focused on the discussion of issues related to breast cancer. The results showed three major dimensions of online communication on the list: (a) exchange of information, (b) social support, and (c) personal empowerment. For example, topics involved political and nonpolitical announcements, informational requests about the disease (i.e., classifications of tumors and diagnoses), medication efficacy and side effects, and patients' concerns about treatments and their relationships with physicians.

Gustafson, McTavish, Hawkins, Pingree, Arora, et al. (1998) studied a sample of patients using the Comprehensive Health Enhancement Support System (CHESS) for obtaining basic information about disease, risk factors, treatment and social support from others. Among 51 elderly women with breast cancer, only 16% of the messages sought treatment information, whereas 71% sought or provided social support. Sheikh (1999) suggested that CHESS could be expanded beyond social and emotional support to include information at the time of diagnosis, information on the prognosis, information on the choice of therapy, and information of a variety of services, such as rehabilitative, cosmetic, occupational therapy, and vocational training services.

Problems With Prior Studies

Prior research that has utilized content analysis of breast cancer online communication suffers from four problems. First, the research was conducted under the assumption that the role of cancer discussion groups or listserves is solely or primarily to provide social support for patients and their friends and family. However, online discussion groups also serve as a cancer information resource on a wide variety of topics (Degner et al., 1997; Rees & Bath, 2000; Sharf, 1997).

Second, prior research has typically described the content from a single discussion group, often sponsored by a formal cancer-related system or list server, rather than cancer discussion groups in general (Gustafson et al., 1998; Sharf, 1997). The individual site may have specific goals and be designed in such a manner as to render the description of its content limited to the context of the site itself.

A third shortcoming of past research on cancer discussion groups is the relatively small sample sizes of postings. Weinberg et al. (1996) examined the messages of only six cancer patients, Gustafson et al. (1998) of only 51 elderly patients, and Alpers, Winzelberg, Classen, Roberts, Dev, et al. (2004) of only nine participants. Also, because the data was collected in the specific setting of a single breast cancer support group for women, generalization to other populations was limited. One study reviewed 10 articles of online cancer support groups (Klemm, Bunnell, Cullen, Soneji, Gibbons, & Holecek, 2003). The researchers confirmed the limitation due to small samples and the fact that the subjects were primarily Caucasian women, thereby limiting the generalizability and thus applicability of the research.

Finally, the published content analyses were not performed systematically and as a result may prove problematic in future replication attempts. Sharf (1997) simply *lurked* on the listserve and described the "flavor of the range and variety of the themes that emerged" (p. 70). Gustafson et al. (1998) did not report their methods to determine the subject matter of the group discussions. Wienberg et al. (1996) reported using two coders to sort the statements into categories, but did not report interrater reliabilities, and provided no theoretical justification for the categories.

The current research avoids the shortcomings of past research. A content analysis of online support groups by Alpers et al. (2004) argued that automatic text analysis may be a powerful tool for helping to understand what is communicated in these groups. They suggested that the discussion patterns would allow moderators to offer new members guidelines for maximizing the benefit they receive from participation. Through the investigation of the content of the messages posted by participants (cancer patients and their friends and families), we can also better determine the subject matter about which individuals seek and provide information. With this knowledge, cancer Web sites may be designed to more closely meet the informational requirements and specific interests of cancer patients and their significant others. New modules (i.e., moderated newsgroups and chat rooms) in health Web sites can be based on the content suggested by participants. Health professionals could then begin to include such sites as part of their information and referral processes. Also, the Internet provides a new opportunity for building patient–provider relationships. Health providers can monitor the accuracy and completeness of the information exchanged online and operate as more effective gatekeepers. The current study demonstrates a reliable and systematic approach for developing a greater comprehension of present and future online communities in the health care industry, specifically cancer support groups.

DATA COLLECTION PROCEDURES

When seeking online health information, the most common places to begin are through a search engine, Internet portal, or hyperlink (Eysenbach & Kohler, 2002; Lazonder, Biemnans, & Wopereis, 2000). Google™ is the most popular search engine. It generates a list of relevant web pages based on keyword search (Brin & Page, 1999). Using Google™, the following search strategy/procedure was performed on October 26, 2004. The key terms "breast cancer discussion groups" were entered, and Google™ identified 625,000 web pages. By default, Google™ only returns pages that include all of the search terms. The first 10 sites listed were inspected to find links to online discussion groups for breast cancer patients and their families.

Because Google™ uses stemming technology, a search includes not only the keyword, but also words that are similar to some or all of those terms. The 10 pages did not all use the same exact keywords, but used related variations of the terms, which were highlighted in the summary of text accompanying each result. The keyword search also generates web directories from Google™ and Yahoo!®. These directories show the search results within a category of interest, allowing users to quickly focus in on the most relevant pages.

In terms of identifying breast cancer discussion groups, the full web address (URL) of each of the 10 Web sites on the list was entered into a browser, and inspected for related links (i.e., support, community, discussion boards, and chat rooms) in each site. The detailed procedures, such as clicking through the hyperlinks and entering the next content page, and descriptions of each site, follow. Six discussion groups were identified and downloaded (two from Cancer Index Menu, and one each from Patient Resources, Le Club Discussion Groups, and BreastCancer.org).

Discussion Group 1: Y-ME National Breast Cancer Organization

The Y-ME National Breast Cancer Organization (www.y-me.org) was founded in 1978 by breast cancer patients Mimi Kaplan and Ann Marcou to provide peer support and fellowship to breast cancer patients. From Google™, the search result links directly to the "national programs and services" page (http://www.y-me.org/programs/default.php). Although several services (i.e., 24-hour hotline, resource links, monthly 1-hour teleconference and quarterly newsletter) are available via the web, the Web site does not have any indication of links to online discussion groups, and therefore was excluded from the study.

Discussion Group 2: CancerIndex Menu: News Groups and Discussion Lists

The URL of Cancer e-mail discussion lists and news groups (http://www.cancerindex.org/clinks10.htm) of the CancerIndex links directly from the Google™ search results screen. The CancerIndex was created by Simon Cotterill to provide a guide to Internet resources about cancer in 1996. Since then, it has provided a directory of key cancer-related sites and resources. The menu of news groups and discussion lists is divided into three categories: e-mail discussion lists, news groups, and interactive chat online. There are eight links under this last subcategory. Among them, the Breast Cancer Chat Room links to a new window of "Cancer Information and International Support." The Web site is extensive and well-organized, with subject headings in alternative medicine, conventional medicine for chemotherapy and radiation, cancer news, and helpful tools for medical symptoms diagnosis. The drop-down menu for support group and cancer boards includes "breast cancer," which connects to the message board (http://www.cancer-info.com/cgi-bin/boards/view.pl?board=breast). Specifically, the messages posted in October, 2004, were downloaded for content analysis. Cancer Survivors OnLine (http://www.cancersurvivors.org/), linked from the CancerIndex menu, was also included in the analysis. The Web site has provided cancer information, resource, and support to all who ask (via e-mail to the Webmaster) since 1997. The site moderates an online community with MSN Groups (CancerSurvivorsOnLine@groups.msn.com) as well as a woman's cancer forum via Microsoft (http://www.groups.msn.com/WomensCancer Forum/_homepage.msnw?pgmarket=en-us), and suggests several useful newsgroups to which users can subscribe. The October messages on MSN Groups were downloaded for the analysis. (The Cancer chat [4-Lane.com] links to OmniChat, an interactive chat system, but messages cannot be downloaded or copied. Cancer Survivors IRC channel [http://www.aoma.com/cs/] currently remains for historical reference, and its online chat service has moved to OncoChat [http://www.oncochat.org], but the messages cannot be downloaded or copied. Of the remaining links on the CancerIndex menu, SarcomaSurvivors could not be located on the server and the Compassionate Friends-Chat room was unrelated to breast cancer.)

Discussion Group 3: Patient Resources: Breast Cancer

Patient Resources: Breast Cancer, from Doctor's Guide (http://www.docguide.com/news/content.nsf/PatientResAllCateg/Breast%20Cancer?OpenDocument), contains hyperlinks for the latest medical news and information for patients or friends/parents of patients diagnosed with breast cancer. The site has the following categories: medical news and alerts; breast cancer information; discussion groups and newsgroups; and other related sites. Under "discussion groups and newsgroups," there are six listed Web links: Alt.support.cancer; sci.med.diseases.cancer; BCANS Discussion Forum; Breast Cancer ListServs; SupportPath.com: Breast Cancer; and TopicA (list directory)—Breast Cancer. Specifically, alt.support.cancer, sci.med.diseases.cancer, and TopicA are newsgroups to which users subscribe for cancer information or newsletters. SupportPath.com could not be found. Breast Cancer ListServs links to Oncolink (http://www.oncolink.upenn.edu/coping/), the web's first cancer resource, founded in 1994 by University of Pennsylvania cancer specialists (Benjamin, Goldwein, Rubin, & McKenna, 1996). However, there are no online discussion groups in OncoLink site.

BCANS discussion forum (http://www.bca.ns.ca/communityforums.html), on the other hand, is primarily an online discussion forum. Breast Cancer Action Nova Scotia (BCANS) was formed in 1994 in Nova Scotia, Canada, to voice the concerns and needs of those affected by breast cancer. The site includes 24/7 online support, user profiles, and biography pages; a breast cancer glossary; "Best of Tips & Hints" from the forum; a searchable archive; online chat; community section; and much more. Specifically, the chat room (http://www.chat.bcans.net/) is a group discussion hosted by any participant who requests and schedules a chat. The messages for October on BCANS were downloaded for analysis.

Discussion Group 4: Online Discussion of Breast Cancer

The Google™ search results linked directly to the Stephens YWCA Encore-Plus Online Discussion of Breast Cancer (http://www.ywcaencore.org/lists.html). This page provides two major services—mailing lists and

Usenet newsgroups. Users can subscribe to the breast cancer mailing list, the IBC (inflammatory breast cancer) mailing list, and the Cancer-L mailing list (a discussion list for patients and families). Usenet offers a list of newsgroups for users to access. Unfortunately, there is no online discussion group on this site. However, the sidebar contains more links for low-cost women's health services, frequently asked questions, ethnic and foreign language breast cancer resources, publications about emotional supports, breast self-examination, and clinical trials.

Discussion Group 5: Le Club Discussion Groups: Coping With Breast Cancer

Le Club Discussion Groups: Coping with Breast Cancer (http://www .womenshealthmatters.ca/cgi-bin/ultimatebb.cgi?ubb=forum;f=2) is an online discussion board of women's health matters. This women's health matters site is based at the Women's College Ambulatory Care Center, which was created in 1998 through an amalgamation of three of Canada's hospitals: Sunnybrook Health Science Centre, Women's College Hospital and Orthopaedic and Arthritic Hospital. It is also an academic center affiliated with the University of Toronto. The Le Club Discussion Groups have several forums involved with different topics, such as "coping with breast cancer." The Le Club Breast Cancer Message Board contained 37 topics with 72 posts (accessed 12/14/04) with posting dates ranging from as early on November 20, 2001 to the latest on November 25, 2004. Participants must register to post and the message board is moderated by two researchers. The messages posted in October, 2004, were downloaded for this study.

Discussion Group 6: BreastCancer.org

BreastCancer.org (http://www.breastcancer.org) is a nonprofit organization dedicated to providing education, information, and community to those touched by the disease. The site is quite extensive and usefully organized into categories such as prevention, symptoms and diagnosis, treatment, research news, ask the experts, recovery and renewal, support and community, and pictures of breast cancer. The chat rooms and discussion boards are listed under "support & community." Users must register or sign in (as a user/member or remain anonymous). There are two open chat rooms available: (1) treatment and beyond, and (2) staying connected. Users choose one of the chat rooms when they first enter, but are able to switch between chat rooms at any time while chatting. However, the chat room messages cannot be downloaded. Online forums, such as "just diagnosed," "help me get through treatment," and "moving beyond cancer," are accessible through the site for patients and their friends and family members to share experiences or concerns in breast cancer. Participants must register to post, but one can enter the discussion boards anonymously for viewing. The messages in October were downloaded for this analysis.

The last four Web sites retrieved with Google™ were extensively inspected but they did not contain any material suitable for the analysis, and were excluded (Google™ Directory—Health > Conditions and Diseases > Cancer > . . . ; Breast Cancer Research—web links; Yahoo!® Directory: Breast Cancer; and Cancer, a list from WebMD).

In summary, the current study collected and analyzed the discussion board messages of (1) Breast Cancer Chat Room (from the Cancer Index); (2) Cancer Survivors OnLine MSN groups (from the Cancer Index); (3) BCANS discussion forum (from Patient Resources); (4) Le Club Discussion Groups; and (5) BreastCancer.org. Due to the extremely large size of the data set compiled by the 6-month-period message downloads from each site, the present study content-analyzed only those messages posted in October 2004. October was chosen because it is National Breast Cancer Awareness Month. Because the population of Web sites with breast cancer discussion groups is not clearly specified, the results from Google™ change over time as new sites are added and others deleted. Thus, there are no standard sampling procedures.

DATA ANALYSIS PROCEDURES

Software

The subject matter of Internet discussion groups concerning breast cancer and the areas of patient concern may be analyzed using computer-based content analysis techniques (for a discussion of these procedures, see Krippendorf, 1980). In particular, the CATPAC program was used to identify and explore the major issues facing cancer patients and their friends and family as discussed in Internet chat rooms (Terra Research and Computing, 1994). CATPAC is best described as a set of programs for analyzing text—such as responses to open-ended question, newspaper articles, transcripts of speeches and broadcasts, or, in this case, textual information expressed in discussion groups concerning breast cancer. CATPAC has been used in various applications to content analyze corporate communication and customer service (Fitzgerald & Doerfel, 2003; Freeman & Barnett, 1994; Jang & Barnett, 1994; Woelfel, 1997), presidential debates or acceptance speeches to their party conventions (Doerfel

& Marsh, 2003), corporate image (Salisbury, 2001), and voice mail (Rice & Danowski, 1993; Sherblom, Reinsch, & Beswick, 2001).

The main advantage of CATPAC is that it does not impose or require the use of *a priori* categories. Instead, word frequency counts, cluster analysis, and multidimensional scaling techniques provide a description of the shared symbols and meanings within a given set of text, which facilitates the identification of categories or themes. In this case, CATPAC was used to determine the main topics of concern for those interested in the treatment of breast cancer. CATPAC performs content analysis through the use of a computer algorithm, and thus is readily replicable. Thus, the reliability of its results are not problematic as is typical for traditional content analysis (Krippendorf, 1980). Also, CATPAC enables the large bodies of discussion messages to be summarized into meaningful conceptual clusters that best present the semantic relations of their constituent words.

Analyses

In this research, CATPAC was used according to the following procedures (see Doerfel & Barnett, 1996, for a detailed discussion). The program first read into memory the text of each of the five sampled Web site's discussion group. CATPAC works by passing a moving window of size *n* through the text file. For example, a window of size 7 (the window size for this study) would read the text seven words at a time (Words 1 through 7), and then slides one word over and reads the next seven (Words 2 through 8). An alternative procedure, not employed in this research, requires the statements for each discussion group to be separated from each other by a delimiter, which allows the analysis of the text in the context of an entire statement, rather than as only single words (Barnett, 1988).

Once read, the program then systematically deletes any cases of a list of "stop" words—including articles, prepositions, transitive verbs, and conjunctions—that over the course of the development and application of the program in past research, have been demonstrated as inconsequential to analysis. Additionally, similar words—for example, two words that share a common root, or the singular and plural forms of the same word—may be combined to facilitate the analysis. For instance, "years" was replaced to "year," "going" was converted to "go," and "weeks" was replaced with "week." The program then counts the occurrences of the remaining words. Words that occur infrequently are ignored to yield a list of the most frequently occurring words present in the sample. CATPAC allows the analyst to determine the number of retained words—in past research (e.g., Jang & Barnett, 1994; Woelfel, 1993) the average number of words used is roughly 100. This figure has proven to consistently allow meaningful analysis of diverse content. From these words, a subset may be selected. For this study, 40 words (56.15% of total words) were retained. CATPAC also allows the user to force the inclusion of infrequently occurring words in the analysis. In this case, the words radiation, tamoxifen, onc (oncology), and mastectomy were included.

The above operation results in a word-by-statement matrix, indicating whether a given word was present in a given statement (or, here, 7-word window) or not. CATPAC then postmultiplies the matrix by its transpose, resulting in a word-by-word matrix. The number in each cell of the matrix represents the number of times each two words have occurred together in the same statement. CATPAC then performs a hierarchical cluster analysis of this cooccurrence matrix (Woelfel, 1997). The program generates a set of outputs denoting the frequency of the most prevalent words (by word frequency and by alphabetic listing), and a visual portrayal of the how these words cluster together (using hierarchical cluster analysis) in symbolic space. Therefore, using this procedure, the major issues discussed by cancer patients and their significant others can be identified and grouped, allowing for interpretation, analysis, and presentation of the results.

A further means of data analysis is to enter the cooccurrence matrix generated by CATPAC into a multidimensional scaling (MDS) algorithm (for a complete discussion of MDS, see Torgerson, 1958). In essence, multidimensional scaling is a mathematical process used to transform numerical distances into spatial representations—the same process that would be required to convert a matrix of inter-city distances into the coordinates (latitude and longitude) of a map. In this way, it is possible to visually portray the relationships among the various issue clusters and the dimensions differentiating the discussants' expressed concerns. This may be accomplished using CATPAC's companion software Thought View (Terra, 1994).

RESULTS

The messages for the month of October for the discussion boards of five Web sites—Breast Cancer Chat Room, Cancer Survivors OnLine MSN groups, BCANS discussion forum, Le Club Discussion Groups, and BreastCancer.org—were downloaded and analyzed. The data set consisted of 12,570 postings or 181,910 lines of text (6.12 Mb). CATPAC was run, retaining the 40 most frequently occurring words in the postings. They are listed in descending as well as alphabetical order in Table 12.1.

TABLE 12.1
Most Frequent Words From Breast Cancer Discussion Groups

Total Words	102151
Total Unique Words	40
Total Episodes	102145
Total Lines	181910

Descending	Frequency List		Alphabetically Sorted List		
Word	Freq	Percentage	Word	Freq	Percentage
I	36282	35.5	AGAIN	1047	1.0
ME	5265	5.2	ANYONE	1048	1.0
CANCER	3524	3.4	BC	1097	1.1
GO	3227	3.2	BEST	1035	1.0
KNOW	3087	3.0	BETTER	1116	1.1
GOOD	2866	2.8	BREAST	2591	2.5
BREAST	2591	2.5	CANCER	3524	3.4
CHEMO	2460	2.4	CHEMO	2460	2.4
YEAR	2206	2.2	DAY	1518	1.5
TIME	2201	2.2	DON'T	2108	2.1
DON'T	2108	2.1	FEEL	1395	1.4
THINK	2040	2.0	GO	3227	3.2
LOVE	1842	1.8	GOOD	2866	2.8
HELP	1662	1.6	GREAT	1056	1.0
HOPE	1648	1.6	HAVING	1058	1.0
WEEK	1594	1.6	HELP	1662	1.6
DAY	1518	1.5	HOPE	1648	1.6
US	1485	1.5	HUGS	1206	1.2
THANKS	1403	1.4	I	36282	35.5
FEEL	1395	1.4	KNOW	3087	3.0
TREATMENT	1337	1.3	LONG	1101	1.1
RIGHT	1307	1.3	LOVE	1842	1.8
PAIN	1303	1.3	MASTECTOMY	775	0.8
HUGS	1206	1.2	ME	5265	5.2
SURGERY	1201	1.2	NEED	1190	1.2
NEED	1190	1.2	ONC	838	0.8
WANT	1171	1.1	PAIN	1303	1.3
BETTER	1116	1.1	RADIATION	1009	1.0
LONG	1101	1.1	RIGHT	1307	1.3
BC	1097	1.1	SURE	1095	1.1
SURE	1095	1.1	SURGERY	1201	1.2
HAVING	1058	1.0	TAMOXIFEN	757	0.7
GREAT	1056	1.0	THANKS	1403	1.4
ANYONE	1048	1.0	THINK	2040	2.0
AGAIN	1047	1.0	TIME	2201	2.2
BEST	1035	1.0	TREATMENT	1337	1.3
RADIATION	1009	1.0	US	1485	1.5
ONC	838	0.8	WANT	1171	1.1
MASTECTOMY	775	0.8	WEEK	1594	1.6
TAMOXIFEN	757	0.7	YEAR	2206	2.2

The most frequent word was "I," which occurred 36,282 times or 35.5% of the total words, and the second most frequent word was "Me" (5,265 occurrences and 5.2% of the total words). This indicates that the individuals who posted message discussed their personal experiences with breast cancer. The next most frequent words were "cancer" (3.4% of the words), and "go" (3.2%). The remaining words were by "know" (3.0%), "good" (2.8%), "breast" (2.5%), "chemo" (2.4%), "year" (2.2%), and "time" (2.2%). These discussions were generally upbeat: frequent words included "good" (2.8% of the individual words), "thanks" (1.4%), "great" (1.0%), and "better" (1.1%), "hope" (1.6%), "hugs" (1.2%), and "love" (1.8%). The only specifically negative term that occurred with some regularity was "pain," which was mentioned 1,303 times or 1.3% of the total.

The cluster analysis revealed two distinctive clusters of content that are represented as icicled dendograms (which are read vertically where the height of the pillars connect the words to represent the strength of their association, see Fig. 12.1). The first cluster focused on medical treatment-related words: "again," "onc" (oncology), "tamoxifen," "surgery," "anyone," "radiation," and "mastectomy." The second, larger, cluster revealed the social support and user's need for affirmation on breast cancer-related information: "bc" (breast cancer), "breast," "cancer," "don't," "think," "good," "I," "me," "love," "year," "know," "thanks," "hope," "go," "time," "right," "us," "long," "day," "week," "chemo," "need," "help," "treatment," and finally words like "feel," "better," "having," and "pain" that showed the emotions the breast cancer patients or families are having or experiencing.

Figure 12.2 displays the results of the MDS of the breast cancer discussions. The MDS revealed the positions that key concepts (discussed by cancer patients and their significant others) occupy in visual space. The stronger the relationship between word clusters, the closer together they are positioned in a multidimensional space, and vice versa. The first primary dimension differentiates social support from medical treatment ("mastectomy" and "surgery"). The second primary dimension differentiates positive words (social support) from breast cancer.

DISCUSSION

This study found that there are extensive resources available online about breast cancer. Web sites provide both medical information about breast cancer and social support for patients and their friends and family. The information and social support is available in many forms, one of which is online discussion groups. During this period, two major subjects were discussed in the online forums: positive social support, and medical treatment information. However, finding and making sense of online cancer

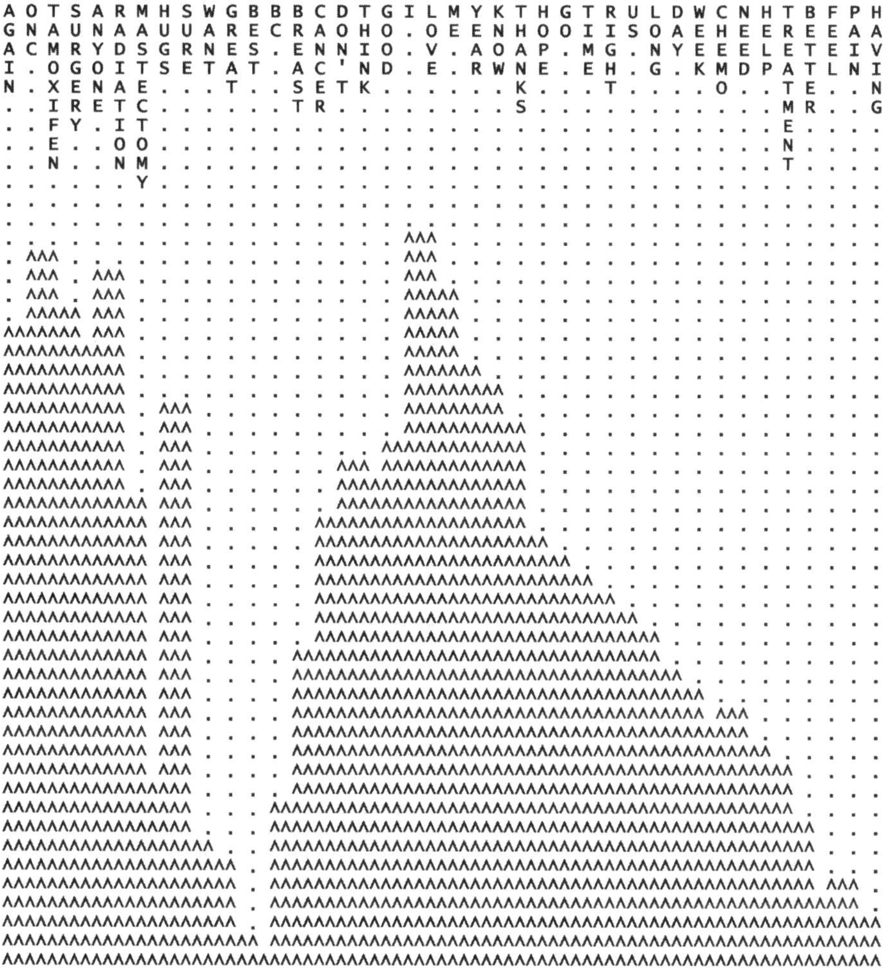

```
A O T S A R M H S W G B B B C D T G I L M Y K T H G T R U L D W C N H T B F P H
G N A U N A A U U A R E C R A O H O . O E E N H O O I I S O A E H E E R E E A A
A C M R Y D S G R N E S . E N N I O . V . A O A P . M G . N Y E E E L E T E I V
I . O G O I T S E T A T . A C ' N D . E . R W N E . E H . G . K M D P A T L N I
N . X E N A E . . . T . . S E T K . . . . . . . K . . . T . . . . O . . T E . . N
. . I R E T C . . . . . T R . . . . . . . S . . . . . . . . . . . M R . . G
. . F Y . I T . . . . . . . . . . . . . . . . . . . . . . . E . . . .
. . E . . O O . . . . . . . . . . . . . . . . . . . . . . . N . . . .
. . N . . N M . . . . . . . . . . . . . . . . . . . . . . . T . . . .
. . . . . . Y . . . . . . . . . . . . . . . . . . . . . . . . . .
```

FIG. 12.1. Hierarchical cluster analysis of most frequent words from breast cancer discussion groups.

discussion groups is not straightforward. The Google™ search results have many pages that did not lead to discussion groups; the five Web sites that contain online discussion boards often require additional navigation through the web; and discussions on the boards may involve extensive postings and text.

The results of this content analysis of breast cancer discussion groups may be applied to the design of web pages. That is, web designers can present information about the topics that breast cancer patients and their

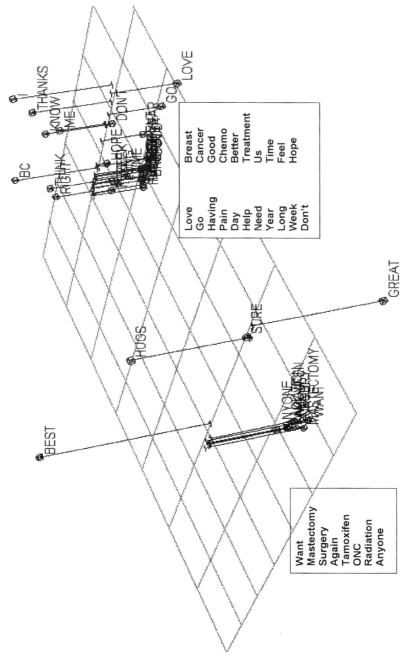

FIG. 12.2. MDS of breast cancer discussion groups.

Love
Go
Having
Pain
Day
Help
Need
Year
Long
Week
Don't

Breast
Cancer
Good
Chemo
Better
Treatment
Us
Time
Feel
Hope

Want
Mastectomy
Surgery
Again
Tamoxifen
ONC
Radiation
Anyone

248

significant others expressed most frequently. For example, key words of the findings specifically expressed participants' concern about surgical procedures, chemo or radiation therapy, and the need for certain information about treatment before and after surgery. Also, the Web site may discuss these subjects using the expressed words of the interested audience rather than using the medical jargon of health professionals. For example, the participants used the symbols "BC" and "ONC" to refer to breast cancer and oncology. Audience- or participant-oriented Web sites should be more effective at communicating cancer treatment information, thus helping patients in seeking proper treatment.

Also, the findings help identify those issues that should be addressed in the communications of health-related agencies, such as the National Cancer Institute, and organizations such as hospitals, managed health care facilities and Women's clinics. These concerns should also be discussed by individual health care professionals who have contacts with patients and their significant others, including nurses, social workers, and counselors and oncologists (Jefford & Tattersall, 2002; Winefield, Coventry, & Lambert, 2004). These topics should be useful in the production of both print and electronic materials designed to inform individuals about breast cancer.

The analytical procedures used in this study may also be performed for other types of cancer and disease, such as discussion groups for male cancers such as prostate and testicular cancer (Pinnock & Jones, 2003; Walling, Maliski, Bogorad, & Litwin, 2004). Males and females seek different types of information online (Wellman & Haythornthwaite, 2002), with women seeking health information to a greater degree. Male disease-oriented discussion groups could be compared with female-disease groups to determine if males and females seek different health information requiring special consideration in Web site design.

As regards the study limitations, the majority of downloaded messages were from the BreastCancer.org (9,513 postings, 75.68%) and BCANS.org (2,944 postings, 23.42%). Future studies should collect more messages from other breast cancer discussion groups for further analysis to facilitate the generalizability of the results. Also, the results were based only on the Google search engine, for 1 month. Future studies should search other Internet resources and search engines (i.e., Netscape Navigator, Alta Vista, Lycos, and Microsoft Internet Explorer) to increase variety in data.

REFERENCES

Alpers, G. W., Winzelberg, A. J., Classen, C., Roberts, H., Dev, P., Koopman, C., & Taylor, C. B. (2004). Evaluation of computerized text analysis in an Internet breast cancer support group. *Computers in Human Behavior, 5, In Press, Corrected Proof.* Retrieved December 5, 2004, from http://www.dx.doi.org, doi:10.1016/j.physletb.2003.10.071

Barnett, G. A. (1988). Communication and organizational culture. In G. M. Goldhaber & G. A. Barnett (Eds.), *Handbook of organizational communication* (pp. 101–130). Norwood, NJ: Ablex.

Benjamin, I., Goldwein, J. W., Rubin, S. C., & McKenna, W. G. (1996). OncoLink: A cancer information resource for gynecologic oncologists and the public on the Internet. *Gynecologic Oncology, 60,* 8–15.

Boman, L., Andersson, J., & Bjorvell, H. (1997). Needs as expressed by women after breast cancer surgery in the setting of a short hospital stay. *Scandinavian Journal of Caring Science, 11,* 25–32.

Braithwaite, D. O., Waldron V. R., & Finn, J. (1999). Communication of social support in computer-mediated groups for persons with disabilities. *Health Communication, 11,* 123–151.

Brennan, P. F., Moore, S. M., Bjornsdottir, G., Jones, J., Visovsky, C., & Rogers, M. (2001). HeartCare: An Internet-based information and support system for patient home recovery after coronary artery bypass graft (CABG) surgery. *Journal of Advanced Nursing, 35*(5), 699–708.

Brennan, P. F., Moore, S. M., & Smyth, K. A. (1992). ComputerLink: Electronic support for the home caregiver. *Advances in Nursing Science, 13,* 14–27.

Brin, S., & Page, L. (1999). *The anatomy of a large-scale hypertextual Web search engine.* Retrieved December 8, 2004, from http://www-db.stanford.edu/~backrub/google.html

Chen, X., & Siu, L. (2001). Impact of the media and the Internet on oncology: Survey of cancer patients and oncologists in Canada. *Journal of Clinical Oncology, 19*(23), 4291–4297.

Degner, L. F., Kristjanson, L. J., Bowman, D., Sloan, J. A., Carriere, K. C., O'Neil, J., Bilodeau, B., Watson, P., Mueller, B. (1997). Information needs and decisional preferences in women with breast cancer. *Journal of the American Medical Association, 277,* 1485–1492.

Dickerson, S. S., Flaig, D. M., & Kennedy, M. C. (2000). Therapeutic connection: Help seeking on the Internet for persons with implantable cardioverter defibrillators. *Journal of Acute and Critical Care, 29*(4), 248–255.

Doerfel, M. L., & Barnett, G. A. (1996). The use of CATPAC for text analysis. *Cultural Anthropology Methods, 8,* 4–7.

Doerfel, M. L., & Marsh, P. S. (2003). Candidate-issue positioning in the context of presidential debates. *Journal of Applied Communication Research, 31*(3), 212–237.

Eysenbach, G., & Kohler, C. (2002). How do consumers search for and appraise health information on the World Wide Web? *British Medical Journal, 324,* 573–577.

Finn, J. (1999). An exploration of helping processes in an online self-help group focusing on issues of disability. *Health and Social Work, 24*(3), 220–231.

Fitzgerald, G., & Doerfel, M. L. (2003). Don't overlook the value of customer communication. *CRM Guru,* Retrieved November 5, 2004, from http://www.crmguru.custhelp .com/cgi-bin/crmguru.cfg/php/enduser/std_adp.php?p_faqid=1152.

Fogel, J. (2004). Internet breast health information use and coping among women with breast cancer. *Cyberpsychology & Behavior, 7*(1), 59–63.

Fogel, J., Albert, S. M., Schnabel, F., Ditkoff, B. A., & Neugut, A. I. (2002). Internet use and social support in women with breast cancer. *Health Psychology, 21*(4), 398–404.

Fogel, J., Albert, S. M., Schnabel, F., Ditkoff, B. A., & Neugut, A. I. (2003). Racial/ethnic differences and potential psychological benefits in use of the Internet by women with breast cancer. *Psycho-Oncology, 12,* 107–117.

Freeman, C. A., & Barnett, G. A. (1994). An alternative approach to using interpretative theory to examine corporate messages and organizational culture. In L. Thayer & G. A.

Barnett (Eds.), *Organizational communication emerging perspectives IV* (pp. 60–73). Norwood, NJ: Ablex.

Granovetter, M. (1973). The strength of weak ties. *American Journal of Sociology, 73,* 1361–1380.

Gustafson, D. H., McTavish, F., Hawkins, R., Pingree, S., Arora, N, Mendenhall, J., & Simmons, G. E. (1998). Computer support for elderly women with breast cancer. *Journal of the American Medical Association, 280,* 1305.

Hilton, B. A. (1993). Issues, problems, and challenges for families coping with breast cancer. *Seminars in Oncology Nursing, 9,* 88–100.

Jang, H., & Barnett, G. A. (1994). Cultural differences in organizational communication: A semantic network analysis. *Bulletin de Methodologie Sociologique, 44,* 31–59.

Jefford, M., & Tattersall M. H. N. (2002). Informing and involving cancer patients in their own care. *Oncology, 3,* 629–637.

Johnson, K. B., Ravert, R. D., & Everton, A. (2001). Hopkins Teen Central: Assessment of an Internet-based support system for children with cystic fibrosis. *Pediatrics, 107*(2), 396.

Klemm, P., Bunnell, D., Cullen, M., Soneji, R., Gibbons, P., & Holecek, A. (2003). Online cancer support groups: A review of the research literature. *CIN: Computers, Informatics, Nursing, 21*(3), 136–142.

Krippendorf, K. (1980). *Content analysis: An introduction to its methodology.* Beverly Hills: Sage.

Kristjanson, L. J., & Ashcroft, T. (1994). The family's cancer journey: A literature review. *Cancer Nursing, 17,* 1–17.

LaCoursiere, S. P. (2001). A theory of online social support. *Advances in Nursing Science, 24*(1), 60–77.

Lamberg, L. (1997a). Computers enter mainstream psychiatry. *Journal of the American Medical Association, 278*(10), 799–801.

Lamberg, L. (1997b). Online support group helps patients live with, learn more about the rare skin cancer CTCL-MF. *Journal of the American Medical Association, 277,* 1422–1423.

Lazonder, A., Biemnans, J., & Wopereis, I. (2000). Differences between novice and experienced users in searching information on the World Wide Web. *Journal of the American Society for Information Science, 51,* 576–581.

Lewis, D., & Behana, K. (2001). The Internet as a resource for consumer healthcare. *Disease Management & Health Outcomes, 9*(5), 214–247.

Lieberman, D. (1992). The computer's potential role in health education. *Health Communication, 4,* 211–225.

Lieberman, M. A., Golant, M., Giese-Davis, J., Winzlenberg, A., Benjamin, H., Humphreys, K., Kronenwetter, C., Russo, S., & Spiegel, D. (2003). Electronic support groups for breast carcinoma: A clinical trial of effectiveness. *Cancer, 97*(4), 920–925.

Marton, C. (2000). Evaluating the Women's Health Matters Website. *CyberPsychology & Behavior, 3,* 747–760.

Michie, S., Rosebert, C., Heaversedge, J., Madden, S., & Parbhoo, S. (1996). The effects of difference kinds of information on women attending an out-patient breast clinic. *Psychology, Health and Medicine, 1,* 285–296.

Murero, M., D' Ancona, G., & Karamanoukian, H. (2001). Use of the Internet in patients before and after cardiac surgery: An interdisciplinary study. *Journal of Medical Internet Research, 3,* e27. Retrieved December 2, 2005, from http://www.jmir.org/2001/3/e27/

Pinnock, C. B., & Jones, C. (2003). Meeting the information needs of Australian men with prostate cancer by way of the Internet. *Urology, 61*(6), 1198–1203.

Rees, C. E., & Bath, P. A. (2000). The information needs and source preferences of women with breast cancer and their family members: A review of the literature published between 1988 and 1998. *Journal of Advanced Nursing, 31*(4), 833–841.

Rice, R. E., & Danowski, J. (1993). Is it really just like a fancy answering machine? Comparing semantic networks of different types of voice mail users. *Journal of Business Communication, 30*(4), 369–397.

Rice, R. E., & Katz, J. E. (2001). *The Internet and health communication: Expectations and experiences.* Thousand Oaks, CA: Sage.

Ritchie, H., & Blank, P. (2003). The promise of the Internet for disability: A study of on-line services and Web site accessibility at Centers for Independent Living. *Behavioral Sciences and the Law, 21*, 5–26.

Rozmovits, L., & Ziebland, S. (2004). What do patients with prostate or breast cancer want from an Internet site? A qualitative study of information needs. *Patient Education and Counseling, 53*, 57–64.

Salisbury, J. G. T. (2001). Using neural networks to assess corporate image. In M. West (Ed.), *Progress in communication sciences, Vol. 17: Applications of computer content analysis* (pp. 65–86). Westport, CT: Ablex.

Santoro, E. (2003). Internet and information on breast cancer: An overview. *The Breast, 12*, 424–431.

Scheerhorn, D., Warisse, J., & McNeilis, K. (1995). Computer-based telecommunication among an illness-related community: Design, delivery, early use, and the functions of HIGHnet. *Health Communication, 7*, 301–325.

Sharf, B. F. (1997). Communicating breast cancer on-line: Support and empowerment on the Internet. *Women & Health, 26*, 65–84.

Shaw, C. R., Wilson, S. A., & O'Brien, M. E. (1994). Information needs prior to breast biopsy. *Clinical Nursing Research, 3*, 119–131.

Sheikh, K. (1999). Computer-based support systems for women with breast cancer. *Journal of the American Medical Association, 281*, 1268.

Sherblom, J. C., Reinsch, N. L. Jr., & Beswick, R. W. (2001). Intersubjective semantic meanings emergent in a work group: A neural network content analysis of voice mail. In M. West (Ed.), *Progress in communication sciences, Vol. 17: Applications of computer content analysis* (pp. 33–50). Westport, CT: Ablex.

Smyth, K. A., & Harris, P. B. (1993). Using telecomputing to provide information and support to caregivers of persons with dementia. *Gerontologist, 33*, 123–127.

Sutter, J. D. (2001). Cancer center web site adds online support group, *Continuum,* March–April, 20–21.

Terra Research and Computing. (1994). *The GALILEO computer program.* Ithaca, NY: Rah Press.

Till, J. E. (1995). Discussion groups on the Internet. *Canadian Journal of Oncology, 5*, 379–380.

Torgerson, W. S. (1958). *Theory and methods of scaling.* New York: Wiley.

Turner, J. W., Grube, J. A., & Meyers, J. (2001). Developing an optimal match within on-line communities: An exploration of CMC support communities and traditional support. *Journal of Communication, 51*, 231–251.

Walling, A. M., Maliski, S., Bogorad, A., & Litwin, M. S. (2004). Assessment of content completeness and accuracy of prostate cancer patients' education materials. *Patient Education and Counseling, 54*, 337–343.

Walther, J. (1996). Computer-mediated communication: Impersonal, interpersonal, and hyperpersonal interaction. *Communication Research, 23*, 3–43.

Wellman, B., & Haythornthwaite (2002). *The Internet in everyday life.* Oxford: Blackwell.

Wellman, B., & Gulia, M. (1999). Net surfers don't ride alone: Virtual communities as communities. In M. A. Smith, & P. Kollock (Eds.), *Communities in cyberspace* (pp. 167–194). London: Routledge.

Wienberg, N., Schmale, J., Uken, J., & Wessel, K. (1995). Computer-mediated support groups. *Social Work with Groups, 17*(4), 43–54.

Wienberg, N., Schmale, J., Uken, J., & Wessel, K. (1996). Online help: Cancer patients participate in a computer-mediated support group. *Health and Social Work, 21,* 24–29.

Wilson, P. (2002). How to find the good and avoid the bad or ugly: A short guide to tools for rating quality of health information on the Internet. *British Medical Journal, 324,* 598–602.

Winefield, H. R., Coventry, B. J., & Lambert, V. (2004). Setting up a health education website: Practical advice for health professionals. *Patient Education and Counseling, 53,* 175–182.

Winzelberg, A. (1997). The analysis of an electronic support group for individuals with eating disorders. *Computers in Human Behavior, 13*(3), 393–407.

Winzelberg, A., Classen, C., Alpers, G. W., Roberts, H., Koopman, C., Adams, R. E., Ernst, H., Dev, P., & Taylor, C. B. (2003). Evaluation of an Internet support group for women with primary breast cancer. *Cancer, 97*(5), 1164–1173.

Woelfel, J. (1993). Cognitive processes and communication networks: A general theory. In W. D. Richards, & G. A. Barnett (Eds.), *Progress in communication science* (pp. 221–242). Norwood, NJ: Ablex.

Woelfel, J. (1997). Attitudes on nonhierarchical clusters in neural networks. In G. A. Barnett & F. J. Boster (Eds.), *Progress in communication science: Advances in persuasion* (pp. 213–228). Greenwich, CT: Ablex.

World Health Organization. (2005). IARC Database. Retrieved February 9, 2005, from http://www-depdb.iarc.fr/ and http://www.who.int/whosis/

Ziebland, S. (2004). The importance of being expert: The quest for cancer information on the Internet. *Social Science & Medicine, 59,* 1783–1793.

Ziebland, S., Chapple, A., Dumelow, C., Evans, J., Prinjha, S., & Rozmovits, L. (2004). How the Internet affects patients' experience of cancer: A qualitative study. *British Medical Journal, 328*(7439), 564–570.

Designing and Implementing Virtual Patient Support Communities: A German Case Study*

Jan Marco Leimeister
Technische Universität München, Germany

Helmut Krcmar
Technische Universität München, Germany

Virtual Communities (VC) can be defined as a group of people who gather because of a common interest, problem, or task and whose members are independent of time and space for interacting (for similar definitions see Armstrong & Hagel, 1996; Mynatt, Adler, Ito, & O'Day, 1997; Preece, 2000; Schubert, 1999). Therefore, virtual communities have great potential to serve ubiquitous needs. Such an omnipresent problem situation exists for instance in health care, when patients develop a desire for information and communication that exceeds the resources of the treating physician. From the characterization of virtual health care communities as ubiquitous information and interaction spaces, we have derived design requirements for VCs as well as for the process of developing a community platform. The results are transferred into the health care domain, particularly into the situation of cancer patients. On this basis, we give an overview of our experiences with the development of a community platform for cancer patients. In closing, we put special emphasis on the possibilities and challenges of mobile technologies for virtual health care communities.

*The research project COSMOS (Community Online Services and Mobile Solutions) is a joint project of the Technische Universität München and O2 (Germany) GMBH & Co. OHG. The project is supported by the Ministry of Education and Research FKZ 01 HW 0107–0110. Further information can be found under http://www.cosmos-community .org

RESEARCH DESIGN AND RESEARCH PLAN

Research design describes the key objectives of the research project, what methods will be used for data collection and analysis, as well as how the research process shall take place. The objective of this venture is to plan, build, introduce, and evaluate IS-platforms for cancer patients (see Fig. 13.1). As usual in pilot projects, the starting-point of this research is a socioorganizational problem—in this case, the situation of cancer patients after they leave hospital.

The objective of the field studies was to study cancer patients' needs and to analyze already available web-based offers for cancer patients. Therefore, we analyzed the situation of cancer patients in general with a standardized questionnaire, followed by in-depth studies in five different cancer self-help groups with approximately 100 active members. Methods applied here were case studies (Yin, 1989), ethnographic analysis, semistructured interviews, observations, and document analysis. After that, web-based information and interaction opportunities were in-

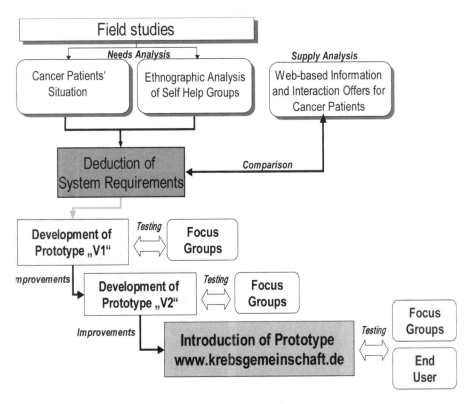

FIG. 13.1.   Research plan.

vestigated. Finally, identified cancer patients' needs and already available interaction opportunities were compared. The results of the analysis were used for designing an IS-platform. This platform was implemented in the field, and improvements in the system were made during the remainder of the project. On this basis, the development of the prototype began, using an iterative process model in order to allow a high degree of user involvement in the development process. After several iterations, the prototype was introduced to public on August 18th, 2002. The platform is being tested continuously by users and additionally by focus groups in controlled settings.

FIELD STUDIES

Needs Analysis of Cancer Patients

Patients' needs and demands for information often increase after a diagnosis of a disease or during medical treatment (Sheppherd, Charmock, & Gann, 1999). These demands can be the result of asymmetric information, for instance between patients and physicians. Patients may seek information to help them make sense of a cancer diagnosis or to provide them with information that assists them in making informed decisions about treatment. Besides demands for factual information, there can be a desire to seek emotional support and to communicate with other patients.

These behaviors, such as participating in self-help groups, can play an important role in dealing emotionally with a disease (for an overview, see Hasebrook, 1993). If we assume that there is a correlation between the threat to quality of life imposed by a cancer diagnosis and the need to seek and obtain knowledge and support (e.g., Eysenbach, 2000), the potential benefit of cancer-related communities becomes evident. However, the diversity of more than 100 types of cancer, the diversity of the presentation of the same disease in two patients, the complexity of treatment modalities coupled with the hardly manageable extensive professional and lay literature in this area, all combine to make coping with cancer, even through participation in virtual communities, extremely difficult.

Recent research on cancer patients' informational demands (e.g., Kaminski, Thomas, Charnley, & Mackay, 2001) demonstrates a strong information interest in the following areas: side effects/"how I will feel"; explanation of disease and prognosis; treatment options and explanations of therapy; logistical issues (transportation, work, etc.); lifestyle issues (exercise, diet, sexuality, smoking); follow-up/"what happens after therapy finishes?"; and support or self-help groups, alternative medicine. Above these information demands, books of cancer survivors such as

Lance Armstrong (2001) and their huge success show that cancer patients also have strong desires for emotional support and empathy.

Many of patients' needs to find answers to perceived and real problems as well as informational needs can be solved through self-help groups. Self-help groups exist in many major cities for a number of different types of cancer. According to information provided by the AOK, Germany's largest health insurance company, only approximately 5 to 10% of cancer patients take part in self-help groups. Reasons for this can be, among others, that interested patients are unable to locate a group in their vicinity or that meeting times of groups do not fit the individual schedules. Very often, integration into a group plays an important role, and, in particular, fear and mistrust in "strangers" are often experienced. Taking part in self-help groups is linked with talking about a very intimate subject like one's disease and symptoms, therefore, is a very uncomfortable situation for most patients.

These circumstances of real-life communities, on one hand, and the demand for information and interaction, on the other, show the great potential of virtual health care communities as ubiquitous information and interaction spaces for solving these problems. Broad-based and enlightening information showing advantages and disadvantages of alternative treatments as well as infrastructure issues such as, where one can obtain what type of treatment is not provided. In order to enable patients to be autonomous in their decision making, a solid basis in prior-related research is necessary.

Empirical Findings of Conducted Field Studies

During the European Week against Cancer (October, 2002) a standardized questionnaire was distributed to approximately 500 visitors, with 116 responding. More than 60% of the cancer patients agree with the question that their physician has a big information advantage. One third of them agree in parts to the statement that they want to look for information on the Internet. Approximately 28.8% of the female cancer patients use mobile phone as well as the Internet; by men, mobile phones are used by 56.3% and the Internet, 43.8%. More than two thirds agreed in part that they want to communicate more with other patients. These statements emphasize the need for web-based or mobile information and interaction services.

Additionally we conducted ethnographic analysis of self-help groups. We conducted narrative interviews with self-help group leaders and several semistructured interviews with the group members. The results showed that there is a lack of information and interaction possibilities for cancer patients and their relatives. The patients want and need information about their specific type of cancer, treatment, or hospital. Most of the members of self-help groups found it important to share information and to speak with other patients in the same or similar situations. They got hope and encouragement when they saw one of the members recovering. Even if the meetings just took place quarterly, the members called each other by telephone very often to get advice from others. Some members traveled a long way to their self-help group meetings. The use of materials and tools like mobile phones, personal digital assistants, or the Internet correlated with the average age of the group and the age of the members. In some groups, almost all members had mobile phones and used the Internet.

Unrestricted access to valid, understandable, and relevant information, as well as the possibility to contact other patients of the self-help group at any time, was considered as very important. But this approach is only possible for members of self-help groups and therefore not for the majority of cancer patients. Thus our results confirm cancer patients' demands for information and interaction services.

Analysis of Web-Based Information and Interaction Offers for Cancer Patients

Until the start of the project (mid-2001) a working virtual community for cancer patients could not be identified on a European level (German- or English-speaking). Only in the United States were we able to find first approaches towards virtual cancer patient communities (Daum, Klein, Leimeister, & Krcmar, 2001). Existing Internet services in German language offered mostly content without user-interaction possibilities. Additionally, hardly any services focused on quality assurance of their content or target-group specific editing of their content (e.g., most offered medical content was almost not understandable by lay people). Concerning mobile services support for access through mobile devices, we could not identify any services in the German-speaking Internet. Therefore, a pilot project for developing a community platform for cancer patients was initiated.

REQUIREMENTS AND THE DEVELOPMENT PROCESS

The Dilemma of Requirements Collection

Although software development is usually done within an organizational framework, many of the developed information systems do not match the needs of the target users. Many orphaned community platforms on the Internet underline this. Traditionally, system development takes place in a linear manner, starting with the conception phase and ending with the phase of the death or substitution of the system. Many alternative models have been developed, as the linear model has many dysfunctional aspects (see Boehm, 1988). The Internet as a possible environment for an information system, especially with its heterogeneous user groups, demands more flexibility, and involves a high degree of uncertainty concerning how hardware and software will be used.

The collection of requirements often takes place very early in the development process and is transferred into a requirements specification. Little attention is paid to the alteration or adaptation of already acquired requirements during the following phases. There is little time and space to pick up on new requirements in most processes. Mistakes within the requirements specification and the management of customer requirements reduce system quality and generate high costs for ongoing system corrections.

Therefore the collection of requirements should be emphasized and the target user should be involved in early stages of the software development cycle. The requirements engineering approach tries to fulfill this request. Requirements engineering is defined by the IEEE Std. 610.12 as "(1) the process of studying user needs to arrive at a definition of . . . requirements; and (2) the process of studying and refining . . . requirements" (1990, cited in Hoffmann, 2000). It also emphasizes the fact that requirements can change during the development process. In order to develop a platform that meets users' needs, requirements engineering addresses many essential success factors for system development and is therefore a suitable framework for the development of a community platform in general. There are many activities and methods reported in the literature that guide and support the discovery of requirements (for an overview see Hoffmann, 2000), but are they applicable for our purpose and can they be combined with a process model for system development?

Although considering many published approaches,[1] we did not find an appropriate model that combined both an applicable process for the development of a platform on the Internet and the inclusion of require-

---

[1]Process models for the development of community platforms in general can either be derived from existing information system development approaches (for an overview, see Boehm, 1989) or from community informatics works with a rather social science perspective on community (platform) building like Preece (2000) or Kim (1999). But none of the existing approaches seems to be appropriate because they are either not detailed or feasible enough or too extensive for being manageable for smaller projects. The development of information and interaction platforms for patients in general, or cancer patients in particular, has special requirements that are hard to integrate in existing process models for system development.

ments engineering activities that involve intense participation of targeted users, and certainly none with a proven track record.

Requirements Deducted From Prior Field Studies

The results of prior field studies about the information and interaction needs of cancer patients (see earlier discussion or Leimeister, Daum, & Krcmar, 2002) and the examination of existing web-based information platforms on the German language market (see earlier discussion and Daum et al., 2001) lead to the general requirements listed in Table 13.1.

Starting with these first requirements, the process model for community platform engineering has to allow the integration of parallel activities of requirements engineering in order to provide the flexibility needed for the development of a platform for cancer patients on the Internet. Therefore, an applicable process model should: be an iterative process; be able to adapt to changes of requirements during the development process; include several builds of prototypes; be easy to apply especially for small and medium size projects; be applicable for different types of services (information as well as interaction); and involve users and/or experts from the beginning. The following suggests a process model that meets these preconditions.

A Community Platform Engineering Process

The objective of this section is to describe a process model for developing an information system, a community platform for cancer patients. Because system requirements are neither completely nor exactly defined, a linear model does not fit the uncertainty that arises from the field. An iterative model seems to be more appropriate. Starting out with general requirements, the system can be built step by step. The outcome of each stage of the iterative development should be evaluated. Within each iteration, however, the type of development should be shaped by the demands of the situation. Figure 13.2 shows the process model COPEP (Community Platform Engineering Process) that was used during the development of the Internet platform http://www.krebsgemeinschaft.de for the target group of breast cancer patients.

The heart of this model is an iterative process, adapted from the generic spiral process model (Boehm, 1988; Wigand, Picot, & Reichwald, 1998). It is combined with a prototyping approach. Each iteration consists of four phases: planning, analysis, engineering, and evaluation. Different from the original spiral model, a much stronger focus has to be put on the building of prototypes and the involvement of users in evaluation. The goal of the engineering phase of each iteration is the building of

TABLE 13.1
Deduced Requirements From Field Studies (Arnold, Leimeister, & Krcmar, 2003)

Results/Section	General Requirements for a Community Platform for Cancer Patients	Implications for a Process Model
Development of Platform	• The envisioned community platform is an *innovation*. No comparable system exists on the German-speaking Internet (none offers interaction possibilities). Therefore all the *requirements cannot be collected in advance* or copied from existing platforms; moreover they appear and change during the development process. Activities should be ongoing throughout the development to collect and evaluate requirements. • The future environment of the system, the Internet itself, opposes a *flexible design of the front end*. Aspects such as size of screen, supported types of browsers, and transfer rates must be taken into consideration within the development process. • The targeted users, patients, are often not familiar with the use of the Internet or information systems in general and therefore are not able to transfer their needs into a concrete design of Web site services. The development must involve representatives for the target users. Groups of experts, for example, can function as representatives at the very beginning of the development cycle until there is something tangible, like a demonstration prototype that can be presented to the patients for evaluation.	• Iterative process necessary. • High degree of user involvement necessary. • Use of prototypes for demonstration purposes and testing on the Internet is necessary.
Target Group	• The *navigation* of the platform should be *intuitive* as most cancer patients are older and unfamiliar with the use of the Internet (for similar findings see, e.g., Binsted, Cawsey, & Jones, 1995). The use of colors, a constant navigation bar, larger font size and the *avoidance of fancy features* (flash-animations, mouse-over, etc.) is advisable. • Trust is a crucial element for target group, therefore access-right structures that support the development of trust and that support real-life situations and interactions are necessary (Leimeister, Ebner, & Krcmar, 2005).	• Use of mock-ups and prototypes for demonstration purposes is necessary. • Process has to include access-right structures development • Process must adapt to changes of requirements during development.
Content for Platform	• The platform should have an *information section* as well as *interaction possibilities*. • The offered *information must be trustworthy and comprehensible* for patients.	• Development process should be applicable for different types of services (information and interaction services).

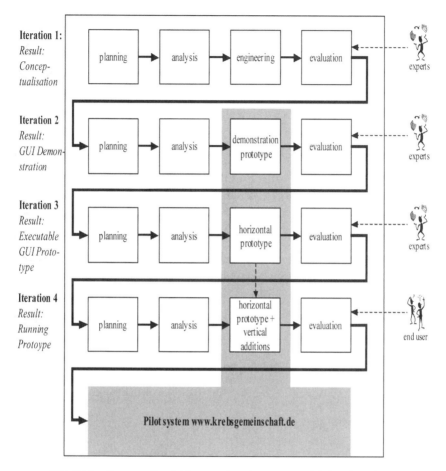

FIG. 13.2. Community platform engineering process with four iterations combining a spiral model with prototyping elements (shaded; Arnold, Leimeister, & Krcmar, 2003).

a prototype in order to get a tangible version of parts or the whole product very early in the development process. After the evaluation phase, the second iteration starts over with planning again, but applying experiences from the previous iteration.

As Fig. 13.2 shows, each prototype undergoes an evaluation at the end of its development cycle. That allows a high degree of involvement of target users, with experts as their representatives. The method used for evaluation was a mixture of interviews and group discussions. We presented the results of each cycle to a group of experts (Iteration 1 to 3) and to a group of patients (Iteration 4 and during the run of the prototype). Their feedback was integrated into the planning of the next iteration. The prototype was introduced to a broader public on August 18th, 2002.

Through an early involvement of various stakeholders in the development cycle and the visualization of parts of the end product through prototyping, COPEP counters the danger of dragging inappropriate requirements, fixed in the beginning, into the end product. General requirements get more detailed as the development process goes on, and mistakes made in the beginning can be redefined.

DESIGN OF AN ONLINE PLATFORM FOR CANCER PATIENTS

Sociotechnical System Design

Our research has shown, so far, that a sociotechnical design for virtual health care communities has to consider (among others) the following issues (see also Leimeister et al., 2002):

- Creation of a virtual information and interaction space with appropriate communication channels according to cancer patients needs.
- Trustworthy operators (no financial interest in the subject, explicit competence in medical issues, etc.) of the community platform and transparency about the source of funds in order to support the development of trust.
- Competent content managers for the quality assurance of centrally provided content.
- Access-right structures that support the development of trust and that also support real-life situations and interactions.
- The provision of tools for working with shared material for supporting group activities that have been successfully used in computer-supported meetings.
- The facility for an active community management to remotely monitor and control the participants' information and interaction spaces and the tools within the system (an equivalent for the role of a self-help group leader in order to avoid problems known from real-life groups like charlatanism, etc.).

Cancer patients migrate between different contexts, such as different hospitals and medical centers, work, and home. Hospitals or medical professionals remain their most important source of information (Kaminski et al., 2001), but information and interaction desires are ubiquitous and are not limited to physicians' office hours. Besides that, there are other needs than just medical knowledge retrieval. The desire for social peer-to-peer interaction, and emotional support is independent of time, cost, or stage of disease and mobility, and also of structures required by self-help groups (Hasebrook, 1993). Opening oneself to others, dealing with very intimate and private issues requires an intimate environment. Trust could be, as always, identified as a very critical issue.

Thus we suggest (in accordance with Gryczan & Züllighoven, 1992) providing useful digital tools and digital materials for cancer patients. Tools allow modification and processing of material. In the tradition of computer-supported collaborative work, tools can enable users to communicate, to coordinate common tasks or to cooperate on shared material (Krcmar & Klein, 2001). Trust-related issues can be approached through a high priority of data security and a highly specialized and scalable authorization concept.

Therefore, we propose an approach using the room metaphor for software design (for details, see also Schwabe & Krcmar, 2000). Its advantages—from the point of view of software engineering—lie in several aspects: It allows an intuitive handling of documents, offers easy-to-access appropriate structures, and supports existing ways of cooperation and coordination in social structures (Schwabe & Krcmar, 2000).

Three types of information and interaction spaces seem to be useful for cancer patients: (a) A "private room," where the user can store private information, documents, links, and have direct communication with others only after having them invited to join; (b) a "public room," where all members and visitors of the virtual community can see all information and documents and search for information; and (c) a "group room," which is restricted to members of a group (e.g., like the self-help groups) and provides all group members access to all documents in this group room and all group-related issues. This is especially supported through the results of our ethnographic studies of self-help groups, where almost all active members stated strong interest in maintaining their usual social group structures combined with the wish for unrestricted access to information and spontaneous interaction with others.

Architecture and System Requirements

In order to fulfill the deduced requirements on a community platform, a client-server solution is utilized, whose architecture consists mostly of three layers (data, application, and presentation layer; see Fig. 13.3). This architecture allows high scalability and flexibility of the system, as well as extensions by context-sensitive elements. It also offers the advantage of making a modular structure of the platform possible. Furthermore,

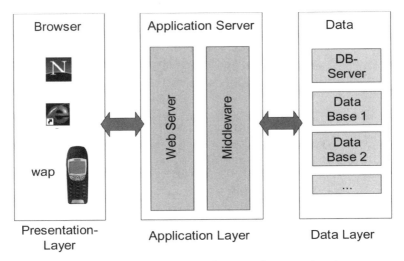

FIG. 13.3.   Three-layer architecture of community-support systems.

different standards (for example XML/XSL, HTML, WML, JDBC, and HTTP(S)) are supported by this system, thus permitting support for any access device using a browser (web-browser, WAP-mobile-browser, etc.).

The presentation layer regulates the communication between client and server. It is possible to spread it over several computers. Because it carries the major part of the load, systems are quite scalable. This layer receives inquiries of users in HTML or WML, converts them in XML, and responds in XML-pages, which are again converted into HTML- or WML-pages. The protocol used for communication between the client and the presentation layer is mostly "http" but other protocols, in particular WAP for mobile devices, may also be used. The application layer responds to inquiries of the presentation layer and takes charge of central functions of the administration. Nearly all the functions of the community are provided on the server side. Typical functions include, for example, calendaring or chat modules.

In the data-retention layer, information is saved permanently. The system provides interfaces that are tied into the data-retention systems and that can be applied to the data storage. SQL-compatible databases are supported. In the ideal case, it is irrelevant for the application layer, which system is used for the data storage. It accesses structures that are reflected on the respectively available data retention system. Thereby, the application components can be developed independently of the system on which they are based. Thus, for example, the integration of existing data sources can be managed.

Applying COPEP: Iterative Development
of http://www.krebsgemeinschaft.de

The following provides a summary of the development steps during each iteration with a focus on the findings from the concluding group discussions either with patients or with experts (for further details, see Arnold et al., 2003).

User Involvement.   COPEP counters the danger of fixating incorrect requirements during the initial phases of development by involving end users early on in the development cycle. Visualization of parts of the end product through mock-ups, scenario discussion, and prototyping induce a high level of transparency. General requirements get more detailed as the development process progresses, and mistakes can be redefined. The targeted users—in our case, breast cancer patients—are often unfamiliar with the use of the Internet or information systems in general. The proposed community platform was somewhat difficult for them to envision. It was also difficult for them to transfer their needs into a concrete design of a Web site from scratch. Further, their fragile medical state prohibited prolonged and unrestricted access to them as collaborative partners. In order to meet the substantial claim of user involvement from the very beginning, representatives for the target users were substituted as consultants for the project. The role of target group representatives is to take up various positions of the system until there are mock-ups or prototypes functioning as visualization that can be presented to the intended end users. We used a group of various stakeholders as representatives (see Table 13.2) in order to work with as many perspectives on the system as possible.

Once the content for the platform is roughly outlined and the case scenarios are conceptualized (in our case, at the end of the third iteration) the target users can more easily get involved. At this point in development, the target users are provided with the intermediate result as a basis for further design, adaptation, and detailing.

Results of the First Iteration.   Based on the general requirements we designed a draft of what kind of services the platform should contain. For the categorization, we used the suggested composition by Brunold, Merz, and Wagner (2000). They work with four main sections: information, communication, participation, and orientation category. As seen earlier, the orientation category is very important because the target group is not so familiar with the use of the Internet.

TABLE 13.2
Representatives During the Development

Representatives	Competence
Two associates of a cancer patient hotline from the German Cancer Research Center (KID), Krebsinformationsdienst Heidelberg	Familiarity with cancer patients' information needs and usual questions asked. Know comprehensible language for patients.
One associate of the largest German public health insurance	Familiarity with cancer patients. Know-how in disease-management programs.
One communication theorist	Communication theory. Computer-mediated communication.
Two associates of the Applied Informatics Department, Technische Universität München	Technical specification. Computer programming.
Two associates of the interdisciplinary tumour centre (ITZ), Tübingen	Execution of information sessions for patients. Medical know-how.
Three associates of the Information Systems Department, at the University of Hohenheim	Community engineering. Human–computer interaction.
Two associates of the collaborative cancer centre (OSP), Stuttgart	Execution of information sessions patients. Medical know-how.

The concept (see Fig. 13.4) was approved in the discussion by the experts. Possible services that match the needs of the patients were collected in a brainstorming session. Moreover, the evaluation lead to the requirement that the platform has to be divided into a public and a private space in order to protect users of the platform from anonymous invasion. Especially the interaction and participation services should only be usable after a previous registration and login.

Results of the Second Iteration. The work in the second iteration focuses on the design of the front end. It is made tangible for evaluation with the help of a demonstration prototype (see Fig. 13.5). Furthermore, the information section is planned in further detail and the color scheme is determined: orange, yellow, and white should mediate warmth, brightness, optimism, and hope. According to the reading habits of web users and the distribution of attention on Web sites, subcategories are placed within the sections. An evaluation by experts lead to the result that some services were put into different categories and aspects that seem to be more important are placed accordingly (for example: soft facts like sports and cancer, or nutrition tips, are summarized in a new subcategory "how to deal with cancer").

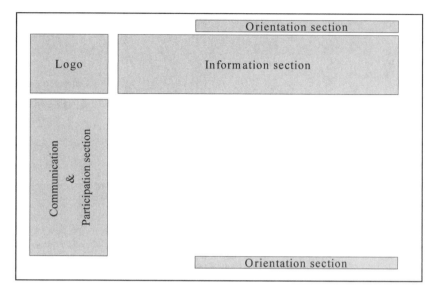

FIG. 13.4.   Division into sections (Arnold et al., 2003).

Results of the Third Iteration.   The third iteration focuses on vertical supplements of the demonstration prototype. A map showing what pages are linked is the base for further development. Furthermore, the communication and participation section is planned in more detail. The evaluation at the end of the third iteration produced only a few new aspects, which showed us that it was time to present the system to real users.

Results of the Fourth Iteration.   At the end of the forth iteration, a runable prototype exists that is shown to end users, a group of patients who have only little knowledge of the use of the Internet. At the beginning, the users somewhat disassociated themselves from the system because of their suspicion against the Internet in general. Throughout the discussion, however, they became excited about the system and had only a few complaints. We implemented their recommendations to emphasize certain categories that are more important than others (e.g., emphasizing the tips from the experts in Iteration 2).

Going Live.   A prototype for the target-group breast cancer patients was introduced to a broader public on August 18th, 2002. An evaluation of the running platform is currently carried out by taking into account click streams, typical behavior of heavy users, and feedback about the design of the platform from users and experts. Based on this evaluation, the

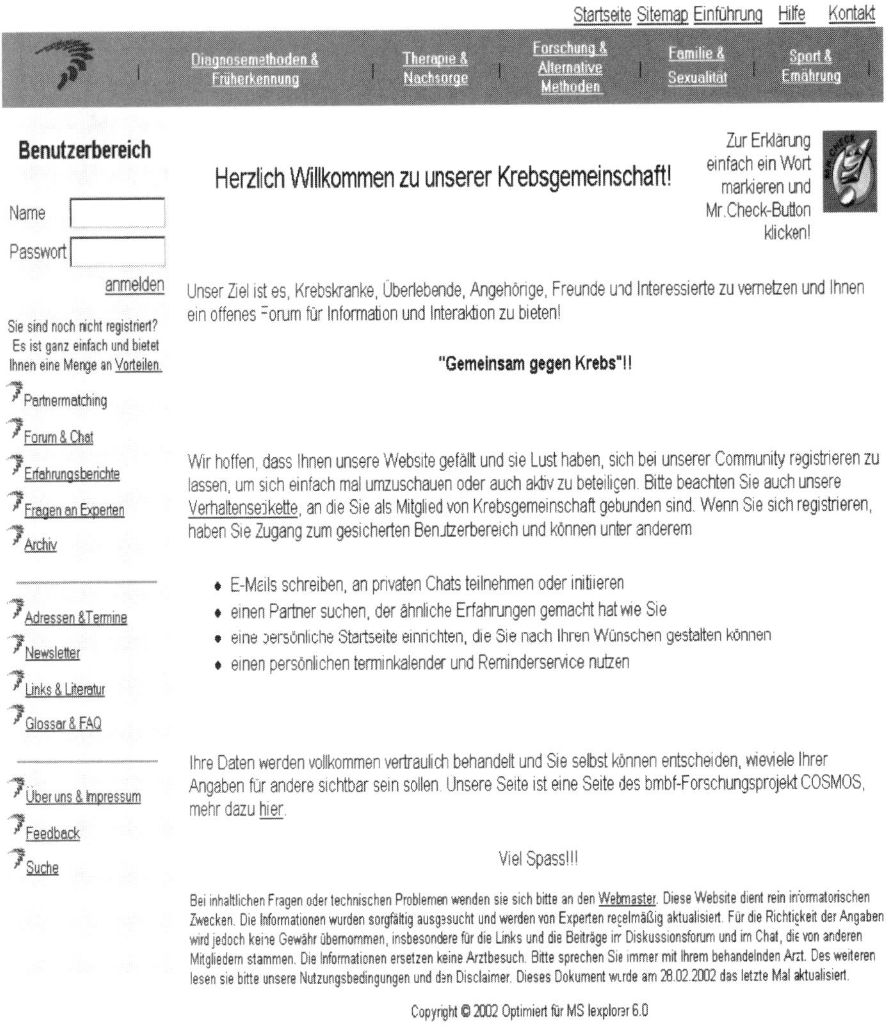

FIG. 13.5.   Demonstration prototype (Arnold et al., 2003).

platform can be considered successful and, thus, COPEP has its first proven track of applicability.

As of early 2005, there are approximately 1,300 registered users on the platform for breast cancer patients, with new registrations daily. Accompanying the continual refinement of the platform, an evaluation of the running platform is conducted, taking into account click streams, typical behavior of heavy users, content analysis of the entries of the personal guest books, feedback about the design of the platform via e-mail, user surveys, and group discussions with cancer patients.

The feedback of the users about the design of the navigation and the structure of the breast cancer community was very positive (for additional details on the evaluation of the platform see Leimeister, 2004; Leimeister et al., 2005). Therefore a second platform—for the target group of leukemia patients—was structured and designed the same way. Only the information area was changed because of the higher variety of diseases within leukemia. This Internet community was introduced to a broader public on May 21st, 2003.

Separation Into Different Areas Should Provide Transparency

It is of great importance in the health care field to identify and segregate scientific and user-generated content. Patients are probably not aware of the difference between facts and opinions. This has legal consequences with respect to liability issues, as well as to quality assurance issues of user-generated content. A possible solution for the problem of separation between centrally provided and quality-assured content and user-generated content is to emphasize the difference through design—here made possible with the use of tabs at the top of the page (all centrally provided content is found here in the horizontal "content bar") and marking all the user-generated content (mostly found under on the vertical "functionality bar") throughout the page with a disclaimer (see Fig. 13.6). This should provide transparency as to the source of the information.

Users can only communicate or generate content as long as they are logged on to the platform. The first registration process is standardized and should guarantee that the identity of prospective users is double-checked before allowing new users access to all functionalities. Taking usability aspects into consideration, another reason for segregation of content and functionality comes into play: Usability of Web sites is considered better when content ("content bar") and functionalities (here aggregated to an interaction area, or "functionality bar") are located on different areas of the page. Components that provide the possibility of communication with each other are placed on the left of the screen within the interaction area. This area is only accessible after registration.

Private Space and Personalization

Parts of a private room as stated earlier are realized within the individual welcome page. This page is only visible to the user after login (see Fig. 13.7).There the user has access to his or her personal mailbox; he or she can modify his or her personal data and decide which part of the data should be visible to other community members. Beyond that, he or she

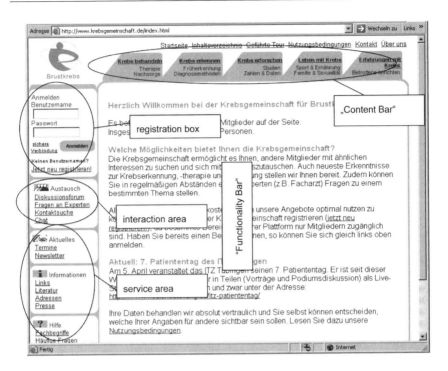

FIG. 13.6. Starting page of http://www.brustkrebs.krebsgemeinschaft
.de—A Platform for Breast Cancer Patients.

can create a list of friends (buddy list) who have access to more of his or her data than the rest of the community. The possibility to give individual recommendations to other users of the community completes the service of the "private" room. Recommendations could be links to other interesting Web sites, addresses of good clinics, helpful literature or references to related events.

Projected Development: Notifications and Rating Possibilities

In order to encourage a more lively community and to intensify the integration of user-generated content there are several projected components, including that the buddy list will be extended by a notification tool. Each time a user logs on or does a certain action on the platform, his or her buddies get a message. Another projected component is the possibility that the scientific content should be rateable by users. They will be able to comment on the user-generated content as well as the centrally provided content, in order to give each other or new users an orientation.

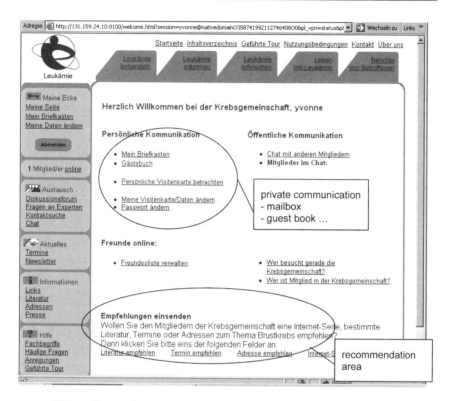

FIG. 13.7. The personal page of http://www.leukaemie. krebsgemeinschaft.de—A Platform for Leukaemia Patients.

ADDING VALUE THROUGH MOBILE SERVICES

Another promising area for the extension and improvement of virtual communities is the sector of mobile devices and mobile services. They can add value to traditional web-based communities for several reasons. They extend and/or improve already existing services. Figure 13.8 visualizes some possibly value-adding services.

Through ubiquitous access to already existing web-based services, community members have the possibility to inform themselves and to interact with others at any place and at any time. The second point concerns secure and easy user authentication. Users of mobile devices normally carry their device with them and their device is technically easy to identify (e.g., via the SIM–Card and/or the device ID). This and a personal PIN allows for easy and feasible possibilities for user identification (e.g., automated log-in procedures, etc.). Another improvement concerns already existing reminder services on the Internet. SMS-based reminder

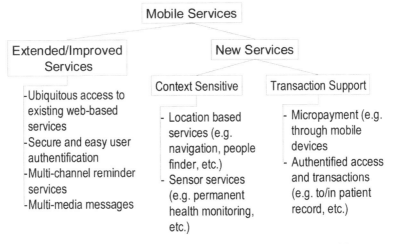

FIG. 13.8.   Mobile services for adding value to virtual communities.

services, for instance for the next medical examination or especially for drugs/pills, are by far more efficient. Most mobile devices are "always on" and close to the user; therefore the reminder reaches its addressee more often and better, in contrast to a mailbox on the Internet.

The other class of advantages refers to new services enabled through new mobile devices. These devices support context-sensitive and location-based services. That means, for instance awareness services of who (buddy) or what (location) is around. These services can be push-or-pull services. Push service means that information is offered by the mobile device that a certain person/location is nearby. If it is a pull service, the user has to take some action to request the information he wants. Furthermore, it is possible to choose context and location attributes for selecting contacts, for example spontaneous matchmaking. Of course, the user can specify rules and parameters such as when, how, and for whom they want to be reachable. Other new services in the medical field are emergency services. It is possible to monitor parameters such as blood pressure, pulse rate, temperature, or electrocardiograms. They can be transmitted to a service center or to a physician. If necessary (life-threatening parameters), an emergency call can be generated automatically and, through the location/ positioning service, the patient can be found easily. Another kind of new mobile services deals with transaction support, such as micropayments through a mobile device. But there are many more possible applications to come. Which services might be valuable to cancer patients, in general, and to members of a cancer patient community, in particular, has yet to be investigated. With the COSMOS project, we hope to clarify some of the issues concerning mobile services for cancer patients.

SUMMARY AND OUTLOOK

Virtual communities are a very promising approach for overcoming information asymmetries and for supporting interaction. Especially for cancer patients, it seems to be a very promising model, because cancer patients have strong and ubiquitous demands for valid and trustworthy information and intensive wishes for empathy and interaction with other peers in similar situations. We outlined how a systematic design of a virtual community for cancer patients in Germany can be achieved. On the basis of in-depth field studies and with the application of an iterative development process, we have shown how requirements for community engineering and system development in this domain look like and what kind of components can be useful for a virtual community for patients. Mobile services have the potential to add significant value to virtual communities and especially the aspects of ubiquitous access to a community and its members and new services enabled through new mobile technologies seems very promising.

REFERENCES

Armstrong, A., & Hagel III, J. (1996). The real value of online communities. *Harvard Business Review, 74*(3), 134–141.

Armstrong, L. (2001). *It's not about the bike: My journey back to life.* London: Yellow Jersey Press.

Arnold, Y., Leimeister, J. M., & Krcmar, H. (2003, June). *COPEP: A development process model for a community platform for cancer patients.* Paper presented at the Eleventh European Conference on Information Systems (ECIS), Naples, Italy.

Balzert, B. (1998). *Lehrbuch der softwaretechnik: Software management, software qualitätssicherung, Unternehmensmodellierung.* Heidelberg: Spektrum Akademischer Verlag.

Binsted, K., Cawsey, A., & Jones, R. (1995). Generated personalized patient information using the medical record. In P. Barahona, M. Stefanelli, & J. Wyatt (Eds.), *Proceedings of the Fifth Conference on Artificial Intelligence and Medicine Europe* (pp. 29–41). New York: Springer.

Boehm, B. W. (1988). A spiral model of software development and enhancement. *Computer, 21*(5), 61–72.

Brunold, J., Merz, H., & Wagner, J. (2000). *www.cyber-communities.de—Virtual communities: Strategie, umsetzung, erfolgsfaktoren.* Landsberg/Lech: mi, Verlag Moderne Industrie.

Daum, M., Klein, A., Leimeister, J. M., & Krcmar, H. (2001). *Webbasierte informations- und interaktionsangebote für onkologiepatienten—ein überblick. Arbeitspapier Nr. 109.* Hohenheim: Universität Hohenheim, Lehrstuhl für Wirtschaftsinformatik.

Eysenbach, G. (2000). Consumer health informatics. *British Medical Journal,* (320), 1713–1716.

Gryczan, G., & Züllighoven, H. (1992). Objektorientierte systementwicklung: Leitbild und entwicklungsdokumente. *Informatik Spektrum, 15*(5), 264–272.

Hasebrook, J. (1993). Krebs-Selbsthilfegruppen—Untersuchungen zu bedarf, funktionen und wirksamkeit. In F. A. H. Muthny, Gunther (Ed.), *Onkologie im psychosozialen*

Kontext—Spektrum psychoonkologischer Forschung, zentrale Ergebnisse und klinishe Bedeutung (pp. 260–275). Heidelberg, Germany: Roland Asanger Verlag.

Hoffmann, H. F. (2000). *Requirements engineering: A situated discovery process.* Wiesbaden, Germany: Deutscher Universitäts-Verlag und Gabler Verlag.

Kaminski, E., Thomas, R. J., Charnley, S., & Mackay, J. (2001). Measuring patients' response to received information. *European Journal of Cancer, 37*(Supplement 6), 387.

Kim, A. J. (1999). *Secret strategies for successful online communities/Community-building on the web.* Berkeley, CA: Peachpit Press.

Krcmar, H., & Klein, A. (2001). Computer supported cooperative work. In P. U. A. Mertens (Ed.), *Lexikon der Wirtschaftsinformatik* (4th ed., pp. 113–114). Berlin: Springer.

Leimeister, J. M. (2004). *Pilotierung virtueller Communities im Gesundheitsbereich—Bedarfsgerechte Entwicklung, Einführung und Betrieb.* Unpublished dissertation, Universität Hohenheim, Stuttgart.

Leimeister, J. M., Daum, M., & Krcmar, H. (2002). Mobile virtual healthcare communities: An approach to community engineering for cancer patients. In S. Wrycza (Ed.), *Proceedings of the 10th European Conference on Information Systems, ECIS* (pp. 1626–1637). Gdansk, Poland.

Leimeister, J. M., Ebner, W., & Krcmar, H. (2005). Design, implementation and evaluation of trust-supporting components in virtual communities for patients. *Journal of Management Information Systems, 21*(4).

Mynatt, E. D., Adler, A., Ito, M., & O'Day, V. (1997). *Design for network communities.* Paper presented at the Computer Human Interaction Conference (CHI 97), Atlanta.

Preece, J. (2000). *Online communities: Designing usability, supporting sociability.* New York: Wiley.

Schubert, P. (1999). *Virtuelle Transaktionsgemeinschaften im Electronic Commerce: Management, Marketing und Soziale Umwelt.* Lohmar, Köln, Germany: Josef Eul Verlag.

Schwabe, G., & Krcmar, H. (2000, July). *Digital material in a political work context: The case of Cuparla.* Paper presented at the Proceedings of the 8th European Conference on Information Systems ECIS 2000, Vienna.

Sheppherd, S., Charmock, D., & Gann, B. (1999). Helping patients access high quality health information. *British Medical Journal,* (319), 764–766.

Wigand, R., Picot, A., & Reichwald, R. (1998). *Information, organization and management: Expanding corporate boundaries.* New York: Wiley.

Yin, R. K. (1989). Research design issues in using the case study method to study management information systems. In J. I. Cash & P. R. Lawrence (Eds.), *The information systems research challenge: Qualitative research methods* (pp. 1–6). Boston, MA: Harvard University Press.

V

PRACTICE AND INFRASTRUCTURE

Technology and Health Information Privacy: Consumers and the Adoption of Digital Medical Records Technology

Kier Wallis
University of California, Santa Barbara

Ronald E. Rice
University of California, Santa Barbara

NATIONAL AND REGIONAL IMPLEMENTATIONS OF DIGITAL MEDIAL RECORDS

This chapter investigates consumer concerns, knowledge, and level of awareness of digital medical records (DMRs) technology, and privacy and identifies those factors most strongly related to consumers' potential adoption or rejection of the technology.

Digital Medical Records

The nature of health care in the United States, largely HMO-based, is driving the implementation of DMRs, also known as electronic health records (EHRs) in response to a demand for data transparency. Gunter and Terry (2005) described the EHR as "a longitudinal collection of elec-

---

*The authors would like to acknowledge, and thank, the six regional health care administrators who shared their thoughts during the stakeholder interviews; the students and employees who participated in the focus groups and surveys; the Arthur N. Rupe endowed Professorship in the Social Effects of Mass Communication, and an Undergraduate Research and Creative Activities grant, for financial support; and especially Mr. Mike Skinner, Executive Director of the SBCCDE, for his guidance, contacts, expertise, and support. Due to space limitations, much detail is missing in this chapter; see http://www.comm.ucsb.edu/faculty/rrice/sbccde.pdf for complete literature review and tables.

tronic health information from individual patients and populations" (p. 2). Concerns about medical mistakes, the widespread occurrence of ambulatory care, and the increasing responsibility among patients for their health care are among the reasons DMRs have become a priority for health care providers. However, providers must also respond to patient demands for privacy, access, correction, and consent, as well as legislative demands for legal compliance (Gunter & Terry, 2005).

DMRs are credited with improving health care by reducing medical errors, eliminating handwritten clinical notes, enabling error-reducing technologies, increasing the consistency of medical records, and providing data for research (Reynolds, 2003). Several studies have also cited benefits for both physicians and patients (Hassol, Walker, Kidder, Rokita, Young, et al., 2004; Joustra-Enquist & Eklund, 2004). For example, Wang, Lau, Matsen, and Kim (2004) developed a web-based personal health record (PHR) for patients to collect and manage their health information (medical history, past surgeries, medications, and allergies), to request self-referrals, and to store a record of their consultations. Thirty-two patients completed a survey in which 85% of respondents were satisfied with the usability and 94% were satisfied with the overall online referral process. Using DMRs in hospital databases was demonstrated to help ensure consistent and correct coding by physicians, as well as context-sensitive treatment (Muller, Burkle, Irps, Roeder, & Prokosch, 2003). A study of the 30% of physicians using DMRs in 2003 reported that 78% saw an improvement in patient satisfaction, 87% said it allowed them to deliver better care, and 89% saw improved compliance with managed care (Harris Interactive, 2003). One health record exchange pilot project involving three Indianapolis hospitals found an average reduction of $27 in costs per patient visit (mostly from reducing waste and duplication; Ferris, 2005b).

Connecting for Health (2005) reported on a series of focus groups and national surveys investigating the public's awareness of and willingness to adopt an EMR. They found that people have a limited understanding of health IT today. When presented with messages about the potential benefits of PHRs, more than half said they had never thought about concepts such as (a) "I should have access to my health information anywhere, anytime," or (b) "My own online medical record would help me get all my doctors on the same page when they treat me." Yet, 72% of the respondents to their 2004 survey strongly or somewhat agreed that they wanted to be involved in medical decisions that affect them, and having their own medical record would help them make better decisions; and 62% strongly or somewhat agreed that they would like to have all their health information in one place, and obtain it with a click of the mouse.

Participants in the 2003 focus groups reported a strong desire to have total control of their personal health information, wanting the power to decide who could and could not access their record and an expectation that they should provide explicit consent to any access. However, preferences for how to access this information varied by age; under 45, the Internet was the most preferred channel (33%), whereas over 45, paper was most preferred (34%). Their 2003 survey of online Americans (Connecting for Health, 2003) found these medical services desired by the respective percents: e-mail my doctor (75%), track immunizations (69%), note mistakes in record (69%), transfer information to new doctors (65%), and get and track test results (63%). Still, 96% were most comfortable with their primary care doctors having access to their medical record (58% preferred their doctor's office to be the host of an online medical record system), and less comfortable with the idea of having family members (69%) and their health insurance company (65%) having access.

The development of the current DMR model in the United States has focused on establishing data interoperability and comparability (Gunter & Terry, 2005), using a system in which patients "pull" or censor certain information in their records, although the exact amount of patient authority remains unclear. Such a pull system is intended to maximize the flow of patient data, enabling valuable research, although some critics worry it may result in a loss of patient privacy and confidentiality.

Regional health information organizations (RHIOs) are responding to this initiative. More than 100 have been formed, comprising community institutions such as hospitals, physicians, government agencies, insurers, laboratories, employers, and consumers. And more than 20 are already exchanging health care information (Ferris, 2005a). But funding and cost recovery for RHIOs is still very uncertain. There is no agreement yet as to whether individuals, insurance companies, government agencies, hospitals, or others who pay medical bills will fund these systems (Ferris, 2005b).

THEORY: DIFFUSION OF INNOVATIONS, TECHNOLOGY AND HEALTH INFORMATION PRIVACY

Rogers's (1983) Diffusion of Innovations theory, and Smith, Milberg, and Burke's (1996) Information Privacy theory will be used to frame the investigation of the relationship between technology and privacy, and their relationship to the implementation of DMRs in Santa Barbara County.

Technology Diffusion

A new technology faces various challenges to successful diffusion within its potential community (Aydin & Rice, 1991; Davis, 1993; Rogers, 1983). Different obstacles apply at every level, influencing adoption and reinvention of an innovation (Johnson & Rice, 1987; Rice & Anderson, 1994), and among prospective consumers (Davis, 1993; Demiris & Eysenbach, 2002; Mandl, Szolovits, & Kohane, 2001; Rogers, 1983). Of particular interest to this study are the characteristics of the diffusion process among the upcoming generation of consumers, as they have greater familiarity and comfort with technology.

Rogers (1983) identified five characteristics of innovations central to the effective diffusion of any new technology: relative advantage, compatibility, complexity, trialability, and observability. Consumers perceiving a new technology to rate high on these characteristics, with the exception of complexity, are more likely to adopt the technology. Other models emphasize the importance of characteristics similar to those established by Rogers. For example, the technology acceptance model (Davis, 1993) recognizes the importance of consumers' attitudes toward a technology as a main determinant of their actual technology use. Davis (1993) identified two main technology components influencing consumers' attitudes—perceived usefulness and perceived ease of use—which correspond with Rogers's (1983) descriptions of relative advantage and complexity, respectively. Also, Mandl et al. (2001) noted six desirable characteristics of DMRs: comprehensiveness, accessibility, interoperability, confidentiality, accountability, and flexibility, all of which reflect the five innovation characteristics.

Relative advantage is the "degree to which an innovation is perceived as better than the idea it supersedes" (Rogers, 1983, p. 15). In the case of individuals' DMRs, relative advantage may be conceptualized as the innovation's benefits in comparison to traditional paper records, such as the improvement of patient care and safety, the reduction of medical errors, and the positive financial return to health care organizations (Chin, 2001; Wang, Middleton, Prosser, Bardon, Spurr, et al., 2003). Some of the qualities that might indicate relative advantage for consumers include accessibility, accountability, and flexibility (Mandl et al., 2001). *Compatibility* is "the degree to which an innovation is perceived as being consistent with the existing values, past experiences, and needs of potential adopters" (p. 15). Innovations inconsistent with the value system of potential adopters are likely to be rejected. Important consumer values may include personal health and health of loved ones, the ability to control their own health care, and privacy (Alpert, 2003; Jeffords, 1999; Mandl et al., 2001). *Complexity* is "the degree to which an innovation is perceived as difficult to understand and use" (p. 15). Not all consumers are equally able to use, understand, and benefit from new technologies. An important consideration under complexity is self efficacy, or one's perceived ability to perform a specific task (Bandura, 1997). Thus, individuals who have greater expertise with Internet technology and use it more frequently are more likely to be comfortable adopting a new Internet-based technology. However, some health care recipients, such as the elderly or individuals with chronic illnesses, may not be as adept at using the Internet, or have functional limitations preventing them from access (Demiris & Eysenbach, 2002). *Trialability* is "the degree to which an innovation may be experimented with on a limited basis" (p. 16). This may pertain to the extent of the commitment required of the consumer, or to the user's ability to release and then later restrict access to a DMR (Mandl et al., 2001). *Observability* is "the degree to which the results of an innovation are visible to others" (p. 15). In diffusing a new technology, publicly displaying an innovation's positive consequences is likely to aid in reducing consumer uncertainty surrounding the new technology. Although uncertainty is an inevitable companion to innovation (Rogers, 1983), consumers' outcome expectations have been found to impact actual technology use (Compeau & Higgins, 1991).

Privacy and Technology

Public opinion has demonstrated the growing importance of privacy in today's information-saturated society (Udo, 2001). Metzger and Docter (2003) reviewed public opinion polls, industry positions, enacted legislation and proposed legislation about online privacy protection, between 1998 and 2001. They considered online privacy concerns to include anonymity, intrusion (spam, data mining), surveillance (individual and public—especially since the Uniting and Strengthening America Act 2001, commonly referred to as the Patriot Act), and autonomy. Over two thirds of one survey's respondents felt that their ability to control the collection of personal information was extremely important (Harris Interactive, 2003). Most (85% to 97%) Web sites collect at least one type of personal information, generally without user consent, whereas other sites also sell customer information to third parties. Averaged across a number of polls, three quarters of respondents (74%) were "very" or "somewhat" concerned about privacy when using Internet, though concerns declined a bit with increased Internet experience, and when using familiar e-commerce sites. Six primary concerns about users' rights emerged from this review with from 60% to 89% supporting or concerned about: Notice, choice, access, security of information, enforcement, and children's online privacy rights. Metzger and Docter (2003) concluded that "existing and proposed Internet privacy legislation fails to address the full range of consumers' concern" (p. 366), with little fulfillment of the six principles. Most sites rely on self-regulation, and there is little prospect of new legislation protecting individuals' privacy being passed, especially after the increased powers of law enforcement agencies after the terrorist attacks of 9/11 in the United States.

The risks and benefits associated with information technology have resulted in tension between the information-collecting organization and the consumer, and the consumer is caught in the position of both victim and beneficiary. As competitors in the marketplace have harnessed information technology to collect and assemble data into usable and marketable forms, the general public is not convinced that the benefits of information technology outweigh its costs (Culnan & Armstrong, 1999). Having lost the ability to control collection and use of personal information raises concerns in accordance with Westin's (1967) definition of privacy as the ability to control the collection and use of personal information. Smith et al. (1996) identified four factors that affect an individual's level of privacy concern: (1) unauthorized secondary use, (2) improper access, (3) collection, and (4) errors.

The traditional realm of information privacy has been affected by the rapid growth of computer and digital technology, leading to an increasing number of medical records stored in a digital or electronic format (Jeffords, 1999; Li & Shaw, 2004; Nasser & Alpert, 1999; Swartz, 2004). The transfer of data from traditional paper to the new digital format has resulted in increased concerns among the patient population, and has prompted at least some new legislation to establish privacy guidelines (Alpert, 2003; Fedorowicz & Ray, 2004; Li & Shaw, 2004; Swartz, 2004). In the Connected for Health (2003) survey of online users, nearly all (91%) were very concerned about privacy and health information security, but most felt that technology provides appropriate protections. People with chronic illness and frequent health care users were less concerned about privacy and security.

The most notable legislation relevant to DMRs is the Health Insurance Portability and Accountability Act (HIPAA), which is designed to ensure the integrity of patient information as it travels between health care providers, insurers, and data-clearing houses (Epstein, 2002; Fedorowicz & Ray, 2004; Health Privacy Project, 2004; U.S. Department of Health and Human Services, 2000; 2001). HIPAA establishes requirements for health care organizations intended to maintain an acceptable level of privacy, to be enforced by severe punishments for the misuse of patient information. Health care entities, specifically health plans, health care clearinghouses, and health care providers who conduct transactions electronically, were required to achieve HIPAA compliance by April 14, 2003 (U.S. Department of Health and Human Services, 2004). Recent public comments (more than 500 responders and more than 5,000 pages) on the National Health Information Network (NHIN) and health records exchanges in the United States, provided to the Department of Health and Human Services, emphasized that such a system must be patient-oriented, with safeguards to protect personal health information privacy (Brewin, 2005).

A recent integrated set of recommendations (Connecting for Health, 2005) argued that such a health information environment must: (a) facilitate effective connectivity for the delivery of high quality health care; (b) provide timely access to information; (c) empower patients to access and control their own information and contribute to the quality of care provided; (d) support the application of "intelligent" tools to improve health and health care; (e) facilitate the appropriate aggregation of data for public health, research, and quality assessment; and (f) enable improvements in the quality of clinical care. Patients must be able to: (a) choose whether or not to participate in sharing personally identifiable information; (b) exercise their rights under HIPAA; (c) control who has access to their records (whether in whole or in part); (d) see who has accessed their information; (e) review, contribute to, and amend their records (without unreasonable fees); (f) receive paper or electronic copies of their information; and (g) reliably and securely share all or portions of their records among institutions. Once patient consent has been granted for a certain type of information access, however, information should be able to be accessed freely in a trusted environment.

Relationship Between Technology Adoption and Health Information Privacy

The factors contributing to privacy concern may be discussed as subsets of many of the technology diffusion characteristics, especially relative advantage, compatibility, and complexity. Privacy concerns corresponding to the proposed security of DMRs are an important factor when evaluating the technology in terms of relative advantage. Several improvements over paper records have been cited, including increased security (Shoesmith, 2001), and improved health care quality (Alpert, 2003; Shoesmith, 2001). Critics of DMRs are concerned that the misuse of information (Alpert, 2003) might ultimately result in a compromised level of patient care, negating any advantage of the digital system in comparison to paper records. The CHCF found that one in six adults reported having done something "out of the ordinary" to prevent the disclosure of their medical information, including avoiding medical care all together (California HealthCare Foundation, 1999). Therefore, improper access, unauthorized use, and error, whether system or human error (Smith et al., 1996), may contribute to a lower evaluation of DMRs in terms of relative advantage.

Similar concerns reverberate in terms of the technology's compatibility with consumers' current value systems and needs. Privacy is an important value to consumers (Alpert, 2003; Jeffords, 1999; Mandl et al., 2001), and it is likely that any privacy violation would reduce consumers' beliefs that DMRs are compatible with their value systems. Also, the collection of information for DMRs, depending on the level of communication between the collecting organization and individual, might be linked to compatibility, as consumers have been found to value control over their personal information and its disclosure to third parties (Milberg, Smith, & Burke, 2000). Errors would indicate that the digital system is overly complex for its intended users, and due to the sensitive nature of personal medical information, the possibility for error is extremely important in determining a consumer's adoption or rejection of DMRs. If an individual is not convinced that the system will store or provide reliable and accurate data, it is unlikely that he or she will spend time with the system, leading to rejection.

METHODS: SITE, STAKEHOLDER INTERVIEWS AND FOCUS GROUPS

The study used a variety of methods to summarize, integrate, and identify factors influencing potential users' responses toward DMRs. First we discuss the site, the stakeholder interviews and focus group discussions, and their results.

Site: SBCCDE

The Santa Barbara County Care Data Exchange (SBCCDE), a major regional health infrastructure project, is in the process of implementing digital medical records (DMRs) technology in Santa Barbara County, California, and is subject to evaluation by the general public and medical community (Care Science, 2005). The SBCCDE cites its mission as "assisting all physicians, caregivers, and consumers in Santa Barbara County to locate and facilitate the sharing of patient data held by multiple health care organizations . . . thereby increasing the quality, safety, and efficiency of care delivery." The SBCCDE, founded in 1998, is currently testing its technology, the Care Data Exchange (CDE), and preparing for its diffusion into local hospitals, health care organizations, and the community at large (McGee, 2003). The SBCCDE project is a small-scale extension of the larger national plan to institute a national electronic health information infrastructure (McGee, 2003; U.S. Dept. of Health and Human Services, 2004). (For an online demonstration/explanation of Healthcare Collaborative Networks, prepared in 2003, using three case studies—preventative care, outbreak alert, and monitoring adverse drug events—see: http://www.connectingforhealth.org/resources/HCN_24.html.)

Stakeholder Interviews

Six interviews were conducted with individuals representing institutions the executive director of the SBCCDE identified as major stakeholders in the CDE project, including Cottage Hospital, Santa Barbara Regional Health Authority, Sansum Medical Foundation, Santa Barbara Public Health Authority, a community business professional, and a participating physician. The interviews, all conducted by the same researcher, lasted approximately 90 minutes, and were tape-recorded to facilitate later analysis. The interviewees answered 12 questions on behalf of their organization, primarily focusing on the organizations' roles within the CDE and their perceptions of the technology in terms of privacy, security, and operability. The stakeholders were also asked to evaluate the CDE's advantages and disadvantages, and estimate the level of consumer participation their organization expected following the system's implementation.

Focus Groups

A focus group is a qualitative data-gathering approach that offers insight into target populations and new concepts, provides a basis for developing questionnaire or survey content, and allows the exploration of categories that would be restricted by quantitative methods (Fuller, Edwards, Vorakitphokatorn, & Sermsri, 1993; Knodel, 1993; Krueger, 1993; Morgan, 1993; O'Brien, 1993; Wolff, Knodel, & Sittirari, 1993). Focus groups are a common method of testing new technologies (Williams, Rice, & Rogers, 1988).

From the stakeholder interviews and the prior literature review, we developed questions for focus group discussions. A pilot focus group was conducted with undergraduate students to identify any problems with the discussion guidelines. The five remaining focus groups consisted of three undergraduate groups, one graduate student group, and one employee group. Of the three undergraduate groups, one group was students who had identified themselves as having a chronic illness, such as diabetes or asthma. This distinction was made based on literature demonstrating that patients' experiences with health technology may differ among healthy and unhealthy patients (Ralston, Revere, Robins, &

Goldberg, 2004; Ziebland, Chapple, Dumelow, Evans, Prinjha, & Roz-movits, 2004).

Each focus group had two main concepts for discussion. The first was a conceptual understanding of DMRs. The moderator read an excerpt from an article in PC Magazine (September 26, 2001) describing the concept and then opened discussion of DMRs by asking questions about the participants' views and concerns regarding the new technology. The second concept was the local implementation of the technology, with the moderator reading a paragraph written by the researchers to introduce the details of the system and concepts.

RESULTS FROM STAKEHOLDER INTERVIEWS AND FOCUS GROUPS

Stakeholder Interviews

The interviews are the statements and opinions of individuals on behalf of the organization or population they represent. Following completion of the interviews, researchers designated the 6 stakeholders as nonprofit or profit organizations with SBPHD, SBRHA, and the community-at-large as nonprofit stakeholders, and Cottage Hospital, SFMC, and clinicians as profit stakeholders. Table 14.1 summarizes these answers, providing those responses that were common to both kinds of organizations, and those unique to each of the two types of organizations.

Focus Groups

Table 14.2 provides the focus groups questions asked, and summarizes the participants' responses to two of these, according to group type. The focus groups' responses were also analyzed according to word frequency. First, all responses within each of the 15 questions were combined across the six focus groups. Then, the 15 questions were grouped into three categories: (a) personal or individual concern (Questions 1, 2, 11 and 12); (b) others' concern (Questions 3, 8, 13, 14, and 15); and (c) advantages and disadvantages of DMRs (Questions 4, 5, 6, 7, 9, 10, 11). "Stop words" ("a," "and," "the," "etc.") were removed, and words were "stemmed" (all variants were converted to one form, such as "patients" and "patient," or "you're" and "you"). Then a computer program went through the text in the three categories, identified and counted each unique word, and sorted the words alphabetically according to decreasing frequency. Table 14.3 lists the words occurring five or more times

TABLE 14.1

Summary of Responses to 12 Questions of Stakeholder Interviews

Question	Common Among Profit and Nonprofit Stakeholders	Unique to Nonprofit Stakeholders	Unique to Profit Stakeholders
1. Years current org 2. Years medical field 3. Role in CDE Possible gains or losses?	Active in CDE's development. Member on CDE board. Contribution of data, resources.	7.1 years 23.9 years One organization serves as insurance company to the CDE. Community is unaware of CDE. Security violation would equal loss.	9.3 years 32.7 years Recognize the benefit to community. Unclear direct benefits to organizations. Previous concern over competitive advantage. Initial implementation requires money and time.
4. CDE's purpose/function within SB community	Improved quality of care. Improved overall health outcomes. Coordination of care, medical programs.	Reduction of test and prescription duplication.	Clinicians will have a single access point to services outside of local network.
5. Involvement with CDE's development	Active participation on CDE board throughout CDE's conception and implementation.	Unaware of general community involvement in CDE (prior to establishment as nonprofit in 03/2004).	Contribution of staff, resources, funding, data.
6a. Advantages of instituting CDE	Improved quality of care. Save time by consolidating medical information into individual digital records.	Reduced labor costs with capabilities of electronic system.	Records available quickly and in a usable format.
6b. Disadvantages of instituting CDE	"Challenges" or "Things to think about." Development and maintenance costs. Issues remain to be resolved.	CDE is not a substitute for personal interaction. Patients' reactions remain unknown. Anxiety over security and privacy issues.	CDE participants have separate and different technology systems. Getting started. Technology is a hurdle; "CDE is not proven state-of-the-art technology."

(Continued)

289

TABLE 14.1
(Continued)

Question	Common Among Profit and Nonprofit Stakeholders	Unique to Nonprofit Stakeholders	Unique to Profit Stakeholders
7. Concerns about CDE's current testing	Adequacy and accuracy of CDE's data.	Good planning and communication between CDE management and testing clinicians is vital. Consumer doesn't have concerns because "out of the loop."	Source of future funding is unclear. Physician must see value in the CDE. CDE needs to have all glitches resolved. CDE must accurately identify individual patients.
8a. Definition of operability	How the system works. System's ability to retrieve correct data.		Accessibility and navigability of CDE to user with standard technology.
8b. Definition of security	Technical protection of data via user authorization.	Can system be hacked into?	Access must have clear guidelines and procedures.
8c. Definition of privacy	Patients to be aware that their medical data is shared with CDE and aware of who has access.	Protection and confidentiality of medical records.	HIPAA compliance.
9a. Operability rating	Seems to be working, but CDE is still in testing phase.	Unsure if data is rich enough.	
9b. Security rating	In theory, CDE is secure, but technology has yet to be implemented.	Outside evaluation passed CDE.	Important to achieve security.
9c. Privacy rating	In theory, CDE seems to be private, but technology has yet to be implemented.	Outside evaluation passed CDE. CDE continuously working on privacy issues.	Important to achieve privacy.

10a. Characteristics advantageous to community acceptance	National attention for Santa Barbara. Improved and safer treatment of patients.	Patients can avoid redundant testing and blood work, saving time and money.	Less effort for patient to coordinate different physicians and specialists. CDE consumer portal.
10b. Characteristics disadvantageous to community acceptance	Not all patients have adequate technology, Internet access, or the skills to use the CDE. Security and privacy concerns over data on Internet.	Paper medical records eliminated. CDE development has lacked community involvement and input.	Security and privacy concerns about insurance companies and employers access to medical records.
11. Consumers' rights to regulate and access medical records	Law dictates consumers' rights. By law, patients have right to access their medical records.	Patients have right to request record be removed from system.	HIPAA provides for those people managing patient's care to have access to medical records. Question of consumers' abilities to interpret data in medical record.
12. Consumer participation in CDE	Consumer portal is on hold. Some organizations are skeptical of consumer use. Patients to use CDE to view test results, get up-to-date medical information. Consumer use will vary according to characteristics of patient population. People are becoming increasingly active in health care.	Low-income and uninsured patients won't be likely to access the CDE. People will review the log of users accessing their medical record.	Chronically ill patients are more likely to use CDE; may participate in disease state management. People to view test and lab results, request appointments and medicine.

TABLE 14.2

Focus Group Topics, and Summary Themes From Two of Them, by Type of Focus Group

Focus Group Topics

Part I: Concept of Individual Digital Medical Records

A. Privacy
1. What information do you think your medical record contains? How would you use such information if you had access to it?
2. What rights do you think you have regarding your medical record?
3. What information from your medical record can doctors share with other health care providers or health institutions?
4. What concerns or questions do you have regarding the availability of your medical records?

B. Read a short description of individual digital medical records on the conceptual level.
5. How do you think digital medical records would compare to current paper-based health care records?
6. What risks or disadvantages come with the implementation of this technology?
7. What benefits or advantages come with the implementation of this technology?
8. How would you feel about having your physician or health care provider implementing such digital records?

Part II: Local Implementation of Digital Medical Records

C. Read a short description of the local implementations of CDE technology in Santa Barbara.
9. In the context of digital medical records' implementation in Santa Barbara County, what risks or disadvantages do the residents of Santa Barbara face following the implementation of this technology?
10. In the context of digital medical records' implementation in Santa Barbara County, what benefits or advantages will the residents of Santa Barbara encounter following the implementation of this technology?
11. Would you access your own medical record if given the opportunity? If so, for what purpose? If not, why? (Remember what they said medical records contained . . . Q1).
12. What do you think about other consumers accessing their medical records? For what purposes might they access their medical records?
13. What do you think about being able to see a list of individuals and institutions that have authorized access to your medical record?
14. What do you think about being able to see a log of individuals who have had authorized access to your medical record?
15. Would you be willing to sign a waiver allowing physicians and other authorized parties to view your medical record?

Q4. Concerns or Questions	Healthy Students	Chronic Illness	Graduate Students	Employees
Are records transferred when a patient changes doctors?			X	
Are you allowed to have access to your records?	X			
Can a child look at her parents' record?	X			
Can parents' view their child's record?		X		
Can responsibility for an individual's record be transferred to a third party if the individual is capable of caring for herself?	X			
Is medical information understandable to avg. person?	X			
Marketing				X
None		X		
Parties should only be able to access the information they need	X		X	
Patient should be able to put medical information in context	X			
Too young to have thought about it	X			
What information is available to insurance companies?			X	X
Who do you have to talk to get old records?	X		X	
Who has access?			X	

(Continued)

293

TABLE 14.2
(Continued)

Q7. Benefits and Advantages of Digital Medical Records	Healthy Students	Chronic Illness	Graduate Students	Employees
Ability to view access log	X			
Accurate diagnoses	X	X		
Benefits patients with illnesses		X		
Brings integrity to medical field		X		
Convenience for doctors	X		X	
Easier to change doctors	X			
Easier to keep track of medication		X		X
Eliminates repeat paper work	X		X	
Ideal for emergency	X			
Ideal for travel	X	X		X
Information used for research		X		
No risk of losing files (in a fire, etc.)	X		X	
Patient access			X	
Quickly accessible	X			
Reliability	X			
Well organized	X			

TABLE 14.3
Focus Groups' Words Mentioned Five or More Times in Responses
to Three Categories of Questions

Personal

I (77, 9.5%), doctor (37, 4.6%), yes 33 (4.1%), people (20, 2.5%), access, check, history (19, 2.3%), don't, might, record, want (17, 2.1%), curious, know (13, 1.6%), information (12, 1.5%), medication (11, 1.4%), need, right (10, 1.2%), family, insurance, look, stuff (9, 1.1%), blood, disease, go, medical (8, 1%), illness, parents, privacy, thing (7, .9%), allergies, ask, good, keep, maybe, visit (6, .7%), company, file, health, patients, think, type, vaccinations, whether, wouldn't (5, .6%)

Others

I (106, 13.4%), yes (62, 7.9%), don't (39, 4.9%), access (29, 3.7%), doctor (25, 3.2%), want (23, 2.9%), people (17, 2.2%), know (16, 2%), long (15, 1.9%), care, information (13, 1.6%), look, record (12, 1.5%), think (11, 1.4%), might, wouldn't (9, 1.1%), good, health, need, thing (7, .9%), fine, interested, list, problem, share (6, .8%), asked, authorization, change, company, consent, definitely, insurance, maybe, permission, right (5, .6%)

Advantages and Disadvantages

record (47, 4.9%), I, easy (42, 4.3%), access (41, 4.2%), people (40, 4.1%), doctor (38, 3.9%), don't (33, 3.4%), paper (27, 2.8%), information (21, 2.2%), computer (20, 2.1%), patient (17, 1.8%), thing (15, 1.6%), go (14, 1.4%), look (12, 1.2%), cost, hacker, health (10, 1%), change, file, know, might, think, wouldn't (9, 9%), ask, Santa Barbara, digital, having (8, .8%), better, good, help, history, lose, medical, problem, transfer (7, .7%), different, emergency, seems, system (6, .6%), advantage, allow, benefit, copy, diagnosis, hard, hospital, long, lot, older, online, outside, privacy, saves, time, want, wrong (5, .5%)

Note. Values are the number of times mentioned, and percentage of the specific word's occurrence within the top 160 words.

within each group of questions. (The words used for both the thematic and word frequency analysis were the text provided by an independent note-taker, and it is possible that some bias may be present among the words. For example, the one person who took all the notes may have summarized participants' comments in ways that systematically emphasized some words and meanings over others.)

Expectations About Use

The prospect of DMRs technology was exciting to the stakeholders and focus groups, with both groups recognizing the technology's advantages in comparison to current paper records and the possible health care improvements. Stakeholders were not in complete agreement as to how consumers would participate in or use the CDE, and the nonprofit stakeholders felt that their lower income and uninsured clientele would not reap the benefits of the CDE's consumer portal. The focus group participants, when asked if they would access their DMRs, were also not in agreement. The majority of participants said that they would, for reasons ranging from curiosity to self-treatment, but the graduate and employee groups exhibited greater hesitancy due to concerns involving health insurance and employment. It is possible that to successfully diffuse the CDE, participants' age and financial independence should be considered when developing appropriate marketing campaigns.

Meanings of "Privacy"

The stakeholders agreed on a general definition of privacy, including patient awareness as a requirement in fulfilling their organizations' obligations to privacy. More generally, stakeholders tended to combine privacy and security, defined as the technological protection of data accomplished through user authorization. Although focus group participants were not asked to define privacy, they identified privacy as a specific concern accompanying the implementation of DMRs, along with the desire to be informed of and exercise discretion over their medical records' authorized users. The general sentiment among stakeholders was that, provided the CDE was in compliance with HIPAA regulations, privacy issues would not be a major problem. In contrast, focus group participants, who were largely unaware of patients' legal rights, overestimated their ability to access and control their traditional medical information, and perhaps as a result were not completely willing to participate in the CDE.

Awareness of Digital Medical Records and CDE

Although the stakeholders discussed the need for patient awareness, the focus group participants confirmed that they had not been properly informed of the technology's implementation and would have appreciated communication between the SBCCDE and the community.

METHODS: SURVEY DEVELOPMENT, MEASUREMENT, AND SAMPLE

Based on central concepts from the literature review, and results from the stakeholder interviews and focus groups, a pilot survey was developed, tested with a small set of respondents, and revised for the formal survey. The final survey contained the following sections and items.

Measures

Individual Characteristics.   Survey respondents were asked to rate their *health status* in comparison to other people of the same age and sex on a scale of 1 = very unhealthy to 7 = very healthy. Respondents were also asked to indicate whether or not they had ever had a *chronic illness or health problem. Age* was measured by the number of years and months since the respondents' birth. Respondents' *year in college* was measured as 1 = freshman to 4 = senior. Respondents were asked to estimate how much of their *annual expenses* (tuition, housing, food, travel) they earn or pay for themselves (1 = none to 5 = all), and whether or not they pay for their own *health insurance.* A 10-item scale from Jerusalem and Schwarzer (1992) was used to measure *general self-efficacy* (1 = not at all true, 2 = hardly true, 3 = moderately true, 4 = exactly true).

Privacy Attitudes.   Eight items measured respondents' *general privacy* attitudes. The items were developed based on frequently cited definitions of privacy, including Warren and Brandeis (1890), "people should have the right to be left alone," and Westin (1967), "people should have the right to control their personal information" (1 = very strongly disagree to 7 = very strongly agree). *Need for privacy* was measured by Buss's (2001) 19-item scale (1 = very strongly disagree to 7 = very strongly agree). Respondents' attitudes toward *organizational privacy* were measured using 11 items from Smith et al.'s (1996) 15-item instrument. The instrument uses four subscales to measure individuals' concerns about collection, errors, unauthorized secondary use, and improper access (1 = very strongly disagree to 7 = very strongly agree). Nine items measured *general concerns about computer privacy,* such as monitoring and hacking (1 = not concerned at all to 7 = very strongly concerned). Twelve items developed from focus group participants' responses to a question about their medical rights, measured respondents' perceptions of patients' medical rights (1 = true, 2 = false), with correct answers identified by the SBCCDE's Executive Director. The number of participants' correct answers was summed.

Technology Use and Expertise.   Respondents were asked to indicate the *frequency of their Internet use* from home, work, school (excluding the library), library, or other locations (each 1 = never to 5 = daily). They were also asked to indicate the number of years that they have been using the Internet (including email, web, chat, downloading, etc.). *Web expertise* was measured by 12 questions taken from the Georgia Tech (1998) web survey that asked whether or not the respondent had performed a variety of activities (such as created a web page). The Georgia Tech survey calculated the total number of activities respondents had completed and grouped respondents according to four levels of expertise: 0–3 activities, novice; 4–6, intermediate; 7–9, experienced; and 10–12, expert. *Web fluency* was measured by 17 items taken from the computer-e-mail-web fluency scale developed by Bunz (2004; 1 = very difficult to 7 = very easy). Fluency, according to the Committee on Information Technology (1999), is defined by three concepts: it (1) entails a lifelong learning process, (2) implies personalization of skills on levels of sophistication, and (3) is composed of three kinds of knowledge: contemporary skills, foundational concepts, and intellectual capabilities.

Innovation Attributes. After the individual characteristics and technology use and expertise sections on the questionnaire, survey respondents read two paragraph-long descriptions of DMRs, identical to those used in the focus groups. The scales used to measure the five primary innovation attributes were developed based on the thematic and word frequency results of the focus groups, Rogers's (1983) research, and feedback from the SBCCDE's executive director. Survey respondents were asked to indicate their agreement with items representing the following attributes (1 = very strongly disagree to 7 = very strongly agree). *Relative advantage* was measured using 13 items comparing paper-based and DMRs. *Compatibility* was measured using eight items representing focus group participants' statements of values and needs, with the most prevalent being access, privacy, security, and quality health care. *Complexity* was measured by eight items derived from focus group participants' questions, and statements of concern, disadvantages, and the likelihood of their own individual use and others' use. *Trialability* was measured by three items indicating the extent to which respondents desired the ability to experiment with digital medical records, or reserving the ability withdraw their participation as well. *Observability* was measured using seven items, focusing on support for the innovation's progress and respondents' desire to participate in its development or obtain some physical representation of their participation in the CDE. These items resulted from collaboration between researchers and the SBCCDE's executive director who identified several ways in which the public might observe or experience the results of DMRs.

Technology Evaluation. To measure survey respondents' likelihood of *adoption* of DMRs, the SBCCDE's executive director identified nine consumer actions that would indicate adoption, such as whether a respondent would be willing to sign a consent form releasing their information to the SBCCDE digital database (1 = very strongly disagree to 7 =

very strongly disagree). When reviewing the focus group data, research-ers noticed a wide variety of statements describing previously unantici-pated consumer and administrative uses of DMRs. These statements were compiled along with statements about anticipated uses of the innovation, resulting in 14 items measuring the ways in which participants antici-pated they or others might *reinvent* the DMRs (1 = very strongly disagree to 7 = very strongly disagree).

Table 14.4 provides descriptive statistics on the scales and subscales used in the analyses, with scale reliabilities, and, where relevant, subscale principal component values. Descriptive statistics and wording for scale items are available from the Web site listed earlier, though illustrative items from each scale are noted below. Figure 14.1 summarizes the hy-pothesized relationships between the explanatory overall scales and subscales, and the outcome measures of adoption and reinvention.

RESULTS: DESCRIPTIVE

Individual Characteristics

The sample, composed of undergraduate students taking introductory communication courses at the University of California Santa Barbara, was 76.8% female, 29.8% of respondents were freshmen, 37.8% were sophomores, 26.9% were juniors, and 3.1% were seniors. The SBCCDE Executive Director was particularly interested in the attitudes and knowl-edge of this population group, as they represent the next generation of medical system users, and have greater familiarity with Internet technol-ogy. The majority of respondents described their *health* as at least aver-age, with no more than 8.5% reporting to be below average, and 67.8% as above average; only 17.9% of respondents had ever had a *chronic illness*. A small 7.7% of respondents were personally *responsible for their own health insurance*, and the remainder received health insurance through their par-ents or a third party. Similarly only 3.1% of respondents were responsi-ble for all of their *annual personal expenses*, whereas 78.5% of respondents were not responsible for any of their expenses. Respondents averaged 3.2 on the *general self-efficacy* scale, indicating a fairly high level of self effi-cacy within the sample.

Technology Use and Expertise

Respondents averaged 7.3 years *Internet use*, with the most experienced re-spondent reporting 15 years of use. Concerning *web expertise* respondents had completed 6 tasks (at the top of "intermediate expertise"), with the

TABLE 14.4
Descriptive Statistics for Individual Items,
Scales and Subscales, With Reliabilities

Demographics	Min	Max	Mean	S.D.
Gender M1F2	1	2	1.8	0.42
Age Years	17	28	19.5	1.39
Age Months	0	12	5.6	3.30
Healthy	1	7	5.1	1.25
Chronic Illness Y1N2	1	2	1.8	0.39
Annual Expenses Responsible for	1	5	2.1	0.99
Health Insurance Coverage Responsibility Y1N2	1	2	1.9	0.27
College Year 1F4S	1	4	2.0	0.84
Use of Internet Number of Years	2	15	7.3	1.91
Web expertise—sum of 12 items	0	12	5.99	2.26
Web expertise—grouped according to GT four levels of expertise: 0–3 activities, novice; 4–6, intermediate; 7–9, experienced; and 10–12, expert	1	4	2.34	.79
Web fluency α = .88	2.9	7.0	5.7	.82
Efficacy α = .86	2.1	4.0	3.16	.39
Need for Privacy α = .81	1.6	6.8	4.0	.78
General Privacy α = .66	3.5	7	5.8	.75
Organizational Privacy α = .85	2.6	7	5.5	.79
Organizational Collection Privacy 4.5 40.9% α = .67	2	7	5.1	1.1
Organizational Personal Privacy 1.3 12.2% α = .74	1	7	4.9	1.0
Organizational Unauthorized Access Privacy 1.2 10.5% α = .82	2.2	7	6.0	.87
General Concerns about Computer Privacy α = .88	1.7	7	4.7	1.2
Number of Accurate Patients' Legal Rights, out of 12	0	11	6.8	1.4
Relative Advantage α = .88	1.7	7	5.1	.84
Compatibility α = .78	1.4	7	4.7	.86
Complexity α = .69	2.1	6.5	4.4	.75
Error Complexity 2.3 32.9% α = .86	1	7	5.6	1.1
Explanation Complexity 1.8 25.3% α = .82	1	7	3.3	1.3
Trialability α = .77	1	7	5.8	1.1
Observability α = .64	1.9	7	4.6	.85
Adoption α = .88	1	7	4.2	1.1
Reinvention α = .89	1.3	7	5.3	.84

Note. N = 403–413; "α =" is Cronbach's alpha; x.x and y.y% are eigenvalue, and percent variance explained, respectively, for principal components analysis of subscales.

least completed task being "Bought a book to learn more about the Web or Internet" and the most completed task being "Ordered a product/service by filling out an online form." When asked how frequently they used the Internet from five different *locations*, the most popular place was respondents' homes, followed, respectively, by the library, school, other places,

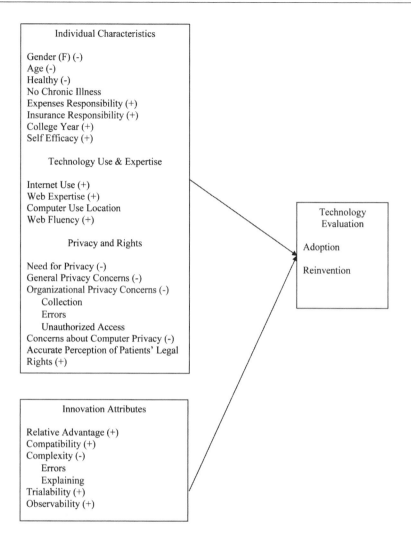

FIG. 14.1. Explanatory model of influences on DMR adoption.

and work. On average, respondents reported a *web fluency* score of 5.7, indicating that most people were at least comfortable in completing the majority of the described tasks. Respondents were most comfortable with such basic web skills as "Using search engines such as Google or Yahoo," and "Using 'back' and 'forward' in your browser to return to pages." The tasks respondents were least comfortable with included "Creating a website using a visual editor," and "Creating a website using HTML."

Privacy and Rights

Respondents did not have a great *need for privacy*, averaging 4, and the area they were most concerned with was personal space. Respondents expressed greatest concern on the items "If I kept a diary, I would never show it to anyone," and "When working or studying, I need lots of elbow room." In contrast, respondents were least concerned with issues of concealment, such as needing to tint car windows or keep shades closed while in their homes.

General privacy concerns had a mean of 5.8, suggesting a fairly high level of concern. Respondents agreed most strongly with the statement "No one should be able to gather or disclose my personal information without my consent." On the contrary, respondents were least in agreement with the statement, "The government should be able to secretly monitor individuals' online activities for national security." The mean of respondents' *organizational privacy concerns* was 5.5, indicating a medium level of concern, with greatest concern about unauthorized access. For example, respondents most strongly agreed with the statements "Companies should never sell the personal information in their computer databases to other companies." Following unauthorized access, respondents were also concerned with the collection of personal information and errors, respectively. Overall, respondents' concerns about *computer privacy* were not as great as their general or organizational privacy concerns, with a mean of 4.7, slightly above "somewhat concerned." Respondents were most concerned with "getting a computer virus attack" and least concerned with "your e-mail will be read by someone besides the person you sent it to."

Respondents' averaged only 6.8 correct responses to 12 statements about *patients' legal rights*. The items respondents scored poorly on concerned physicians' and health care providers' abilities to share medical information without consent, demonstrating that respondents believed they had greater control over their medical information than is actually true.

Innovation Attributes

DMRs' *relative advantage* (compared to paper medical records) had a mean of 5.1, somewhat favorable. Respondents felt that DMRs' most advantageous characteristics were the records' availability in a emergency situations and the added convenience for doctors. The only statement that received below a neutral level of agreement involved DMRs' ability to save people money in comparison to paper records. *Compatibility* had a mean of 4.7, indicating that respondents at least somewhat agreed with the majority of statements. The statement receiving the highest score was "The individual patient should decide who has the authority to view the information in his or her medical record," whereas "My digital medical record would remain private" received the lowest level of agreement. In terms of *complexity*, DMRs were perceived to be most complex in susceptibility to both human and computer error, and respondents felt slightly more comfortable in their ability to understand or explain the technology. Respondents tended to agree with statements indicating DMRs' *trialability*, averaging 5.8. Respondents most agreed they would like the option to remove their medical record from the system in the future. The mean for *observability* was 4.6, indicating basic recognition of DMRs' observability. Respondents agreed most strongly with statements of action, such as viewing a list of those authorized to view their medical record, and less strongly with statements of support, such as their willingness to participate in a community forum on DMRs.

Technology Evaluation

On average, respondents agreed with statements of *adoption* with a score of 4.2, slightly above neutral. The statement with the highest level of agreement was "I would access my digital medical record if given the opportunity," and the lowest level of agreement was "I would participate in a consumer oversight committee to advise health administrators about recommendations for the SBCCDE." Respondents averaged 5.3 on the *reinvention* scale; respondents were most likely to agree with instances of patient reinvention (e.g., they would use their medical records to learn their medical history), and slightly less likely to agree with instances of doctors' and others' reinvention of DMRs, respectively.

RESULTS: BIVARIATE AND MULTIVARIATE

The overall model (Fig. 14.1) proposed directional predictions of individual characteristics, technology use and expertise, privacy and patients' legal rights, and innovation attributes' influences on an individual's likelihood to adopt and reinvent DMRs. Table 14.5 presents correlations between the variables—separate individual characteristics, and scales and subscales of *technology use* and *expertise*, *privacy* and *medical rights*, and innovation *attributes*—and the two outcome measures of *adoption* and *reinvention*. The bivariate analysis provided support for several of those predictions.

Multiple regressions were run to identify unique explanatory variance in adoption and reinvention explained by the variables, because of possible intercorrelations among the explanatory variables. All of the scales,

TABLE 14.5
Correlations of Explanatory Influences
With Adoption and Reinvention

Explanatory Influences	Adoption	Reinvention
Individual Characteristics		
Gender	−.08	−.05
Age total months	.01	.00
Healthy	−.06	.02
Chronic Illness	.00	−.03
Annual Expenses Responsible for	.10*	.11*
College Year	−.00	.01
Health Insurance Responsibility	−.11*	.01
General Self-Efficacy	.06	.17**
Internet Use and Expertise		
Internet Use	.04	−.02
Web Expertise sum	.09*	.13**
Web Fluency	.18**	.19**
Privacy Concerns and Medical Rights		
Personal Privacy Needs	−.02	−.02
General Privacy Concerns	−.01	.16**
Organizational Policy	.06	.22**
Concerns about Computer Privacy	.14**	.16**
Patients' Medical Rights #correct	.08*	.04
Innovation Attributes		
Relative Advantage	.47**	.41**
Compatibility	.49**	.32**
Complexity	−.19**	−.01
Trialability	−.07	.22**
Observability	.54**	.47**

Note.   *$p < .05$ level; **$p < .01$ level (1-tailed). $N = 402$–413.

subscales, and individual measures with significant bivariate correlations were included, stepwise within three blocks (individual characteristics, privacy concerns and medical rights, and then innovation attributes). About 40% of the variance in adoption and a third of the variance in reinvention of the SBCCDE system was explained.

Adoption and *reinvention* of DMRs were significantly influenced by the percentage of annual expenses respondents were responsible for. No Internet use or expertise were significant influences on adoption or reinvention. The *collection* subscale of organizational privacy concerns and concerns about computer privacy were significant influences on

TABLE 14.6
Final Summary Multiple Regressions
Explaining Adoption and Reinvention

Explanatory Influences	Adoption	Reinvention
Individual Characteristics		
Annual Expenses	.08*	.10**
Privacy Concerns and Medical Rights		
Organizational privacy—collection	−.12**	—
Organizational privacy—unauthorized access	—	.12**
Concerns about computer privacy	.10*	—
Innovation Attributes		
Relative advantage	—	.17***
Observability	.44***	.32***
Compatibility	.25***	—
Trialability	−.13***	—
Complexity—explanation	−.12**	−.16***
Complexity—error	—	.15***
Adjusted R^2	.41	.33
F-ratio	40.5***	32.8***
N	393	394

Note.   *$p < .05$; **$p < .01$; ***$p < .001$.

adoption. The *unauthorized access* subscale of organizational privacy was a significant influence on reinvention. *Observability, compatibility, trialability*, and *explanation complexity* were significant influences on adoption. *Relative advantage, observability*, and both *explanation complexity* and *error complexity* were significant influences on reinvention.

DISCUSSION AND IMPLICATIONS OF SURVEY RESULTS

Individual Characteristics

The percentage of *annual expenses* that individuals were responsible for was the most significant individual characteristic related to both adoption and reinvention, whereas other characteristics, such as age and health status, were not significant. Responsibility for *health insurance* and *self efficacy* were also related to adoption, although their influence was not as prominent, and disappeared in the regressions. These results imply that those individuals with a heightened awareness of their financial obligations, such as health insurance, may be more likely to see benefits in

DMRs, and subsequently adopt the technology. Also, financially responsible respondents may possess greater *self-efficacy* as a result of their ability to maintain a sustainable income, and consequently may feel more confident in their personal ability to understand and use their DMRs. Therefore, when introducing DMRs to the public, it may prove useful to identify community segments according to financial independence, and develop programs to foster understanding of the new technology according to each group's specific needs. In general, materials presenting and emphasizing different aspects of DMRs should be developed in anticipation of a diverse consumer population.

Internet Experience and Expertise

Respondents who scored higher on measures of *web expertise* and *web fluency* were more supportive of DMRs and their own ability to successfully use the application, although both disappeared as unique influences in the regressions. Although the current study's sample of college respondents averaged 7.3 years of Internet use, such familiarity with the Internet may not be representative of other populations. For example, as focus group participants and SBCCDE stakeholders voiced, those community members with lower technology expertise will not be able to take advantage of DMRs, and, as the survey results demonstrate, may be less likely to adopt DMRs. To combat the large obstacle of deficits in computer skills among different segments of the population, whether they are senior citizens, minorities, or low-income families, regional health infrastructure organizations (RHIOs), such as the SBCCDE, may consider outreach programs to introduce people to the Internet. Indeed, the first of three primary recommendations by the Working Group on Policies for Electronic Information Sharing Between Doctors and Patients (2004) was to increase public understanding of the value of connectivity in health care through a coordinated, public–private communications campaign.

Also, as many RHIOs are concerned with establishing stable funding for their projects, continued community outreach, in terms of education programs introducing increasingly sophisticated technology into the community, may further their ability to obtain grants, federal funding, and overall public support. Disparities in computer skills should also be taken into consideration when developing materials or publications explaining DMRs and the SBCCDE. Although a discussion of peer-to-peer technology may reassure computer technicians that DMRs are secure, populations less web-fluent would most likely be confused and turned off to DMRs. Those groups whose fall toward the middle of the technologically savvy spectrum may benefit from a simple explanation of the technology that utilizes analogies of web terms and functions with which they are more likely to be acquainted.

Privacy Concerns and Medical Rights

Respondents with a more accurate perception of *patients' legal medical rights* were more likely to adopt DMRs, but this influence disappeared in the regressions. Respondents averaged only 6.8 correct responses out of 12 statements regarding patients' legal rights, demonstrating that these college students were largely misinformed about their medical rights. This may well be true of most population segments, so any implementation of DMRs needs to take into account that consumers' concerns about new health technologies may be confounded by inaccurate assumptions about their actual medical rights. The SBCCDE should consider taking steps toward educating their potential consumers regarding their medical rights as mandated under HIPAA, and the manner in which the CDE strictly complies with those rights. Developing informative pamphlets, presentations, or videos for patients, constructed in a patient-friendly format avoiding legal and medical jargon, may facilitate consumer education. Also, as doctors are often seen as credible authority figures, it may be helpful to have doctors discuss medical rights with their patients, both privately in their offices and publicly in community forums, to reinforce the information and clarify any questions patients may have. Finally, Santa Barbara County, like much of California, has a large Latino population, and it would be wise to have all patient education materials available in both English and Spanish.

Concerns about computer privacy and the *collection aspect of organizational privacy* concerns were also related to the adoption of DMRs. Respondents with lower levels of privacy concerns were more likely to adopt the technology. Similarly, *general privacy concerns, concerns about computer privacy*, and the *unauthorized access aspect of organizational privacy* were related to reinvention. The relationship between organizational privacy concerns to both outcome measures points to the value of future efforts to establish stronger patient–organization relationships, whether it be through the organizations' outreach into the community, or other means that increase the visibility and accountability of the organization within the community. In creating a consumer education program, it might be helpful to explicitly address those issues respondents were especially uncomfortable with, such as the sale of personal information to other companies, the use of personal information for reasons other than stated, or the use of personal information without obtaining consent. Addressing consumers' specific concerns in a privacy pamphlet or video describing exactly how and for what purposes patients' medical information will and will not be used, might reduce consumers' privacy concerns. Also, it may be helpful to inform consumers about how they may engage in 'safer web practices;' for example, learning to look for Web sites' privacy policies and eliminating cookies from the hard drive. By educating consumers on how to better protect themselves from what they consider to be privacy violations, their self efficacy may increase and overall privacy concerns may be reduced, leading to the greater likelihood of adoption of DMRs.

Innovation Attributes

The innovation attributes were, out of all variables, the most strongly related to both outcome measures. In the case of *adoption*, *observability*, *compatibility*, *trialability*, and the *explanation* aspect of complexity were the most significant influences.

Relative advantage, observability, and the *explanation* and *error aspects of complexity* were significantly related to *reinvention*. Whereas *relative advantage* did not play as significant a role in adoption, respondents who saw significant benefits of DMRs in comparison to paper medical records were more likely to acknowledge various reinventions of the new technology. Therefore, in developing consumer strategies, the SBCCDE would benefit from enumerating the differences between DMRs and paper records, and by presenting the paper records as outdated or inefficient. Respondents reacted most positively to advantages focusing DMRs' abilities to enable better health care, especially by facilitating care in emergency situations, providing convenient information access for doctors, and by alleviating the pains of transferring paper records between physicians' offices and medical clinics. Such a focus on treatment is a positive result for the SBCCDE, as it reaffirms its stated dedication to improving health care by facilitating access to medical records at the point of patient care. Creating a variety of opportunities for individuals to interact with their DMRs, such as viewing a list of users authorized to view their record, will help them view the technology as compatible with their everyday needs and values.

REFERENCES

Albisser, A., Albisser, J., & Parker, L. (2003). Patient confidentiality, data security, and provider liabilities in diabetes management. *Diabetes Technology and Therapeutics*, 5(4), 631–640.

Alpert, S. A. (2003). Protecting medical privacy: Challenges in the age of genetic information. *Journal of Social Issues*, 59(2), 301–322.

Aydin, C. E., & Rice, R. E. (1991). Social worlds, individual differences, and implementation: Predicting attitudes toward a medical information system. *Information & Management*, 20, 119–136.

Bandura, A. (1997). *Self-efficacy: The exercise of control*. New York: Freeman.

Brewin, B. (2005). Public wants open health records standards. *Government HealthIT, June 3*. Retrieved July 21, 2005, from http://www.govhealthit.com/article89070-06-03-05-Web

Bunz, U. (2004). The computer-email-web (CEW) fluency scale: Development and validation. *International Journal of Human–Computer Interaction, 17*(4), 477–504.

Buss, A. (2001). *Psychological dimensions of the self*. Thousand Oaks, CA: Sage.

California HealthCare Foundation. (1999). Medical privacy and confidentiality survey: Summary and overview. January 28. Retrieved October 14, 2004, from http://www.chcf.org/documents/ihealth/survey.pdf

Care Science, Inc. (2005). *Santa Barbara County Care Data Exchange*. Retrieved July 21, 2005, from www.Carescience.com

Chin, T. (12 March, 2001). Peer to peer: Sharing patient data online. *American Medical News*, 1–6.

Committee on Information Technology. (1999). *Being fluent with information technology*. Washington, DC: National Academy Press.

Compeau, D. R., & Higgins, C. A. (1995). Computer self-efficacy: Development of a measure and initial test. *MIS Quarterly, 19*(2), 189–212.

Connecting for Health. (2003, June). *Personal health working group survey*. Retrieved July 21, 2005, from http://www.connectingforhealth.org/resources/phwg_survey_ 6.5.03 .pdf

Connecting for Health. (2005, January). *The collaborative response to the ONCHIT* [Office of National Coordinator for Health Information Technology] *request for information*. Retrieved July 21, 2005, from http://www.connectingforhealth.org/resources/ collaborative_response/collaborative_response.pdf

Culnan, M. J., & Armstrong, P. K. (1999). Information privacy concerns, procedural fairness, and impersonal trust: An empirical investigation. *Organization Science, 10*(1), 104–115.

Davis, F. (1993). User acceptance of information technology: System characteristics, use perceptions and behavioral impacts. *International Journal of Man–Machine Studies, 38*, 475–487.

Demiris, G., & Eysenbach, G. (2002). Internet use in disease management for home care patients: A call for papers. *Journal of Medical Internet Research, 4*(2), 6–12, e6.

Epstein, R. A. (2002). HIPAA on privacy: Its unintended and intended consequences. *Cato Journal, 22*(1), 13–32.

Fedorowicz, J., & Ray, A. W. (2004). Impact of HIPAA on the integrity of healthcare information. *International Journal of Healthcare Technology & Management, 6*(2), 142.

Ferris, N. (2005a). Regional health information networks gain traction. *Government HealthIT, June 9*. Retrieved July 21, 2005, from http://www.govhealthit.com/article 89134-06-09-05-Web

Ferris, N. (2005b). Health nets seek sound financial footing. *Government HealthIT, June 9*. Retrieved July 21, 2005, from http://www.govhealthit.com/article89146-06-09-05-Web

Finkelstein, J. B. (9 August, 2004). HHS outlines plan to increase national adoption of health information technology. *American Medical News*. Retrieved December 2, 2005, from http://www.hhs.gov/news/press/2004pres/20040721.html

Fuller, T. D., Edwards, J. N., Vorakitphokatorn, S., & Sermsri, S. (1993). Using focus groups to adapt survey instruments to new populations: Experience from a developing country. In D. L. Morgan (Ed.), *Successful focus groups: Advancing the state of the art* (pp. 89–104). Thousand Oaks, CA: Sage.

Georgia Tech's GVU's 10th WWW user survey. (1998). Retrieved July 16, 2003, from http://www.gvu.gatech.edu/user_surveys/survey-1998-10/

Gunter, T. D., & Terry, N. P. (2005). The emergence of national electronic health record architectures in the United States and Australia: Models, costs, and questions. *Journal of Medical Internet Research*, 7(1), e3.

Harris Interactive. (2003). eHealth's influence continues to grow as usage of the Internet by physicians and patients increases. *Health Care News*, 3(6), 1–7.

Hassol, A., Walker, J. M., Kidder, D., Rokita, K., Young, D., Pierdon, S., Deitz, D., Kuck, S., & Ortiz, E. (2004). Patient experiences and attitudes about access to a patient electronic health care record and linked web messaging. *Journal of the American Medical Informatics Association*, 11(6), 505–513.

Health Privacy Project. (2004). *HIPAA privacy check-up*. Washington, DC: Author.

Jeffords, M. J. (1999). Confidentiality of medical information: Protecting privacy in an electronic age. *Professional Psychology: Research and Practice*, 30(2), 115–116.

Jerusalem, M., & Schwarzer, R. (1992). Self-efficacy as a resource factor in stress appraisal processes. In R. Schwarzer (Ed.), *Self-efficacy: Thought control of action* (pp. 195–213). Washington, DC: Hemisphere.

Johnson, B., & Rice, R. E. (1987). *Managing organizational innovation: The evolution from word processing to office information systems*. New York: Columbia University Press.

Joustra-Enquist, I., & Eklund, B. (2004). SUSTAINS: Direct access for the patient to the medical record over the Internet. *MEDINFO 2004*(CD), 1673.

Knodel, J. (1993). The design and analysis of focus group studies: A practical approach. In D. L. Morgan (Ed.), *Successful focus groups: Advancing the state of the art* (pp. 35–50). Thousand Oaks, CA: Sage.

Krueger, R. A. (1993). Quality control in focus group research. In D. L. Morgan (Ed.), *Successful focus groups: Advancing the state of the art* (pp. 65–85). Thousand Oaks, CA: Sage.

Li, J., & Shaw, M. J. (2004). Protection of health information in data mining. *International Journal of Healthcare Technology & Management*, 6(2), 210.

Mandl, K. D., Szolovits, P., & Kohane, I. S. (2001). Public standards and patients' control: How to keep electronic medical records accessible by private. *British Medical Journal*, 322, 283–287.

McGee, M. K. (3 November, 2003). Collaborate and conquer. *InformationWeek*.

Metzger, M., & Docter, S. (2003). Public opinion and policy initiatives for online privacy protection. *Journal of Broadcasting & Electronic Media*, 47(3), 350–374.

Milberg, S. J., Smith, H. J., & Burke, S. J. (2000). Information privacy: Corporate management and national regulation. *Organization Science*, 11(1), 35.

Morgan, D. L. (Ed.). (1993). *Successful focus groups: Advancing the state of the art*. Thousand Oaks, CA: Sage.

Muller, M. L., Burkle, T., Irps, S., Roeder, N., & Prokosch, H. U. (2003). The diagnosis related groups enhanced electronic medical record. *International Journal of Medical Informatics*, 70(2–3), 221–228.

Nasser, C., & Alpert, S. (1999). *Protecting the privacy of medical records: An ethical analysis*. Lexington, MA: National Coalition for Patient Rights.

O'Brien, K. (1993). Improving survey questionnaires through focus groups. In D. L. Morgan (Ed.), *Successful focus groups: Advancing the state of the art* (pp. 105–117). Thousand Oaks, CA: Sage.

PC Magazine. (September 26, 2001). *A healthier CHIN*. Ziff Davis Publishing, Inc.

Ralston, J. D., Revere, D., Robins, L. S., & Goldberg, H. I. (2004). Patients' experience with a diabetes support programme based on an interactive electronic medical record: Qualitative study. *British Medical Journal*, 328(7449), 1159.

Reynolds, S. (2003). Making sense of information technology. *British Journal of Midwifery*, 11(3), 178–183.

Rice, R. E., & Anderson, J. G. (1994). Social networks and health care information systems: A structural approach to evaluation. In J. Anderson, C. Aydin, & S. Jay (Eds.), *Evalu-*

ating health care information systems: Methods and applications (pp. 135–162). Newbury Park, CA: Sage.

Rogers, E. M. (1983). *Diffusion of innovations* (3rd ed.). New York: Free Press.

Shoesmith, J. (2001). Privacy matters: As the healthcare sector and high-tech worlds converge, governments and service providers are scrambling to ensure that the benefits of ehealth don't come at the expense of personal privacy. *Canadian Healthcare Manager, 8*(2), 21.

Smith, H. J., Milberg, S. J., & Burke, S. J. (1996). Information privacy: Measuring individuals' concerns about organizational practices. *MIS Quarterly, 20*(2), 167–196.

Swartz, N. (2004). A prescription for electronic health records. *Information Management Journal, 38*(4), 20.

U.S. Department of Health and Human Services. (2000). 45 CFR Parts 160 and 164. Standards for privacy of individually identifiable health information; Final rule. *Federal Register, 65,* 82462–82829.

U.S. Department of Health and Human Services. (2001). *Fact sheet: Protecting the privacy of patients' health information. July 6.* Retrieved February 10, 2005, from http://www.hhs.gov/news/press/21001pres/01fsprivacy.html

U.S. Department of Health and Human Services. (2004). *OCR letter to healthcare providers.* May 17. Washington, DC: US DHHS Office for Civil Rights.

Udo, G. J. (2001). Privacy and security concerns as major barriers for e-commerce: A survey study. *Information Management and Computer Security, 9*(4), 165–174.

Wang, M., Lau, C., Matsen, F. A. III, & Kim, Y. (2004). Personal health information management system and its application in referral management. *IEEE Transactions on Information Technology in Biomedicine, 8*(3), 287.

Wang, S. J., Middleton, C., Prosser, L. A., Bardon, C. G., Spurr, C. D., Carchidi, P. J., Kittler, A. F., Goldszer, R. C., Fairchild, D. G., Sussman, A. J., Kuperman, G. J., & Bates, D. W. (2003). A cost-benefit analysis of electronic medical records in primary care. *The American Journal of Medicine, 114,* 397–403.

Warren, S., & Brandeis, L. (1890). The right to privacy. *Harvard Law Review, 4,* 193–220.

Westin, A. (1967). *Privacy and freedom.* New York: Atheneum.

Williams, F., Rice, R. E., & Rogers, E. M. (1988). *Research methods and the new media.* New York: The Free Press.

Wolff, B., Knodel, J., & Sittirari, W. (1993). Focus groups and surveys as complementary research methods: A case study. In D. L. Morgan (Ed.), *Successful focus groups: Advancing the state of the art* (pp. 118–136). Thousand Oaks, CA: Sage.

Working Group on Policies for Electronic Information Sharing Between Doctors and Patients. (July, 2004). *Connecting Americans to their healthcare. Executive summary.* Retrieved July 21, 2005, from http://www.connectingforhealth.org/resources/eis_exec_sum_final_0704.pdf

Ziebland, S., Chapple, A., Dumelow, C., Evans, J., Prinjha, S., & Rozmovits, L. (2004). How the internet affects patients' experience of cancer: A qualitative study. *British Medical Journal, 328*(564).

Web-Based Computer-Tailored Feedback on Alcohol Use: Motivating Excessive Drinkers to Consider Their Behavior

Suzanne Brunsting
University of Amsterdam, The Netherlands

Bas van den Putte
University of Amsterdam, The Netherlands

According to the World Health Organization, more than 76 million people worldwide (mostly in developed countries) suffer from alcohol use disorders. In Europe and the Americas, the level of alcohol-related death, disease, and disability ranges from 8% to 18% for males and 2% to 4% for females (Institute of Alcohol Studies, 2004). In the Americas, alcohol-related death and disability account for even greater costs to life and longevity than those caused by tobacco use, at least in terms of lost years of healthy life (Murray & Lopez, 1996).

Attempts to reduce this level of alcohol-related problems are hindered by the fact that most of the people who drink excessively are not aware they are at risk. Most of them feel just as healthy as moderate drinkers, and even when experiencing mild problems, they often do not attribute these to their alcohol consumption. Therefore, they are not inclined to seek help or treatment (NIGZ, 2004). Reducing consumption among this large group of people would result in a great reduction in the total alcohol-related harm caused to society (Heather, 2001). It is therefore important to identify these excessive, nontreatment seeking drinkers, convince them that their behavior could be harmful to their health, and encourage them to reduce consumption to sensible limits.

Over the last two decades, brief or minimal interventions have become a popular means to this end (Heather, 1996). In their most simple form,

313

brief interventions only last 5 to 10 minutes. They start with a screening, which often consists of an interview or a questionnaire, to identify excessive drinkers and to gather information about them. This information is used to discuss the respondent's alcohol use, often in a face-to-face setting with the person who performed the screening. The respondent is offered several courses of action to change his or her behavior, and is motivated to set goals for lowering consumption. Nontreatment seeking excessive drinkers are approached in primary care settings while they are seeking help for another problem (Heather, 1995; 1996). There is strong evidence for the effectiveness of this type of intervention (Moyer, Finney, Swearingen, & Vergun, 2002).

However, restricting the use of brief interventions to excessive drinkers in primary health care settings would mean that a lot of them are not reached. Many excessive drinkers never visit a doctor or medical institution, and when they do they are often not screened (Heather, 1996; Roche & Freeman, 2004). Over the past 15 years, researchers and practitioners have therefore been exploring the use of the Internet to screen and educate excessive drinkers, a process known as computer tailoring (Dijkstra & De Vries, 1999). Central to this chapter is a discussion of the effectiveness of computer-tailored interventions targeting nontreatment seeking excessive drinkers.

The content of this chapter is as follows. First, we describe the term *computer tailoring* and give examples of computer-tailored interventions that have recently been developed. Second, we describe the theoretical basis underlying computer-tailored interventions. We also describe a recent example of a web-based computer-tailored intervention to illustrate how this theory is used in practice and to give an example of the type of computer-tailored intervention discussed here. Third, we discuss issues raised by the theory and the example, and we further examine these issues in a small-scale study. Finally, we discuss the results of this study and directions for further research.

COMPUTER-TAILORED INTERVENTIONS ON ALCOHOL USE

Tailoring is a process of designing messages to reflect individual's needs, interests, abilities, and motivations, which are derived from an individual assessment (Kreuter, Farrell, Olevitch, & Brennan, 2000). In computer tailoring, the screening is performed online and a computer program registers the respondent's answers. This program contains a variety of possible responses. Based on the screening data, the program chooses the most suitable responses, which are then integrated into an advice and displayed to the respondent. An advice generated this way is called a computer-tailored advice. In contrast, the term *general advice* refers to pieces of information that are not tailored to the individual, like a brochure. For a more extensive description of computer tailoring and the development of computer-tailored interventions, see Brug, Oenema, and Campbell (2003) and Dijkstra and De Vries (1999).

In recent years, the Internet has become a very popular means among the general public to obtain health information (Powell, Darvell, & Gray, 2003; Rice & Katz, 2001; Roche & Freeman, 2004; Toll, Sobell, D'Arienzo, Sobell, Eickleberry-Goldsmith, et al., 2003). Furthermore, research shows that excessive drinkers who are not experiencing severe problems nevertheless take interest in health information if and when it is offered to them (Brug et al., 2003). This indicates that these people lack awareness of the problem rather than interest in information about it. Therefore, computer-tailored interventions potentially reach a large group of excessive drinkers, especially those unmotivated to seek treatment. Evaluations of various alcohol intervention Web sites show that these Web sites attract many visitors, a lot of whom are people who drink excessively but have never sought treatment (Cloud & Peacock, 2001; Cunningham, Humphreys, & Koski-Jannes, 2000; Linke, Brown, & Wallace, 2004; Saitz, Helmuth, Aromaa, Guard, Belanger, et al., 2004).

Computer-tailored interventions can be seen as a kind of brief intervention, but they are much more flexible. Once developed, they can be implemented inside as well as outside of primary care settings. They can be used at the local level by primary health care organizations or general practitioners, but in order to reach the general public they can also be made available through the Internet. Excessive drinkers can take the online screening and receive advice any time they want, from any place they choose while remaining anonymous. Also, updating computer-tailored advice, for instance, to include new insights, is easy and cheap as the advice can be rewritten as often as necessary. If updated regularly, computer-tailored interventions can be used for many years, making them very cost-effective (Dijkstra & De Vries, 1999).

The Dutch Web site http://www.drinktest.nl is an excellent illustration of the development in computer-tailored interventions. At this Web site, visitors are screened by a self-administered questionnaire resulting in an advice that is directly displayed on screen. In similar online interventions in The Netherlands, the respondent has to give his or her address to receive the advice by mail. In contrast, no registration is required for the drink test because the advice is displayed immediately. The drink test Web site is comparable to the recently evaluated U.S. Web site Alcoholscreening.org (Saitz et al., 2004). The fact that the entire intervention takes place online also opens up new possibilities to integrate the drink test with other forms of support. After receiving the tailored advice, visitors of the drink test have the possibility to call the help-desk or ask further questions about the advice by e-mail.

Launched in December 2002 and receiving more than 100,000 visitors in just the first 2 weeks, the drink test is one of the most recently developed and most popular tools. Throughout 2003, the drink test Web site attracted an average of 10,000 visitors per month, of whom about 40% completed the test (NIGZ, 2004). There are plans to connect the drink test to other Dutch online self-help modules targeting problem drinkers who need more intensive treatment, like the Web site www.minderdrinken.nl (Cuijpers, Riper, & Kramer, 2003; Riper, Kramer, & Cuijpers, 2003), which has been launched in November 2004. In time, the organizations participating in this project aim to develop a complete online stepped-care model (NIGZ, 2003).

The previous example shows that online brief interventions have important advantages over brief interventions in offline settings. However, evaluations of the effectiveness of computer-tailored interventions are still limited, especially with regard to alcohol use. The Dutch drink test is based on experiences with earlier developed computer-tailored interventions for smoking (Dijkstra, De Vries, & Roijackers, 1998), dietary behavior (Oenema, Brug, & Lechner, 2001), and exercising (Bull, Kreuter, & Scharff, 1999). In the next sections of this chapter, we review this literature to formulate expectations about the effectiveness of interventions targeting excessive drinkers who are not aware of their possible health problem, and who are hence unmotivated to cut down their drinking.

THEORETICAL BASIS OF COMPUTER-TAILORED INTERVENTIONS

The computer-tailored interventions discussed in this chapter use the transtheoretical model to tailor health messages (Prochaska & Velicer, 1997). According to this model, behavioral change occurs in five stages. People in the first stage, precontemplation, see no reason to change their behavior. People in the second stage, contemplation, are aware of their health problem and consider taking action some day in the future. In the preparation stage, they actively plan to change their behavior in the near future. In the action stage, they actively attempt to change their behavior. If they retain the new behavior over a longer period of time, they reach the maintenance stage. In interventions using the transtheoretical model, the main intervention objective is not a change from unhealthy to healthy behavior, but a transition from one stage to the next in the process of behavior change.

It is supposed that people in different stages have different intentions, thoughts, and feelings with regard to a particular type of healthy behavior. Therefore, they are thought to need different advice and resources (Armitage & Conner, 2000). More specifically, the transtheoretical model argues that people in the first stage, precontemplators, are unmotivated to change their behavior because they see more disadvantages (cons) than advantages (pros) of the healthy behavior. Interventions tailored to these people should therefore contain information aimed at shifting the balance from seeing more disadvantages to seeing more advantages of the healthy behavior (attitude change). Only when an individual sees more advantages than disadvantages will he or she move on to contemplation and beyond. In contrast, once people have formed a positive attitude towards changing their behavior, the need for information on how to change (self-efficacy) becomes relatively more important than attitudinal information to motivate them to progress from contemplation to preparation and onwards.

Intentions, attitude, self-efficacy and social influence are thought to be the main predictors of stage change. In Dutch computer-tailored interventions, measures of attitude and self-efficacy are often derived from social cognitive theory (Bandura, 1986) and the theory of planned behavior (Ajzen, 1991). According to the theory of planned behavior, behavioral intention is the most proximal determinant of actual behavior. The three main determinants of intention are attitude, subjective norm, and perceived behavioral control or self-efficacy. Attitudes are a function of beliefs about the pros and cons of performing the behavior, subjective norms are based on beliefs about what significant others think of the behavior, and self-efficacy is based on beliefs about the extent to which the behavior is under one's control. The strength of the relationship between each of these predictors and the target behavior might vary per behavior. In contrast, social cognitive theory states that self-efficacy is the most important determinant of behavior. This theory distinguishes between a person's perceived self-efficacy to perform the desired behavior in social situations, for example, not drinking at parties, and in various emotional states, for example, not drinking when depressed.

The assumption that attitudinal information is most relevant to precontemplators is based on two consistent findings in research on smoking cessation (De Vries & Mudde, 1998; De Vries, Mudde, Dijkstra, & Willemsen, 1998; Dijkstra, De Vries, & Bakker, 1996; Dijkstra, Roijackers, & De Vries, 1998) and health related food choice (Brug, Glanz, & Kok, 1997; Brug, Hospers, & Kok, 1997). First, when comparing mean scores on behavioral determinants of people in various stages using analyses of variance, contemplators score significantly higher than precontemplators on attitude toward or on perception of advantages of the healthy behavior. Furthermore, the difference between precontemplators and contemplators is usually larger than differences between other pairs of consecutive stages. Second, in most studies the opposite has been found with regard to self-efficacy. Differences between precontemplators and contemplators are relatively small and often not significant, whereas larger differences are found between other consecutive stages.

With regard to the third component in the theory of planned behavior, subjective norm, and related social influence variables (e.g., descriptive norms: perceptions of behavior of important others), findings are less consistent. In some studies, no variables of this type have been included (Dijkstra et al., 1996; Dijkstra, Roijackers, et al., 1998). Other studies have included measures of perceived behavior of self versus others (Brug, Glanz, et al., 1997), perceived social support (Brug, Hospers, et al., 1997; De Vries & Mudde, 1998; De Vries et al., 1998), or perceived behavior of others (Brug, Hospers, et al., 1997; De Vries et al., 1998). It has been found that contemplators sometimes score higher than precontemplators and sometimes equal to precontemplators on these variables. Due to the many different conceptualizations of social influence, it is difficult to draw strong conclusions, but results indicate that contemplators have stronger perceptions of social support from people in their environment then do precontemplators.

Although most of these results are derived from cross-sectional studies that do not allow causal inferences, findings lead to the conclusion that interventions aimed at excessive drinkers who are not yet aware of their problem—from now on referred to as *precontemplators*—should emphasize the advantages of reduced drinking. However, some scholars have criticized this suggestion (Armitage & Arden, 2002; Armitage, Povey, & Arden, 2003; Malotte, Jarvis, Fishbein, Kamb, Iatesta, et al., 2000). Based on their findings, they have concluded that both types of information should be included in advice tailored to precontemplators. We argue that this difference in opinion is not due to actual differences in research findings, but to differences in the way the data were analyzed. Instead of looking at differences in mean scores between stages using analyses of variance, the researchers examined relationships between behavioral determinants as independent variables and stage of change as dependent variable. They reported linear increases in the scores on both attitude and self-efficacy across stages. However, in two of the articles, the mean differences between the stages were also reported (Armitage & Arden, 2002; Armitage et al., 2003). In both studies, the researchers found a significant difference between precontemplators and contemplators on self-efficacy with regard to eating a low-fat diet, but this difference was small compared to the differences between other successive stages. In contrast, they found that contemplators scored significantly higher than precontemplators on attitude and subjective norm, and the differences were much larger than between other successive stages.

These findings suggest that the relationships between attitude, efficacy, subjective norm, and stage are not entirely linear. We believe that the method of analysis the authors used was just not sensitive enough to register this. It must be noted, though, that there is evidence that relationships between stages and determinants might differ per behavior type. In their 2003 study, Armitage, Povey and Arden also included measures with regard to another type of dietary behavior, that is, eating fruit and vegetables. With regard to self-efficacy, results were in line with earlier findings. However, increases in attitude and subjective norm across stages were found to be linear.

In sum, it appears that three findings have consistently emerged from the literature: (1) contemplators score higher on attitude than precontemplators, and the difference between these stages is usually larger than between other consecutive stages; (2) there is a relatively small difference, if any, between precontemplators and contemplators in self-efficacy compared to other consecutive stages; and (3) contemplators experience higher levels of social support than precontemplators. However, it is possible that this pattern is not found for every type of healthy behavior. It is therefore important to investigate differences in behavioral determinants across stages specifically for the behavior under study, in this case, drinking less alcohol.

PUTTING THEORY INTO PRACTICE:
THE DRINK TEST

The primary target group of the drink test consists of adults from 35–55 years in precontemplation. About one in five people in this age group drinks excessively, but does not experience any problems and has never sought help. The drink test aims to increase knowledge about the disadvantages of alcohol among members of this group, knowledge about guidelines for sensible alcohol use, and their intention to follow these guidelines.

The screening consists of two parts. The first part registers demographic information, drinking behavior, and stage of change. A short response providing advice follows, discussing the respondent's drinking and giving information about the sensible limit of alcohol use. This is meant to improve the risk perception of those people who exceed this limit. Definitions of excessive and sensible drinking are usually expressed in standard drinks. In The Netherlands, excessive drinking is defined as drinking at least 21 standard drinks a week for males and 14 standard drinks a week for females. People who engage in binge drinking, defined as drinking 6 (males) or 4 (females) standard drinks in a row at least once a week, are also called excessive drinkers. The definition of a standard drink differs by country (Miller, Heather, & Hall, 1991). A Dutch standard drink contains about 10g of pure alcohol (NIGZ, 2003).

Excessive drinkers are advised to take the second part of the test. This test includes measures of beliefs about the physical advantages and disadvantages of alcohol use (attitude), for example, "if I drank less alcohol, my concentration would improve." Furthermore, the test includes questions that measure the control beliefs underlying self-efficacy. These items determine in which situations the respondent finds it difficult to stay within the limit of sensible alcohol use. A distinction is made between social situations, for example, "when you are at a party or in a restaurant," and negative emotional states, for example, "when you feel lonely." Social influence is addressed to a much lesser extent. The drink test contains only two questions regarding this variable. The first question concerns the subjective norm—expected reactions from others if the respondent should drink less. The second question is whether the respondent expects to be a better example for others if he or she drinks less.

A final piece of advice is then tailored to the respondent's answers. People can print the advice or e-mail it to themselves for later reference. Those who need more information and support are encouraged to call the help line, or ask further questions by e-mail. Although the amount of calls to the help line has neither increased nor decreased since the launch of the drink test, the number of callers who selected the option from the voice-response system to talk to a health counselor increased from 47% in 2002 to 55% in 2003. Although it is not possible to attribute this increase exclusively to the drink test, it is a fact that, in 2003, the help line was only promoted in the drink test campaign. Furthermore, the number of questions asked by e-mail and through a form on the Internet increased by 55% (1,942 questions in 2003), illustrating the growing popularity of the Internet as a means of obtaining information.

With regard to attitude, the respondent's beliefs about the advantages and disadvantages of alcohol are discussed in the advice. Correct beliefs are confirmed, and with regard to incorrect beliefs extra information is given to increase knowledge about the consequences of alcohol. For instance, if the respondent thinks that alcohol will help him or her sleep better, it is explained why alcohol will in fact make the respondent sleep badly. With regard to self-efficacy, the advice discusses the social situations and emotional states in which the respondent has trouble drinking moderately. The advice offers the respondent some tips to help him or her stay away from alcohol at these difficult moments.

With regard to social influence, regardless of what the respondent answered in the questionnaire, he or she is told that other people will appreciate it if the respondent drinks less. The respondent is told that other people, for instance one's children, often model the behavior of others, for instance their parents. Therefore, he or she will be a better example if he or she drinks less. As stated previously, little is known about differences between precontemplators and contemplators in their perceptions of various types of social influence. Therefore, in the drink test, the social influence part of the advice always appears, regardless of the respondent's answer. Further research is needed to investigate if and how social influence information should be tailored to precontemplators. This question will be the focus of the next section in this chapter. After that, we discuss if and how interventions should be tailored to precontemplators in the way suggested previously, that is, accentuating attitude information.

THEORETICAL ISSUES

This section elaborates on the two issues just described. First we discuss the role of social influence. Next, we extend the discussion about the relevance of attitude and self-efficacy by reviewing evidence for the proposition that precontemplators benefit most from attitude-enhancing information. After addressing these issues, we present results of a small-scale research of our own in which we studied these issues. Afterwards, we discuss the implications of the results for these issues.

Normative Social Influence

We have showed that, in theory as well as in practice, the social influence component of the theory of planned behavior receives little systematic attention. Research on the theory of planned behavior has shown that attitude and self-efficacy are usually the strongest predictors of behavior (Godin & Kok, 1996), which would justify the emphasis on these variables in the drink test. Nevertheless, when designing tailored advice for excessive drinkers it is important to consider the presence and possible effects of social influence. Research using other theories has shown a relationship between drinking and various social influence variables (Borsari & Carey, 2003). It has also been suggested that the relatively weak performance of the subjective norm as defined in the theory of planned behavior might be due to its conceptualization (Conner & Armitage, 1998; Terry, Hogg, & White, 1999).

We found the role model perception measure in the Dutch drink test especially interesting because it fits an approach that has been used for some time now in the United States at school campuses, known as the *social norms marketing approach*. Research has shown that people unconsciously adapt their drinking pattern to that of others, a process better known as modeling (Bandura, 1986). Problems arise when people overestimate the amount other people drink, which is often the case among students (Berkowitz, 2003) as well as adults (Wild, 2002). Social norms marketing means that people are made aware of the possibility that they misperceive the attitudes and behavior of their peers who function as their role models (Perkins, 2003). This method has been shown to work among students (Lederman & Stewart, 2004; Mattern & Neighbors, 2004) as well as adults (Cunningham, Wild, Bondy, & Lin, 2001).

If the social norms approach works, the opposite might also work: Instead of pointing out that one is possibly misperceiving norms of others, a campaign might make people aware that they communicate certain norms themselves through their behavior, which are perceived, and possibly misperceived, by others. Therefore, we performed a study in which we not only investigated changes in attitude and self-efficacy, but also whether the advice of the drink test was capable of influencing people's perceptions of their example-setting function.

Cause and Effect

Three consistent findings have emerged from the literature on computer-tailored interventions. First, contemplators score higher on attitude than precontemplators. Second, precontemplators and contemplators do not differ in self-efficacy. Third, contemplators experience higher levels of social support than precontemplators. Based on these findings, it has been concluded that precontemplators should receive mainly attitude-enhancing information. However, findings from evaluations of stage-tailored interventions do not support the proposition that in terms of stage transition, precontemplators would benefit most from attitude-enhancing information. We found one study in which the researchers compared the effects of attitude and self-efficacy information versus attitude-only, efficacy-only, and no information for people in various stages of change. In contrast to their predictions, they found the greatest amount of stage transitions among precontemplators who received an intervention including both attitude- and self-efficacy-enhancing information, and among those receiving self-efficacy-enhancing information only (Dijkstra, De Vries, Roijackers, & Van Breukelen, 1998).

The question whether precontemplators indeed benefit most from attitude-enhancing information is only relevant if a stage transition from precontemplation to contemplation is really a consequence of attitude change. However, all of the aforementioned studies had cross-sectional instead of longitudinal designs, making it impossible to conclude that increasing attitude will lead to stage transition. We encountered only two studies with a longitudinal design (De Vries & Mudde, 1998; Prochaska, DiClemente, Velicer, Ginpil, & Norcross, 1985), and even these studies left room for the hypothesis that it is not attitude change that causes a stage change, but that stage change actually causes a more positive attitude. This is due to the fact that both studies were evaluations of computer-tailored interventions that were not online. Respondents could not take the screening online, but had to fill out a pencil-and-paper questionnaire. This questionnaire was scanned into a computer, which created advice tailored to the survey responses. This advice was printed and was sent by mail to the respondents. The time interval between the screening and the advice varied from a couple of days to several weeks, and the time between receiving the advice and taking the posttest was also at least another week (Brug et al., 2003). It is still possible in such a design that changes found in behavioral determinants in the posttest preceded a found change in stage, and not the other way around.

We want to investigate if a stage change and a change in determinants might occur simultaneously, meaning that one does not necessarily cause the other. Because our study on the drink test was conducted entirely online, we were able to record reactions from respondents immediately after they read the online advice, without having to put them into an experimental setting. We measured stage of change and several determinants of behavior prior to the intervention. The posttest took place immediately after the respondent had read the advice. This way, we can determine immediate changes in stage and if they are accompanied by any changes in attitude, self-efficacy, and perceptions of social influence. Furthermore, we can assess the difference between precontemplators and contemplators prior to exposure to the drink test, and see if we find similar differences between these groups as in previous research.

ANALYSIS OF THE DRINK TEST: METHOD

Procedure

The study was conducted entirely online, from July through August 2003, and consisted of a pretest–posttest design without a control group. An assisting student recruited respondents by e-mail, starting in her personal network of acquaintances. Respondents were asked to participate in the research if they thought they fit the specified criteria with regard to alcohol use; drinking 14 or more glasses a week, or drinking four or more glasses on one occasion at least once a week. Furthermore, they were asked to send the Web site address to all of their acquaintances who possibly fit the criteria. At the research Web site, respondents were invited to fill out the pretest questionnaire. After completing this questionnaire, a link in our Web site sent the respondents to the drink test in a new window. The respondents participated in the drink test, read the advice, and then closed the window, after which they immediately completed the posttest questionnaire of our study.

Respondents

Although our method of respondent selection has disadvantages, it resulted in a sample with characteristics largely resembling those of the real visitors of the drink test. About 200 people visited the research Web site, of whom 103 people participated. The sample consisted of 74 males and 29 females, with a mean age of 30 years. At www.drinktest.nl, the mean age is 33 years, meaning our respondents were slightly younger, but the male–female ratio is representative.

Measures

Behavior was measured with the following question: "How many drinks did you have last week?" Respondents were explicitly asked to report the amount of standard drinks per day. Instructions and a conversion table were given. For instance, a bottle of wine contains about seven standard drinks. The drinks were summed up to a week total.

Stage of change was determined by asking people to indicate which of five statements fitted them best: "I do not plan to reduce my alcohol intake," "I plan to reduce my alcohol intake within 6 months," "I plan to reduce my alcohol intake within 1 month," "I am currently taking action to reduce my alcohol intake," and "I reduced my alcohol intake more than 6 months ago." Similar statements were previously used in research on smoking (De Vries et al., 1998; Prochaska & diClemente, 1983).

Attitude was measured on a set of seven-point bipolar evaluative adjective scales ($\alpha = .70$), derived from the theory of planned behavior (Ajzen, 1991): "For me, reducing my alcohol intake is good–bad, harmful–beneficial, pleasant–unpleasant, foolish–wise and desirable–undesirable." All items were coded in such a way that a higher score represented a more positive attitude towards reducing alcohol intake.

Self-efficacy was measured with two items. First, the perceived difficulty of the behavior was asked: "Do you find reducing your alcohol intake difficult or easy?" Answers ranged from 1 (very difficult) to 5 (very easy). The next question was about perceived self-efficacy in general: "If you wanted to reduce your alcohol intake, would you be able to do so?"

Answers ranged from 1 (definitely not) to 5 (definitely so). The items scaled, $\alpha = .75$.

We derived the *role model perception* measure in our questionnaire from the drink test; "If I should drink less alcohol, I would be a better example for people who are important to me". Answers varied from 1 (totally disagree) to 5 (totally agree).

The posttest contained measures of attitude ($\alpha = .75$), self-efficacy ($\alpha = .67$) and role model perception identical to those used in the pretest.

RESULTS

Drinking Behavior and Stage of Change

On average, people in the sample consumed 20.1 standard drinks in the week before the survey. Fifty-six (54.4%) of the respondents exceeded the limit of sensible alcohol use. This is slightly more than among visitors of the Dutch drink test Web site. With 27.2 against 11.6 standard drinks a week, excessive drinkers differed significantly from moderate drinkers, $t(70.17) = 8.35$, $p < .001$ (two-tailed, equal variances not assumed). Of all respondents, 77 (74.8%) reported to be in precontemplation, 8 (7.8%) were in contemplation, 2 (1.9%) in preparation, 11 (10.7%) in action, and 5 (4.9%) in maintenance. Precontemplators are overrepresented in this sample, because at the national drink test, only 65% of the visitors report to be in precontemplation. Although the main goal of the study was to find out how excessive drinkers respond to the advice, we decided to include moderate drinkers in the analyses due to the small sample size and the uneven distribution across stages. To assure this would not lead to different conclusions, however, all analyses were also executed with excessive drinkers only. These analyses yielded similar results.

Stage Transitions From Precontemplation to Contemplation

In the posttest, we found that of the 77 people in our sample who were in precontemplation in the pretest, 20 (19%) had moved to the contemplation stage in the posttest. Next, we investigated whether these people, hereafter called *ex-precontemplators*, differed from those who stayed in precontemplation. Two people were excluded from these analyses because they reported transitions to the action and maintenance stages. In the group of ex-precontemplators, 55% of the people were excessive drinkers against 37.5% in the group of precontemplators. Both groups differed significantly on alcohol use, with precontemplators on average drinking 16.4 standard drinks and ex-precontemplators drinking 21.8,

$t(73) = -2.0, p < .05$. This indicates that mainly excessive drinkers were influenced by the advice, as was the purpose.

Between-group comparisons were made for pretest and posttest variables, using two-tailed independent samples t tests. Table 15.1 shows that in the pretest, no differences were found. In the posttest, one significant difference was found. Ex-precontemplators and precontemplators differed in role model perception; ex-precontemplators tended to believe they are a better example for other people if they drink less, but precontemplators did not.

We used GLM Repeated Measures to explore within-group differences in pretest and posttest. A significant interaction effect was found between role model perception and stage of change, $F(1,73) = 3.88, p < .05$. The role model perception of precontemplators did not change significantly, $t(54) = -.41, p = .68$. In contrast, the role model perception of ex-precontemplators became significantly more positive, $t(19) = -2.99, p < .01$. Their attitude and self-efficacy also became more positive, although not significantly, whereas the attitude and self-efficacy of precontemplators barely changed. Exploring the data further, we discovered another difference between precontemplators and ex-precontemplators. Among ex-precontemplators 45% had children whereas among precontemplators only 25% had children. Clearly, among ex-precontemplators, people with children were overrepresented. Ex-precontemplators might become more aware of their role model function because they realize they are an example for their children.

TABLE 15.1
Means, Standard Deviations and t Values
for Precontemplators Versus Ex-Precontemplators

	First Two Stages Only					
	Precontemplators *(n = 55)*		*Ex-Precontemplators* *(n = 20)*			
	M	*SD*	*M*	*SD*	*df*	*t*
Pretest						
Attitude	4.23	.85	4.25	.69	73.00	−.08
Self-efficacy	4.05	1.00	3.77	.95	73.00	1.05
Role model perception	2.27	1.10	2.35	.67	55.43[a]	−.37
Posttest						
Attitude	4.17	.81	4.37	.81	73.00	−.96
Self-efficacy	3.95	.81	3.95	.58	73.00	−.02
Role model perception	2.35	.93	3.15	.93	73.00	−3.32**

Note.   **$p < .01$.
[a]Equal variances not assumed.

We also found some evidence that differences in attitude between precontemplators and contemplators come to exist some time after a stage change. Because in the pretest only eight people reported to be in contemplation, results from comparisons with precontemplators have to be interpreted with caution. Results showed that precontemplators differed significantly from contemplators on attitude, with contemplators having a significantly higher score (5.30) than precontemplators (4.25), $t(83) = -3.47$, $p < .001$. No significant differences were found in self-efficacy and role model perception. This is a tentative suggestion that differences in attitude emerge some time after a stage shift.

DISCUSSION

Normative Social Influence

In our review of the literature on the effects of computer tailoring, we showed that the role of social influence in particular stages of change has not been as thoroughly investigated as the role of attitude and self-efficacy. We therefore found it important to measure the influence of social information in the advice of the drink test, more specifically one's perception of being a role model. After filling out the drink test and reading the advice, 19% of the people in our sample reported a stage transition and a more positive role model perception. At the same time, they did not report any significant changes in attitude or self-efficacy, whereas these variables receive more attention in the drink test than role model perception. A possible explanation for our results is that role model perception is a relatively new concept, about which people have not previously thought. It is therefore possible that the drink test guided their opinion formation about the importance of being a role model. In contrast, attitudes and self-efficacy with regard to drinking less alcohol are more likely to be well shaped and stable, and are therefore harder to change by a single exposure to a persuasive message.

Our study was intended as a first exploration of the added value of the role model question. On the basis of the results, we think it is worth considering that role model perception plays an important role in moving precontemplators to contemplation. Previous research has shown the effectiveness of making people aware of the possibility that they misperceive the attitudes and behavior of their peers who function as their role models (Perkins, 2003; Wild, 2002). Our research suggests that the opposite also holds. Instead of pointing out that one is possibly misperceiving norms of others, an intervention might make people aware that they communicate certain norms themselves through their behavior, which are perceived, and possibly misperceived, by others (for in-stance, one's children). As research has already indicated that perceptions of social support also differ across stages, we argue that future research should pay more attention to this variable as well.

Cause and Effect

Our study shows that, apparently, it is possible to find no significant changes in attitude and self-efficacy while still finding a stage transition immediately after the advice has been read. As said before, none of the previous studies on differences between precontemplators and contem-plators has provided strong evidence that the fact that contemplators have a more positive attitude towards a particular health behavior than precontemplators means that a more positive attitude causes precon-templators to move to contemplation. Although our research design does not allow for inferences about causality as well, our data seem to suggest that a stage shift does not have to be accompanied by an in-crease in attitude, at least not in the short term. Our data suggest that it might be the other way around, meaning that precontemplators' atti-tudes increase after their stage transition to contemplation. Results from a comparison between people who were in precontemplation and those who were in contemplation in the pretest tentatively suggest that differences in attitude between these stages might emerge some time af-ter the stage shift.

Furthermore, other research has shown that a simple cue might be enough to move people from precontemplation to contemplation. In their study on how to motivate people to reduce their fat intake, Armitage and Conner (2001) showed that it might be enough just to confront people with normative feedback, that is, display the norm of what most people do so that people compare that to what they do themselves. In the drink test, people receive this type of feedback immediately after the screening in the short advice that follows. This short advice might serve as a simple cue to motivate people to think about their behavior. Furthermore, some studies have found that it does not matter whether the advice is tailored to precontemplators' answers. For instance, Sobell and colleagues (2002) tested a general versus a tailored intervention among people with alcohol problems. In the 1-year follow-up, they found that both interventions, tailored or not, had been equally effective in reducing alcohol consump-tion. Similar findings were reported by Dijkstra and colleagues (1998), who found that precontemplators responded equally well to stage-matched versus unmatched information. Based on their findings, the au-thors suggest that perhaps it does not matter what type of information precontemplators receive, as long as they receive something. A possible explanation is that precontemplators have a low motivation to process information, causing the advice to work as a simple cue to action.

It has even been suggested that screening in itself can encourage some people to consider behavior change (Freemantle, Gill, Godfrey, Long, Richards, et al., 1993). This implies that precontemplators have moved to contemplation just because they have taken a test. Some support for this statement is found in a study of Dijkstra, De Vries, and Roijackers (1999). Four groups were compared who, after taking a test, either received multiple tailored interventions, a single tailored intervention, a nontailored intervention or no intervention. Among precontemplators, the greatest number of stage transitions was reported in the no intervention condition. A possible explanation is that the test itself triggers people to think about its subject. Because the test offers no clues with regard to what to think about, people will think about those aspects that are most relevant to them. This way, the test itself functions as a cue that invites people to actively think about the subject.

An example of this principle is found in a study of Hoogstraten, De Haan, and Ter Horst (1985). In their study, half of the participants received an application form for dental treatment and a message based on the theory of planned behavior. The other half received the application form without a message. In the group that received the message, more application forms were filled in. But remarkably, the authors found that in the group that received no message, more subjects actually went to the dentist than from the group that did receive a message.

CONCLUSION

One of the most interesting questions for future research is whether a change in determinants precedes a stage change or whether a change in determinants is actually a consequence of stage change. Longitudinal research is needed to establish this. We suggest that effects should be measured at least at three points in time: (1) directly after the intervention, (2) some weeks later, and (3) several months later. This can be easily achieved if evaluations of computer-tailored interventions take place on the Internet. This way, the respondent can participate in the research from within his or her natural environment.

The answer to the cause–effect question has large implications for the theoretical basis and the content of computer-tailored advice. If stage change precedes a change in determinants, tailoring the advice to people in precontemplation becomes less relevant. In that case, it becomes more relevant to investigate if it is actually the content of the advice that causes the stage shift, simply the fact that an advice has been given, or even just the fact that a test has been taken. The results just discussed, as well as our study, suggest that taking a test or receiving an advice might function as a cue to move from one stage to the next. Furthermore, our results with respect to role model perception suggest that it can be effective to give respondents social information, which will probably contain new arguments about which they have not thought before.

Although a lot of work needs to be done, for the moment we can conclude that online self-testing and a single piece of advice, whether it is tailored or not, can succeed in making precontemplators aware that they might have a problem with alcohol and motivating them to become contemplators. This makes Internet screenings a valuable tool to increase awareness among nontreatment seeking excessive drinkers of possible health problems.

REFERENCES

Ajzen, I. (1991). The theory of planned behavior. *Organizational Behavior and Human Decision Processes, 50,* 179–211.

Armitage, C. J., & Arden, M. A. (2002). Exploring discontinuity patterns in the transtheoretical model: An application of the theory of planned behaviour. *British Journal of Health Psychology, 7,* 89–103.

Armitage, C. J., & Conner, M. (2000). Social cognition models and health behaviour: A structured review. *Psychology & Health, 15*(2), 173–189.

Armitage, C. J., & Conner, M. (2001). Efficacy of a minimal intervention to reduce fat intake. *Social Science & Medicine, 52*(10), 1517–1524.

Armitage, C. J., Povey, R., & Arden, M. A. (2003). Evidence for discontinuity patterns across the stages of change: A role for attitudinal ambivalence. *Psychology & Health, 18,* 373–386.

Bandura, A. (1986). *Social foundations of thought and action: A social cognitive theory.* Englewood Cliffs, NJ: Prentice-Hall.

Berkowitz, A. D. (2003). The social norms approach: Theory, research and annotated bibliography. Higher Education Center for Alcohol and Other Drug Prevention. Retrieved December 2, 2005, from www.edc.org/hec/socialnorms

Borsari, B., & Carey, K. B. (2003). Descriptive and injunctive norms in college drinking: A meta-analytic integration. *Journal of Studies on Alcohol, 64*(3), 331–341.

Brug, J., Glanz, K., & Kok, G. (1997). The relationship between self-efficacy, attitudes, intake compared to others, consumption, and stages of change related to fruit and vegetables. *American Journal of Health Promotion, 12*(1), 25–30.

Brug, J., Hospers, H. J., & Kok, G. (1997). Differences in psychosocial factors and fat consumption between stages of change for fat reduction. *Psychology & Health, 12*(5), 719–727.

Brug, J., Oenema, A., & Campbell, M. (2003). Past, present, and future of computer-tailored nutrition education. *American Journal of Clinical Nutrition, 77*(4), 1028S–1034S.

Bull, F. C., Kreuter, M. W., & Scharff, D. P. (1999). Effects of tailored, personalized and general health messages on physical activity. *Patient Education and Counseling, 36,* 181–192.

Cloud, R. N., & Peacock, P. L. (2001). Internet screening and interventions for problem drinking: Results from the www.carebetter.com Pilot Study. *Alcoholism Treatment Quarterly, 19*(2), 23–44.

Conner, M., & Armitage, C. J. (1998). Extending the theory of planned behavior: A review and avenues for further research. *Journal of Applied Social Psychology, 285*(15), 1429–1464.

Cuijpers, P., Riper, H., & Kramer, J. (2003). Evaluation of the effectiveness of an online self-help module for problem drinkers. In G. M. Schippers & T. G. Broekman (Eds.), *Alcohol, drugs, and tobacco research 2001–2002: Register of research in The Netherlands and Flanders on the use, the users, and the effects of alcohol, drugs, and tobacco in 2001–2002* (p. 226). Nijmegen, The Netherlands: Bureau Bêta.

Cunningham, J. A., Humphreys, K., & Koski-Jannes, A. (2000). Providing personalized assessment feedback for problem drinking on the Internet: A pilot project. *Journal of Studies on Alcohol, 61*(6), 794–798.

Cunningham, J. A., Wild, T. C., Bondy, S. J., & Lin, E. (2001). Impact of normative feedback on problem drinkers: A small-area population study. *Journal of Studies on Alcohol, 62*(2), 228–233.

De Vries, H., & Mudde, A. N. (1998). Predicting stage transitions for smoking cessation applying the attitude social influence efficacy model. *Psychology & Health, 13,* 369–385.

De Vries, H., Mudde, A. N., Dijkstra, A., & Willemsen, M. C. (1998). Differential beliefs, perceived social influences, and self-efficacy expectations among smokers in various motivational phases. *Preventive Medicine, 27,* 681–689.

Dijkstra, A., & De Vries, H. (1999). The development of computer-generated tailored interventions. *Patient Education and Counseling, 36,* 193–203.

Dijkstra, A., De Vries, H., & Bakker, M. (1996). Pros and cons of quitting, self-efficacy, and the stages of change in smoking cessation. *Journal of Consulting and Clinical Psychology, 64,* 758–763.

Dijkstra, A., De Vries, H., & Roijackers, J. (1998). Computerized tailored feedback to change cognitive determinants of smoking: A Dutch field experiment. *Health Education Research, 13,* 197–206.

Dijkstra, A., De Vries, H., & Roijackers, J. (1999). Targeting smokers with low readiness to change with tailored and nontailored self-help materials. *Preventive Medicine, 28,* 203–211.

Dijkstra, A., De Vries, H., Roijackers, J., & Van Breukelen, G. J. P. (1998). Tailored interventions to communicate stage-matched information to smokers in different motivational stages. *Journal of Consulting and Clinical Psychology, 66,* 549–557.

Dijkstra, A., Roijackers, J., & De Vries, H. (1998). Smokers in four stages of readiness to change. *Addictive Behaviors, 23,* 339–350.

Freemantle, N., Gill, P., Godfrey, C., Long, A., Richards, C., Sheldon, T., Song, F., & Webb, J. (1993). Brief interventions and alcohol use. *Effective Health Care Bulletin, 7,* 1–13.

Godin, G., & Kok, G. (1996). The theory of planned behavior: A review of its applications to health-related behaviors. *American Journal of Health Promotion, 11*(2), 87–98.

Heather, N. (1995). Interpreting the evidence on brief interventions for excessive drinkers: The need for caution. *Alcohol and Alcoholism, 30*(3), 287–296.

Heather, N. (1996). The public health and brief interventions for excessive alcohol consumption: The British experience. *Addictive Behaviors, 21*(6), 857–868.

Heather, N. (2001). Brief interventions. In N. Heather, T. J. Peters, & T. Stockwell (Eds.), *International handbook of alcohol dependence and problems* (pp. 605–626). Chichester, UK: Wiley.

Hoogstraten, J., De Haan, W., & Ter Horst, G. (1985). Stimulating the demand for dental care: An application of Ajzen and Fishbein's theory of reasoned action. *European Journal of Social Psychology, 15,* 401–414.

Institute of Alcohol Studies. (2004). *IAS factsheet—Alcohol and health*, Retrieved September 13, 2004, from http://www.ias.org.uk/factsheets.html

Kreuter, M., Farrell, D., Olevitch, L., & Brennan, L. (2000). *Tailoring health messages: Customizing communication with computer technology*. Mahwah, NJ: Lawrence Erlbaum Associates.

Lederman, L., & Stewart, L. (2004). *Changing the culture of college drinking: A socially situated health communication campaign*. Cresskill, NJ: Hampton Press.

Linke, S., Brown, A., & Wallace, P. (2004). Down your drink: A Web-based intervention for people with excessive alcohol consumption. *Alcohol and Alcoholism, 39*(1), 29–32.

Malotte, C. K., Jarvis, B., Fishbein, M., Kamb, M., Iatesta, M., Hoxworth, T., Zenilman, J., Bolan, G., & The Project RESPECT Study Group. (2000). Stage of change versus an integrated psychosocial theory as a basis for developing effective behaviour change interventions. *AIDS Care-Psychological and Socio-Medical Aspects of AIDS/HIV, 12*(3), 357–364.

Mattern, J. L., & Neighbors, C. (2004). Social norms campaigns: Examining the relationship between changes in perceived norms and changes in drinking levels. *Journal of Studies on Alcohol, 65*(4), 489–493.

Miller, W. R., Heather, N., & Hall, W. (1991). Calculating standard drink units: International comparisons. *British Journal of Addiction, 86*(1), 43–47.

Moyer, A., Finney, J. W., Swearingen, C. E., & Vergun, P. (2002). Brief interventions for alcohol problems: A meta-analytic review of controlled investigations in treatment-seeking and non-treatment-seeking populations. *Addiction, 97*(3), 279–292.

Murray, C. J. L., & Lopez, A. D. (1996). *The global burden of disease: A comprehensive assessment of mortality and disability from diseases, injuries, and risk factors in 1990 and projected to 2020*. Cambridge, MA: Harvard University Press.

NIGZ. (2003). *Project Alcohol Voorlichting en Preventie Jaarverslag 2002*. [Project Alcohol Education and Prevention Annual Report 2002]. Woerden, The Netherlands: NIGZ.

NIGZ. (2004). *Jaarverslag alcoholvoorlichtingscampagne 2003: Drank maakt meer kapot dan je lief is*. [Annual report alcohol education campaign 2003: Alcohol destroys more than you care for]. Woerden, The Netherlands: NIGZ.

Oenema, A., Brug, J., & Lechner, L. (2001). Web-based tailored nutrition education: Results of a randomized controlled trial. *Health Education Research, 16*, 647–660.

Perkins, H. W. (Ed.). (2003). *The social norms approach to preventing school and college age substance abuse: A handbook for educators, counselors, and clinicians*. San Francisco, CA: Jossey-Bass.

Powell, J. A., Darvell, M., & Gray, J. A. M. (2003). The doctor, the patient and the worldwide web: How the internet is changing healthcare. *Journal of the Royal Society of Medicine, 96*(2), 74–76.

Prochaska, J. O., & diClemente, C. C. (1983). Stages and processes of self-change of smoking: Toward an integrative model of change. *Journal of Consulting and Clinical Psychology, 51*, 390–395.

Prochaska, J. O., DiClemente, C. C., Velicer, W. F., Ginpil, S., & Norcross, J. C. (1985). Predicting change in smoking status for self-changers. *Addictive Behaviors, 10*, 395–406.

Prochaska, J. O., & Velicer, W. F. (1997). The Transtheoretical Model of health behavior change. *American Journal of Health Promotion, 12*, 38–48.

Rice, R. E., & Katz, J. E. (Eds.). (2001). *The Internet and health communication: Expectations and experiences*. Thousand Oaks, CA: Sage.

Riper, H., Kramer, J., & Cuijpers, P. (2003). Development of an online self-help module for problem drinkers. In G. M. Schippers & T. G. Broekman (Eds.), *Alcohol, drugs, and tobacco research 2001–2002: Register of research in The Netherlands and Flanders on the use, the users, and the effects of alcohol, drugs, and tobacco in 2001–2002* (p. 243). Nijmegen, The Netherlands: Bureau Bêta.

Roche, A. M., & Freeman, T. (2004). Brief interventions: Good in theory but weak in practice. *Drug and Alcohol Review, 23*(1), 11–18.

Saitz, R., Helmuth, E. D., Aromaa, S. E., Guard, A., Belanger, M., & Rosenbloom, D. L. (2004). Web-based screening and brief intervention for the spectrum of alcohol problems. *Preventive Medicine, 39*(5), 969–975.

Sobell, L. C., Sobell, M. B., Leo, G. I., Agrawal, S., Johnson-Young, L., & Cunningham, J. A. (2002). Promoting self-change with alcohol abusers: A community-level mail intervention based on natural recovery studies. *Alcoholism-Clinical and Experimental Research, 26*(6), 936–948.

Terry, D. J., Hogg, M. A., & White, K. M. (1999). The theory of planned behavior: Self-identity, social identity and group norms. *British Journal of Social Psychology, 38,* 225–244.

Toll, B. A., Sobell, L. C., D'Arienzo, J., Sobell, M. B., Eickleberry-Goldsmith, L., & Toll, H. J. (2003). What do Internet-based alcohol treatment websites offer? *Cyberpsychology & Behavior, 6*(6), 581–584.

Van Der Laan, N. (2003). *Evaluatie 'advies op maat': Een onderzoek naar overmatig alcoholgebruik.* [Evaluation 'tailored advice': Investigating excessive alcohol use]. Amsterdam: NIPO.

Wild, T. C. (2002). Personal drinking and sociocultural drinking norms: A representative population study. *Journal of Studies on Alcohol, 63*(4), 469–475.

Telehealth in Indigenous Communities in the Far North: Challenges for Continued Development

Lorna Heaton
Université de Montréal, Canada

This chapter reports on a pilot project for telehealth in Nunavut, Canada's newest and northernmost territory. Technologically, the Internet plays a peripheral role in Nunavut's telehealth network, which centers primarily on synchronous communication using videoconferencing technology but also incorporates asynchronous, "store-and-forward" components. However, the Internet is becoming a viable solution for linking remote sites to each other and to specialist services and information sources outside the territory. Indeed, this chapter argues that the Internet can be a vital component in the way health services are delivered in remote northern communities and that its significance is likely to increase as infrastructure and technological issues are resolved.

The analysis is grounded in qualitative data gathered through interviews with health service providers, telehealth project managers, health system administrators and government officials. It adopts a systemic, organizational perspective to examine how various technologies and their availability both enable and constrain the organization of health care delivery. The chapter focuses on changes in the practices of health care professionals that are being brought about by telehealth and on the role the Internet is, or will soon be, called on to play in providing support for continuing medical education and administrative activities, as well as its potential for transferring clinical information between sites in a health system that is, by nature, highly distributed. The chapter addresses how health care workers are inventing new ways of doing things with this connective technology and how relationships between different professional groups and institutions are changing. It also examines some of the infrastructural, organizational and policy issues involved in ensuring coordination across multiple provincial/territorial jurisdictions and organizations.

For the purposes of this chapter, *telehealth* is defined as the use of information and communication technologies for mediating distance in health care delivery. As such, it encompasses the use of a variety of telecommunication technologies such as telephone, computers, e-mail, fax, and interactive video transmissions for the purpose of transfer and/or exchange of information and data between two or more users. This includes health care provider–patient consultations, continuing medical education, consultations between professionals and the transfer of medical data. In contrast, *e-health* is generally defined as Internet-based information activities. The distinction between telehealth and e-health is increasingly blurred as more and more telehealth activities are migrating to an Internet platform, however (Canada, 2003). Here, the term telehealth will be used to refer also to those activities that are Internet-based, although in our case, patients are not directly involved in using the Internet for health purposes.

The chapter begins with a description of the situation in Nunavut and the challenges of delivering health care across a large number of remote, isolated communities. It describes how telehealth is changing medical practices and the health system in this context and these practices and the relationships between the various parts of the system. The chapter then discusses lessons learned from this case and considers how the Internet may help meet a number of challenges for continued development. At this point, insights from telehealth programs in other Northern contexts are introduced in support of our argument.

NUNAVUT AND ITS TELEHEALTH PROGRAM

The territory of Nunavut was created in 1999 to respond to the realities of a distinct society and the political aspirations of the Inuit people, who make up 85% of its population. The vast size (2 million square kilometers—roughly the size of Western Europe) and sparse population (29,000 in 25 communities in three regions—Baffin, Kitikmeot, and Kivalliq) of Nunavut make the provision of quality health services particularly challenging.

Although the scope of the challenge facing Nunavut may be particular, a number of issues facing the territory are common to health service delivery in remote and rural contexts. In fact, over the past 30 years, many countries have explored telehealth for linking remote villages with hospital centers (Mitka, 1997). Scandinavia, especially Norway, was one of the first areas to widely deploy telemedicine. Extensive projects using telemedicine to deliver health care in remote areas have also been established in the northern United Kingdom, Japan, Australia, and Canada. Lesser-developed nations have also shown a keen interest in using telemedicine to improve access to high quality health care but often lack either a telecommunications infrastructure or the resources to pay for such access (Mitka, 1997; Vassallo, Hoque, Roberts, Patterson, Swinfen, & Swinfen, 2001; Wootton, 2001).

Telehealth has been examined in a broad spectrum of applications in rural and remote communities. A systematic review (Health Telematics Unit, 2003) of 35 articles specifically on rural and remote telehealth found good evidence that interactive video consultation is effective and efficient, and increases access to health care (Jennett, Hall, Morin, & Watanabe, 1995; Minister of Research, 1999; Nesbitt, Hilty, Kuenneth, & Siefkin, 2000) across a number of specialties such as radiology and cardiology, colposcopy, neuropsychology, and dermatology. The utility of telehealth in remote areas for outpatient follow-up (Boulanger, Kearney, Ochoa, Tsuei, & Sands, 2001), nutrition counseling (Johnson & Jones, 2001; Stiles, Boosalis, Thompson, Stinnett, & Rayens, 1998), and increasing access to specialty care for high-risk or rare disease patients (Lamb, Eydmann, & Boddy, 1997; Tsilimigaki, Maraka, Tsekoura, Agelakou, Vekiou, et al., 2001; Woods, Johnson, Kutlar, Daitch, & Stachura, 2000) has also been demonstrated. There are implications for access to health care, avoidance of travel, quality of care, and cost savings to the health system. Inter-jurisdictional or telehealth policy voids are among the immediate challenges identified. In particular, there are implications for the integration of telehealth into mainstream rural health care, particularly with regard to human factors outweighing technology issues (Monrad Aas, 2002; Swanson, 1999).

Most Nunavut communities have a health center, which is staffed by nurses and clinical technicians. The territory's only hospital is located in Iqualuit, the capital (hospitals are being built in Rankin Inlet and Cambridge Bay, the administrative centers of the other regions). With basic health infrastructures, a limited number of doctors and chronic staff shortages, the volume and severity of cases that can be treated are limited. Nurses and site technicians handle the bulk of non-urgent medical care. Generalist physicians travel to the communities approximately every 6 weeks, and clinics are organized for major specialties (dermatology, ophthalmology, internal medicine, pediatrics, etc.) once or twice a year. Patients with serious illnesses or injuries, or those requiring specialist consultations, are typically flown out of their communities to hospitals thousands of miles to the south (see Fig. 16.1). Clinical referral patterns tend to flow north–south, with patients in the western Arctic going to either the Northwest Territories or Alberta in Western Canada, Kivalliq dealing with Manitoba in Central Canada, and the Baffin region referring cases it cannot treat in its hospital to sites in Eastern Canada. There are, thus, five Canadian jurisdictions involved in the Nunavut health and social services system, and a number of independent institutions participate within each jurisdiction.

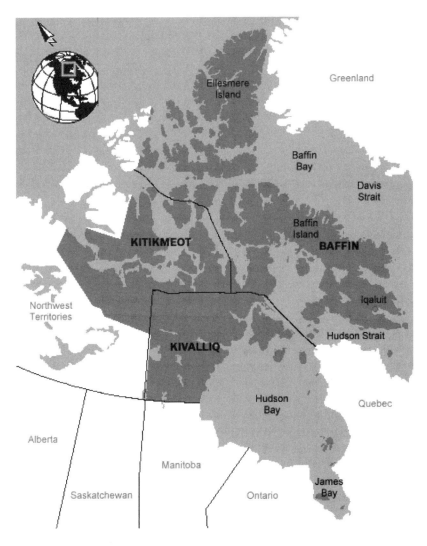

FIG. 16.1.   Map of Nunavut Territory.

In this context, telemedicine seems a logical, if not the only, choice. This is particularly so in the context of the Canadian policy environment. Since 1994, the federal government has invested massively in information technology in the health sector. This movement has been influenced by recommendations of the Canadian Institute for Health Information (CIHI), the Information Highway Advisory Council (IHAC), the Canadian Network for the Advancement of Research, Industry and Education (CANARIE), the Office of Health and the Information Highway (OHIH), and the National Forum on Health. The influential Romanow Report (2002) argued for the increased use of telehealth as a means of mitigating time and distance in order to improve access to health care services and information, especially to rural areas.[1] It also noted a lack of coordination between provincial and territorial governments in addressing telehealth implementation in rural communities and encourages a "coherent national approach" (p. 163) for addressing such issues.

The implementation of a telehealth network throughout Nunavut posed special challenges, many of which had never been encountered in the development of telehealth throughout Canada. Major among these are those imposed by the physical nature of the territory: extreme geographic isolation (communities are only accessible by air or sea), a vast, sparsely populated territory, and difficult and unpredictable weather conditions. These are linked to a relative lack of necessary support and resources: limited technological and telecommunications infrastructure, and limited and often short-term health and technical personnel. Additionally, at the time of implementation, the short history of the territory meant that many administrative procedures were relatively new or still being developed, and that information systems related to the health care system were either not yet available or covered a very short period.

---

[1]The ability to control space and overcome the barriers of geography has always been a key area of interest to Canadian policymakers. In the 19th century, the construction of the Canadian National Railway was heralded as "the National Dream," a means of creating national unity by linking the country from East to West (Babe, 1990). Similarly, with the creation of a public broadcaster, the CBC, to promote a Canadian identity and Canadian unity, came the obligation, and expectation, that Canadians everywhere would be able to receive these broadcasts. In the 1960s, parallels to the railway were made in promoting Canada's leadership in developing and using satellite technology. Babe refers to this idea that the Canadian nation exists by way of its communication structures as *technical nationalism*. He also argues that *technological dependence* is a second, complementary mythology in Canadian telecommunications policy: the position that Canada has little choice but to encourage the implementation of various telecommunication technologies. It is not surprising, then, that the latest connective technology, the information highway and Internet, has been embraced enthusiastically (Canada, 1997). Indeed, the 2001 Report of the National Broadband Task Force is entitled "The new national dream: Networking the nation for broadband access."

Over and above these challenges, the integration of telehealth services within mainstream health service delivery is highly dependent on intricate and sustained cooperation among several key players, often across several provincial/territorial jurisdictions and organizations. These include various Nunavut government departments, the supplier of the telecommunications (satellite) infrastructure in Nunavut, the last-mile telecommunications service supplier, the health centers and their staff in each community, and the remote locations delivering health services using telehealth, including not only health professionals and educators, but also the administrative and managerial levels of their organizations.

THE IIU TELEHEALTH NETWORK PROJECT

Supported by the Canadian Health Infostructure Partnerships Program (CHIPP) and the Government of Nunavut, the objective of the Ikajuruti Inungnik Ungasiktumi (IIU; "a tool to help people who are far away") Telehealth network program is to "improve the access to, and delivery of health, social services and health education in Nunavut using electronic networks and to integrate these tools into the Health and Social Services delivery system" (Nunavut, 2001a).

The IIU Telehealth Network uses interactive video technology to link the health centers of 15 Nunavut communities among themselves and with service providers, typically hospitals in southern Canada. Deployment of the system began in mid-2002 and the system began full operations in January 2003. Funding was later found to extend the network to all of Nunavut's 25 communities by the end of 2004.

The basic communications infrastructure of the IIU utilizes satellite channels to provide 768 kbps (kilobits per second) bandwidth to each site across the region. Each site is equipped with videoconferencing equipment customized with software to facilitate the transfer of patient files, and a general examination camera that can be used, for example, for close-up viewing of sites of clinical interest and to transmit video images of the radiograph on a light box. (This is less than optimal for transmitting radiographs since it results in poorer resolution than the use of x-ray film scanners.) Communication between multiple sites within the region and with individual sites outside the territory is facilitated by the use of an MCU bridge that can connect up to four sites simultaneously. It also facilitates the linking of the H.323-based facilities in Nunavut to sites outside the territory that are using the older H.320 protocol for transmission of video signals. At the time of implementation, this was a high-quality technical solution.

EVALUATION METHODOLOGY

The implementation of the IIU was preceded by a pilot project initiated in 1999–2000 by the Northwest Territories (NWT) involving six remote northern communities. Implications from this pilot were further refined through a community-based needs assessment conducted in 2001 (Nunavut, 2001b). Three broad categories of use were defined for tele-health in Nunavut: administrative uses, continuing medical education, and clinical activity. This chapter reports briefly on the status of each as it stood after 6 months of use, based on data gathered during an external evaluation of the IIU Nunavut Telehealth Network (Infotelmed Communications, Inc., 2003).

The evaluation assessed the impacts of the network over the period from March to September 2003. It gathered qualitative and quantitative data from a broad cross-section of stakeholders including patients and health service providers in all participating Nunavut regions and communities, health service administrators and government officials. The evaluation was guided by both Government of Nunavut requirements and the national CHIPP framework, which focused on the following issues and criteria: quality of care/services, integration of health services, health and related impacts and effects, cost effectiveness, transferability or lessons learned, and technology performance.

Qualitative and quantitative data were gathered from a variety of information sources using a variety of tools and instruments: session monitoring forms ($n = 267$) that recorded information about telehealth activities in four categories (patient care, continuing education, group/community/ public education, and other activities); patient satisfaction surveys following the telehealth sessions; a patient trajectory study; cost savings estimates; and assessment questionnaires to gauge reactions of health professionals to continuing education sessions. Finally, the analysis in this paper draws primarily on face-to-face, video, or telephone interviews with 76 persons towards the end of the evaluation period. Table 16.1 below lists the nine categories of respondents from which respondents were selected (Infotelmed Communications, Inc., 2003, p. 16). The interviews were 30 minutes to 1 hour in length and were conducted by senior evaluators following a structured interview guide. The majority of interviews were taped, transcribed, and analyzed using NUD*IST software.

INTEGRATING TELEHEALTH IN THE HEALTH AND SOCIAL SERVICES SYSTEM

Administration

Administratively, Nunavut's Department of Health and Social Services is highly distributed within the territory. Given the enormous distances in-

TABLE 16.1
Interviews by Respondent Type

Type of Respondent	Number of Individuals Participating in Interviews
IIU central staff[1]	6
Health service providers: physicians	12
Nurses, physiotherapists, psychologists, nutritionists[2]	14
Government officials and staff	9
Health service administrators[3]	5
Social service and community health providers[4]	7
Site techs/operators	11
Have-not community nurse in charge or equivalent	4
Patients[5]	8
Total Individuals Interviewed	76

[1]Includes consultants, project management, regional telehealth coordinators, project support team, technical development/implementation team. Some individuals had more than one function; only their main role vis-à-vis the telehealth system is counted.

[2]Includes Nurses in Charge (NIC's), Community Health Nurses (CHN's), public health nurses, physiotherapists, psychologists, and nutritionists.

[3]Includes public health, social service and community health service administrators.

[4]Includes social workers, community mental health, and environmental health.

[5]Includes patients who used telehealth and family members/friends of patients who used telehealth for televisitations with patients.

Source: Infotelmed Communications, Inc. (2003, p. 16).

volved and the difficulty of traveling (weather, plane schedules, being short-staffed makes it difficult to get away), using the IIU Network is an unconventional solution to an obvious need. In fact, administrative or professional meetings accounted for some 15% of the Network's use, with another 17% of network time spent on education (but not continuing education, which is described in the next paragraph; Infotelmed Communications, Inc., 2003, p. 20). Thus about a third of the system's use was for planning, coordinating, discussing budgets, helping nurses new to the North deal with something they had never before come across, and so on. The bulk of this traffic was between different communities within Nunavut, but some had been for planning upcoming clinics with physicians from the South. This type of use might in Nunavut indicates a real need that other media, such as telephone or fax, do not meet well, and one that the Internet might help fill. Although videoconferencing was available, given the costs involved, it is unlikely it was used when a simple telephone call could suffice. Sample uses included meeting with a nurse who had just arrived in a small, distant community from down south, or for environmental health professionals to meet to develop a strategic plan for the territory.

Continuing Medical Education

Continuing medical education proved to be an extremely popular use of the Network. "They're starved for it. So let me tell you, the educators are going nuts for this . . . , we can't keep up with the requests, it has been a total enhancement" (interview Aug 27, p. 7). The telehealth coordinator in each region made a schedule of sessions offered by third-party content providers on various subjects, that health and social service providers could then request. The level of use was approximately 20 sessions per month, typically with as many sites connected as technically possible. Table 16.2 lists the session themes (Infotelmed Communications, Inc., 2003, pp. 42–43).

Delivery of continuing education over the IIU Telehealth Network is best interpreted as an additional service that would not have been available otherwise (two thirds responded that the Telehealth session represented their only access to this content; Infotelmed Communications, Inc., 2003, p. 44). Some of those interviewed present the sessions as the only way to get current information, whereas others suggest that the same information could be obtained with a lot of searching over the Internet. Given time constraints and the additional effort involved, distance delivery by content specialists was a preferred method. Some 34% (50) of participants indicated that they would be willing to receive continuing education exclusively via the telehealth system while 58% (85)

TABLE 16.2
Continuing Education Session Topics, March–September 2003

• Alzheimer's and dementia	• Fetal alcohol spectrum disorder
• Antipyretic therapy	• Fever syndrome in children
• Asthma	• Headaches
• Brain injury & substance abuse	• Headaches—pediatric
• Breastfeeding initiative	• Intrapartum protocols for TX group B strep
• Carbohydrate counting	• IUD
• Cervical cancer screening	• Letting go of control: letting your patient live at risk
• Child protection	• Nursing leadership
• Childhood obesity	• Nutrition aids/frostbite/atherosclerosis
• Client reviews	• Nutritional management
• Cognitive tools	• OB/Gyn rounds
• Depression	• Physical assessment of child abuse
• Diabetes & hypertension	• Psychiatry
• Diabetes type II and insulin resistance	• Professional networking
• Diagnosis of FASD	• Protocols for TX group B strep
• Dietary internship for cirrhosis/COPD	• Retinopathy of prematurity
• Drug therapy in diabetes	• SARS update
• Ethical issues	• Suicide and suicide prevention

indicated that they would participate regularly in continuing education over telehealth and 8% (11) said they would use it only occasionally. Of course, sessions delivered by teleconference cannot replace professional and in-service training that involves a hands-on, physical component, such as BTLS (Basic Trauma Life Support; p. 44).

The synchronous character of teleconferencing raised a number of issues, however. Scheduling a convenient time across three time zones, or finding a time when staff could be freed of other obligations to attend a session during working hours was not easy, particularly in a context of chronic understaffing. The inflexibility of booked videoconferencing time also made scheduling a challenge, such as when a session was late in starting and the satellite connection had to be cut before it ended. Staff demonstrated great creativity in getting around such obstacles, faxing PowerPoint slides to sites that could attend only on audio, or videotaping sessions to be shown to other staff or other sites at a later date for instance.

None of the participants interviewed in the evaluation broached the subject of interactivity, leading the evaluators to conclude that it was not a significant limiting factor for acceptance and use of continuing education (p. 44). Seen in this light, the Internet might provide an invaluable complement to ongoing professional education. They also found evidence that continuing education sessions helped minimize the sense of personal and professional isolation that practitioners in remote communities face (p. 47).

Clinical Use

In terms of clinical use, the IIU Network allows for real-time transmissions (audio/visual/data) via satellite among Nunavut communities and provides communication links to health care service providers at the main hospital in Iqaluit and outside the territory. Medical professionals can conduct "virtual visits" with patients. Using the network, physicians can often evaluate the severity of a medical situation prior to actually seeing the patient. In many cases, telehealth can eliminate non-urgent travel and a number of preliminary or follow-up visits, thus enabling patients to stay in their communities and with their families during treatment. At an average cost of $2,000 per trip, travel costs are a major expense for the health and social services system in addition to imposing major strains on families. During the evaluation period, half of the telehealth patient care sessions reported that, had telehealth not been used, either a patient or a professional or both would have had to travel. In all cases but one, patient travel would also have involved the travel of at least one other person such as a professional, one or more family members, or an escort (Infotelmed Communications, Inc., 2003, p. 48). When patients have no alternative but to "go south" for care, the IIU Network has been used to connect them with their families in the community from the attending hospital. Family support and the ability to communicate in their own language can have a tremendous impact on patients' psychological well-being and on their recovery time.

Although the IIU Network has been successful, at the end of the evaluation period it had not yet lived up to the high expectations it had raised. In particular, the provision of clinical services was limited by two main barriers: the implementation of functioning service agreements, and the buy-in of health professionals, particularly those on contract to provide in-person services within Nunavut. Delays in signing contracts with outside organizations—especially specialists—destined to provide either face-to-face or telehealth-enabled clinical services had slowed or even blocked the use of the network for patient care.

Regional Commonalities

Although local circumstances and characteristics of the three Nunavut regions introduced variety in the picture, the evaluation outlined a number of recurrent themes. In all three regions, there were questions as to the role and place of telehealth in health service delivery, and a lack of buy-in by clinicians that is at least partially attributable to changes it may require in their practices. Some stakeholders had questions or uncertainties as to how the system would affect their roles and tasks, and clinicians were not all convinced of the utility of telehealth (Infotelmed Communications, Inc., 2003, p 61). The reasons for disliking telehealth are multiple: Some see it as a misguided investment in a context of scarce resources; others clearly don't see the advantage in terms of improving patient care or patient outcomes. A recurrent theme was lack of time and overwork: "everybody is kind of just running around and trying to cope with the things that come up, emergency or urgency" (focus group, Aug. 27, p. 2).

Contingencies of Practice

We suggest that some of what appear to be technical, organizational, or logistical obstacles are in fact *contingencies of practice*. The introduction of a new element, telehealth, into the existing system, requires the adjustment of practices around it. This requires negotiation, both at the systems level (provider agreements) and at the practical level (health professionals' work practices). The introduction of distance between provider and patient in the medical encounter represents a significant disruption of existing and entrenched practices. For instance, medical work is strongly organized around the convention of physical co-presence of the parties involved (Good, 1994; May, Gask, Atkinson, Ellis, Mair, & Esmail, 2001), which has a cultural and practical significance as well as legal importance. Being with the patient implies accepting responsibility for the organization and conduct of care (Jacob, 1999). Direct observation and distinguishing nuances constitute two fundamental resources of diagnostic practice and prognosis (Cicourel, 1990, 1999; Hunter, 1991; Sinclair, 1997), whereas nurses' professional identity is based partially on the assumption that direct human interaction has a therapeutic effect (May, 1992; Mort, May, & Williams, 2003).

What is more, in the case of Nunavut, legal issues in practicing telemedicine, particularly the problem of crossing jurisdictional lines between various provinces and the territory of Nunavut, proved difficult to resolve. Is a physician using telehealth for remote consultations practicing medicine in Nunavut or in the province providing the service? This situation prevented the development of clinical policies and protocols governing telehealth, whose role is to protect and reassure all those involved in patient care.

A number of reasons for clinician resistance to using telehealth are concrete, organizational issues, however. The present network is not organized to be well integrated into the health care system; it is an add-on. Using telehealth is seen as time consuming and not as convenient as the telephone. For example, the inconvenience of having to book or schedule sessions or even having to move to another office to participate in a telehealth session is a deterrent. Additionally, clinicians might be more inclined to use telehealth if sessions were organized around their schedules, and not the other way around.

TELEHEALTH AND THE INTERNET: IS THERE AN OPPORTUNITY HERE?

Is there an opportunity here for the Internet? The speculative discussion focuses on adjusting to practice, both in terms of individual acceptance and adoption and of organizational accommodation. It addresses the interrelationship between infrastructural possibility, technological affordances (particularly the notions of synchronous and asynchronous communications), and possible use. Extrapolations are based on comments from interviews as well as on experiences in other Northern contexts.

Infrastructure: Adequate Connectivity

A precondition for the success of telehealth in Nunavut is adequate connectivity. In order for new programs to function and flourish, a broadband network must be accessible in order to enable data transmission. This was noted as a major obstacle by a number of those interviewed: "It's just that we are sitting on an OC48 terrestrial network here—it's all satellite based and we're talking about some communities having only 64K and 128K in and out. Another world here" (interview Sept 12, p. 6).

The connectivity problem is now being addressed. Following the recommendations of the National Broadband Task Force (Canada, 2001), Industry Canada provided funding under a variety of programs and with various partners in order to guarantee equitable, affordable broadband access all Canadian communities, including those "unlikely to be served by market forces" by 2004. In the case of Nunavut, thanks to funding from Industry Canada, Department of Indian and Northern Affairs, Government of Nunavut's Department of Sustainable Development, high-speed wireless Internet connections should arrive sometime in 2005. As of December, 2004, the Nunavut Broadband Development Corporation had installed the technology in 20 of Nunavut's 25 communities and was about to begin a 5-year training and capacity-building program both on how to use various ICT tools and on content creation and application development. The connectivity problem would appear to be resolved and Nunavut communities should be poised to reap the benefits of the Internet on an equal footing with the rest of Canada.

There is still a piece of the puzzle missing, however. Although communities will soon be able to talk to their local neighbors using wireless technology, all communication coming in or out of the communities must travel by satellite. Each community will soon be connected to the national backbone network through a point of presence (a single drop for sending and receiving from the satellite). Buying satellite time is costly, however. Despite approval in principle by Industry Canada, there have been delays in finalizing the contract for financial assistance under the National Satellite Initiative (press release on the Nunavut Broadband Development Corporation Web site: http://www.nunavut-broadband.ca/newsdec0904.htm). Once the numerous government instances sort out their split responsibilities and bureaucratic politics, expectations of cost-effective satellite communications for the last mile seem reasonable, thanks to a new satellite, Anik F2, which is commercializing the KA frequency band for the first time and using spot beam antennas and smaller ground-based antenna dishes (http://www.space.gc.ca/asc/eng/apogee/2004/07_anikf2.asp).

It would be illusory to assume that increased connectivity will solve all Nunavut's telehealth problems, however. At the moment, there are three parallel networks in use by the health system. All are public: one handles government traffic of all types; another, less secure, network is directed to community uses while the teleconferencing equipment used for telehealth operates on a third, independent network.

Somehow, telehealth is not part of the government's core operations—despite the desire to have it integrated with the rest of the health care system. This is perceived by some as a duplication of effort or waste of resources, but combining telehealth with other community services introduces questions of security and confidentiality of patient data. Such concerns become particularly salient when dealing with patients across jurisdictions. In concrete terms, this means that the videoconferencing channel has to be booked (at great cost) in order to send digital images to physicians. Were the health system allocated its own, secure (especially broadband) network, these images could be transmitted directly to the physicians' desks. This would certainly make it easier to fit telehealth into existing medical routines and practices.

On the other hand, the evaluation report (Infotelmed Communications, Inc., 2003) concluded that, although videoconferencing technology is vital in the communities, the volume of traffic makes it difficult to justify a dedicated network for health care alone. Multiple users could take advantage of the technology if it were made available to others in the community. To this end, discussions are underway with the Departments of Education, Justice and Sustainable Development, as well as Arctic College, all of whom recognize the need for integrating this service into their service delivery.

"Appropriate" Technologies: Synchronous and Asynchronous

The present IIU Network is based on videoconferencing, a synchronous technology. Given the connectivity problem, cost factors, and the problem of fitting within medical routines and schedules, other solutions might be more viable, or at least complementary. In particular, *store and forward* was often mentioned by the physicians interviewed.

The term *store and forward*, when used to describe telemedicine, refers to the concept that data (such as images, video and sound clips, and other patient information between personal computers, such as between a local health professional and a distant specialist) can be stored electronically and retrieved at a later time (often at a distant location) by another health care provider. If bandwidth is sufficient and both ends have compatible software, patient information can travel using an Internet protocol over standard channels. Security measures built into the software ensure the confidentiality of patient information.

In Nunavut, the entire health system is distributed, and sending information between points is central to its operations. Physicians' desktop computers are being equipped with a store and forward application that features conferencing capabilities, integrated security measures, annotation tools, and a customizable database. "Eventually we'll have it loaded on all the PCs and work out a way to send that signal through the regular pipe without having to book a call, but they just can't do it yet" (interview Aug 27, p. 12).

Store and forward has been used successfully in other Northern contexts. For instance, Jong, Horwood, Robbins, and Elford (2001) reported on consultation between nurses in a remote nursing station and a general practitioner in a regional hospital in Labrador using a 56K microwave link and dedicated software. They found positive impacts on patient management, particularly the need for travel outside the community, and the confidence of the remote nurse, as well as on the quality of care. Interoperability, privacy, and security were not concerns in this case, but they gain in importance when, as in the case of Nunavut, communication is occurring across health systems and jurisdictions.

The Alaska Federal Health Care Access Network (AFHCAN) began working in 2000 to provide health care to Aboriginal villages and military installations in 248 sites across Alaska. The AFHCAN Office developed a software application to allow telehealth cases to be created and read by providers. A key innovation was the adaptation of web-based technologies over satellite links to provide an easy-to-use interface at village clinics (http://www.afhcan.org/about). As in Nunavut, satellite connectivity is always a problem. The web-based store and forward software is designed for a low-connectivity environment, however. It essentially stores all user input at the server until a case is sent. If a user is in the midst of creating a case and loses connectivity (or the computer crashes), that information is still available the next time the user logs in from another machine. Using a combination of small transmission packets and multiple retry attempts, in a recent experience AFHCAN software continued to send cases from a remote village clinic on the Aleutian Islands over satellite connectivity that was too poor to permit phone, fax, or e-mail connections. This project, which won the American Telemedicine Association's Award for the Advancement of Telemedicine in 2004, illustrates the potential of Internet use in telemedicine and foreshadows a time when a majority of telehealth transmissions may be sent using an Internet protocol. The advantages are enormous: connectivity between multiple points in a variety of configurations, standard, interoperable, and less expensive applications, and increased accessibility through standard (browser) technologies.

Compatibility With Work Practices and Possible Use

Administration. As noted earlier, some 15% of the IIU Network's use was for meetings. Ensuring that collaborators can meet periodically is an important consideration in the context of a health system that is, by definition, distributed. With adequate connectivity, much of this activity could take place using Internet conferencing applications that are becoming common in organizations. This would represent a much cheaper solution than full scale videoconferencing and would likely be more convivial in both individual and organizational terms. Sessions are easily initiated and can be attended from virtually any room with a computer, eliminating the need to book the equipment and satellite time and to ensure the availability of a site technician. Depending on various considerations such as available bandwidth, an Internet-based solution could be viable across a range of media, from text-based messaging to audio conferencing with shared visual materials to video discussions.

Education. Access to continuing medical education is particularly important in a context such as Nunavut, where personnel must possess multiple skills: "Why it's been really good for our health centers is that they deal with everything, so a nurse is doing joint assessments, nutrition counseling, she is doing everything instead of just being a nurse" (interview Aug. 27, p. 8). This observation is consistent with a major Australian study that found that remote health providers have extensive experience, considerable demands for travel, and feel professionally isolated (Australian Commonwealth Department of Health and Family Services, 1996). The real-time, synchronous nature of content delivery by videoconference was problematic in some respects, however, particularly in terms of ensuring availability of staff to attend in a context of chronic understaffing. Given that few of those interviewed placed high priority on the interactive aspect of education sessions, we suggest that the Internet could play an important role in delivering medical education in Nunavut. Some educational content could be delivered using video streaming over the Internet. Alternately, a hybrid model where traces of the sessions' content are posted would enable those unable to attend to benefit from the sessions' information. Thus far, educational content has come principally from providers outside the territory. With the arrival of broadband services and the Nunavut Broadband Development Corporation's 5-year training and capacity-building program, there is an increased opportunity to create and distribute local content. Plans are underway for developing in-service training within the region, as well as sessions for non professionals on topics such as such medical terminology in native languages for clerk interpreters.

Finally, Internet communication such as chats or an online repository of useful information and frequently asked questions specific to health care in the North could help develop and strengthen a sense of professional and social community among health care workers who share a unique work context.

Clinical Use. In terms of clinical care, the project evaluation report (Infotelmed Communications, Inc., 2003) noted considerable dissatisfaction with, and lack of buy-in to, telehealth among the physicians serving Nunavut. Increased use of the Internet may not do much to resolve staff shortages and overwork, or resistance that results from conflicts with deeply ingrained practices and professional frames of reference, such as confidence in distant diagnosis. However, an Internet-based component to telehealth, such as store and forward between PCs on the doctors' desks, may help resolve some more organizational problems. For instance, if clinical use were organized around the clinicians' schedule, physicians might be more receptive. If there were a way make it so easy to set up sessions that the physicians could do it themselves rather than having to rely on a technician, they might be more inclined to use it. If the communication channel were less time-sensitive, a 20-minute delay might not be so dramatic.

If licensure questions can be resolved, an Internet-based solution might also go a long way to satisfying physicians' needs for direct, immediate access to a specialist. "It's not the actual watching the thing on the screen, it's the availability of the person. . . . Imagine picking up the phone anytime, one simple phone call. Life would be easy" (focus group, Aug. 27, p. 5). For specialists down South, too, a desktop solution would be preferable. "Now there are some specialists that don't want anything to do with it because they have to go to another office for the session" (Infotelmed Communications, Inc., 2003, p. 54). Although the telehealth station is never far away in a Northern Health Center, it can be situated at some distance in an urban hospital.

For all their reticence with using videoconferencing to delivering care, the physicians interviewed were very positive about the use of e-mail and the exchange of digital images. They had developed extremely innovative solutions for transmitting images and X-rays using the technology they have. For example,

I remember I had two nurses call from Up Island, a child with a strange rash that they were very concerned and the parents were very concerned. The father had a digital camera, took a picture of the child and e-mailed it to me. I looked at the rash, diagnosed it, and was able to communicate both with the parents by e-mail and with the nurse. (focus group, Aug 27, p. 3)

Physicians would appear to prefer a more modest, lower tech program for delivering telehealth—as in using e-mail, or store and forward—compatible with Internet-based applications, which would represent a better fit with local practices and the organization of the health and social services system. The notion of the organizational fit of an information technology typically implies the possibility of an optimal technological solution in a given situation (Knoll & Jarvenpaa, 1994). In our view, however, the "fit" of a technology is influenced by the degree to which it is malleable or constraining (see Law & Mol's [2002] notion of *fluid object*; and Majchrzak, Rice, Malhotra, King, & Ba, 2000). Also related is the idea that if a technology is relatively close to something that is already known (Orlikowski & Gash's [1994] notion of *technological frame*) it can be more easily integrated and appropriated. Fit is thus something produced in the *meeting* between something within the technology and something in the cognitive and organizational context.

LESSONS LEARNED AND IMPLICATIONS

The case of the IIU Network highlights four primary lessons.

Connectivity

The technical challenge of connectivity in the Canadian Arctic cannot be overstated. Reliable broadband access via satellite is a prerequisite to meaningful, sustained use of the Internet for health purposes. Nunavut is now poised to begin receiving high-speed Internet services, but widespread accessibility of such services for individuals from their homes is probably several years away. In the meantime, the major role of the Internet in Nunavut's health system is likely to be in facilitating doctor-to-doctor communication and in the consultation of professional databases. This is in keeping with the findings of market analysis of telehealth in the European Union (Hämäläinen, 2003, cited in Anderson & Jennett, 2003).

The bandwidth-intensive, real-time nature of videoconferencing creates considerable technical barriers to use. A store and forward telehealth solution would reduce the amount of bandwidth required and would allow images and data to be sent and seen at a time convenient to both clinicians and specialists (Infotelmed Communications, Inc., 2003; US Dept. of Commerce, 2003). Technologically simple telehealth solutions have proven effective in many cases. For example, there is reasonable evidence for the utility and potential value of the simple telephone for teletriage/telecare (Hunkeler, Meresman, Hargreaves, Fireman, Berman, et al.,

2000; Liesenfeld, Renner, Neese, & Hepp, 2000). Similarly, Vassallo, Hoque, Roberts, Patterson, Swinfen, and Swinfen (2001) illustrate that low-technology approaches such as Internet-based exchange of images and consult requests can be effective in the context of developing countries.

Aligning Technology With Practice

The early experience of the IIU Network points to the importance of adapting technology to the context in which it is introduced. The less disruptive a technology, the more chance it likely has of being incorporated into daily routines, and of being appropriated by its users. The IIU Network was not organized to be well integrated into the health care system: It was an add-on, both technically and organizationally. The telehealth network could not talk to the network that the Health Centers and the rest of the health system share. What is more, it was difficult for health practitioners to fit telehealth into their existing routines. The equipment was located in a separate room, and its use required conscious effort and series of actions that had to be planned well in advance. This lack of flexibility stands in sharp contrast with a medical environment characterized by urgency and quick reaction.

Managing Expectations

The IIU experience also points to the importance of managing expectations. Rather than saving time, an expectation expressed by several physicians, telehealth consultations took longer than face-to-face consultations, and the relative advantages of telehealth over other technologies were not readily apparent in most cases. This produced a lack of buy-in, particularly by physicians. The situation was further aggravated by perceived barriers stemming primarily from deeply ingrained assumptions about the practical and legal importance of physical co-location in practicing medicine.

Health Policy

Finally, the Nunavut experience raises some interesting questions in terms of health policy. Strong momentum for technologically mediated care has been reflected in federal policy documents and funding initiatives. Despite this enthusiasm, there is a major gap between reported plans for telehealth and actual policy and policymaking bodies needed to create a telehealth system. The IIU Network is unique in that it involves clinical referral patterns that extend to a number of Canadian jurisdictions. The lessons learned by the IIU Telehealth Project should be examined closely in any initiative to develop a cross-jurisdictional network. Among them is the need for consistent policies, protocols, and guidelines governing not only standards and clinical activity, but also the liability that is assumed by any organization conducting a telehealth session. Such policies have to be negotiated between jurisdictions and integrated into the organizations' operational structures.

CONCLUSION

The integration of telehealth in Nunavut is an ongoing process. It is the product of a series of trade-offs, some of them technical—between ease of use and technical performance, for example—and others human or organizational, such as negotiating jurisdiction, or developing new ways of practicing medicine. The Internet is an increasingly important part of this complex system which is, by definition, highly distributed. As the practices of health care professionals evolve, so will the role it can be expected to play in supporting coordination and communication among the various parts of the health system.

REFERENCES

Alaska Native Tribal Health Consortium. *The AFHCAN Solution*. Anchorage Alaska. Retrieved October 14, 2004, from http://www.afhcan.org/about

Anderson, C., & Jennett, P. (2003). *Industry partners and market opportunities in e-Health: An EU-Canada Industry Workshop final report*. March 6 & 7, 2003, National Research Centre Ottawa, Ontario, Canada. Retrieved October 14, 2004, from http://www.stakes.info/eucan/Industry%20Workshop.htm

Australian Commonwealth Department of Health and Family Services. (1996). *TeleHealth in rural and remote Australia: Report of the Project for Rural Health Communications and Information Technologies(PRHCIT)*. Traralgon, Australia: Monash University. Retrieved February 22, 2005, from http://www.med.monash.edu.au/mrh/resources/telehealthreport/tele_t.htm

Babe, R. E. (1990). *Telecommunications in Canada*. Toronto: University of Toronto Press.

Berg, M. (1999). Accumulating and coordinating: Occasions for information technologies in medical work. *Computer Supported Cooperative Work, 8*, 373–401.

Boulanger, B., Kearney, P., Ochoa, J., Tsuei, B., & Sands, F. (2001). Telemedicine: A solution to the follow up of rural trauma patients? *Journal of the American College of Surgeons, 192*, 447–452.

Canada. (2003). *First nations and Inuit telehealth research project: Future opportunities*. Ottawa: Health Canada.

Canada. (2001). *Report of the National Broadband Task Force: The new national dream: Networking the nation for broadband access*. Ottawa: Industry Canada. Retrieved January 17, 2005, from http://www.broadband.gc.ca/pub/program/NBTF/table_content.html

Canada. (1997). *Preparing Canada for a digital world: Final report of the Information Highway Advisory Council*. Ottawa: Industry Canada.

Cicourel, A. V. (1990). The integration of distributed knowledge in collaborative medical diagnosis. In J. Galegher, R. Kraut, & C. Egido (Eds.), *Intellectual teamwork: Social and technological foundations of co-operative work* (pp. 221–242). Hillsdale, NJ: Lawrence Erlbaum Associates.

Cicourel, A. V. (1999). The interaction of cognitive and cultural models in health care delivery. In S. Sarangi & S. Roberts (Eds.), *Talk, work and institutional order: Discourse in medical, mediation and management settings* (pp. 183–224). Berlin/New York: de Gruyter.

Good, B. J. (1994). *Medicine, rationality and experience*. Cambridge, UK: Cambridge University Press.

Health Telematics Unit. (2003). *Socio-economic impact of telehealth: Evidence now for health care in the future. Volume one: State of the science report*. Canada: University of Calgary.

Hunkeler, E. M., Meresman, J. F., Hargreaves, W. A., Fireman, B., Berman, W. H., Kirsch, A. J. et al. (2000). Efficacy of nurse telehealth care and peer support in augmenting treatment of depression in primary care. *Archives of Family Medicine, 9,* 700–708.

Hunter, K. M. (1991). *Doctors' stories: The narrative structure of medical knowledge*. Princeton, NJ: Princeton University Press.

Infotelmed Communications Inc. (2003). *IIU Nunavut telehealth project impact evaluation report*. Montreal, Canada.

Jacob, J. M. (1999). *Doctors and rules: A sociology of professional values* (2nd ed.). New Brunswick, NJ: Transaction.

Jennett, P. A., Hall, W. G., Morin, J. E., & Watanabe, M. (1995). Evaluation of a distance consulting service based on interactive video and integrated computerized technology. *Journal of Telemedicine and Telecare, 1,* 69–78.

Johnston, D., & Jones, B. N. (2001). Telepsychiatry consultations to a rural nursing facility: A 2-year experience. *Journal of Geriatric Psychiatry and Neurology, 14,* 72–75.

Jong, M. K. K., Horwood, K., Robbins, C. W., & Elford, R. (2001). A model for remote communities using store and forward telemedicine to reduce health care costs. *Canadian Journal of Rural Medicine, 6*(1), 15–20.

Knoll, K., & Jarvenpaa, S. L. (1994). Information technology alignment or "fit" in highly turbulent environments: The concept of flexibility. SIGCPR'94 Alexandria, VA: ACM. Retrieved February 23, 2005, from http://www.delivery.acm.org/10.1145/190000/186286/p1-knoll.pdf

Lamb, A., Eydmann, M., & Boddy, K. (1997). Remote maternity clinics. *British Journal of Healthcare Computing & Information Management, 14,* 22–24.

Law, J., & Mol, A. (Eds.). (2002). Complexities: Social studies of knowledge practices. Durham, NC: Duke University Press.

Liesenfeld, B., Renner, R., Neese, M., & Hepp, K. D. (2000). Telemedical care reduces hypoglycemias and improves glycemic control in children and adolescents with Type 1 diabetes. *Diabetes Technology Therapy, 2,* 561–567.

Majchrzak, A., Rice, R. E., Malhotra, A., King, N., & Ba, S. (2000). Technology adaptation: The case of a computer-supported inter-organizational virtual team. *MIS Quarterly, 24*(4), 569–600.

May, C. (1992). Individual care? Power and subjectivity in therapeutic relationships. *Sociology, 26,* 589–602.

May, C., Gask, L., Atkinson, T., Ellis, N., Mair, F., & Esmail, A. (2001). Resisting and promoting new technologies in clinical practice: The case of telepsychiatry. *Social Science and Medicine, 52,* 1889–1901.

Minister of Research, Science and Technology of Quebec, & Minister of Health and Social Services of Quebec. (1999). *Telehealth and telemedicine in Quebec: Current issues*. (Rep. No. I-81). Canada.

Mitka, M. (1997). Developing countries find telemedicine forges links to more care and research. *Journal of the American Medical Association, 280*(15), 1295–1296.

Monrad Aas, I. H. (2002). Changes in the job situation due to telemedicine. *Journal of Telemedicine and Telecare, 8,* 41–47.

Mort, M., May, C. R., & Williams, T. (2003). Remote doctors and absent patients: Acting at a distance in telemedicine? *Science, Technology and Human Values, 28*(2), 274–295.

Nesbitt, T. S., Hilty, D. M., Kuenneth, C. A., & Siefkin, A. (2000). Development of a telemedicine program. *Western Journal of Medicine, 173,* 169–174.

Nunavut. (2001a). *IIU telehealth network project document.* Iqaluit: Government of Nunavut.

Nunavut. (2001b). *IIU telehealth project: Needs assessment summary report,* Version 2.6. Iqaluit: Government of Nunavut.

Orlikowski, W., & Gash, D. C. (1994). Technological frames: Making sense of information technology in organizations. *ACM Transactions on Information Systems, 12*(2), 174–207.

Romanow, R. J. (2002). *Building on values: The future of health care in Canada.* Report of the Commission on the Future of Health Care in Canada, Saskatoon, SK.

Sinclair, S. (1997). *Making doctors: An institutional apprenticeship.* Oxford, UK: Oxford University Press.

Stiles, N., Boosalis, M., Thompson, K., Stinnett, D., & Rayens, M. K. (1998). Nutrition telemedicine consultation for rural elders. *Journal of Nutrition for the Elderly, 18,* 47–55.

Swanson, B. (1999). Information technology and under-served communities. *Journal of Telemedicine and Telecare, 5*(2), S3–10.

Tsilimigaki, A., Maraka, S., Tsekoura, T., Agelakou, V., Vekiou, A., Paphitis, C., & Thanopoulos, V. (2001). Eighteen months' experience with remote diagnosis, management and education in congenital heart disease. *Journal of Telemedicine and Telecare, 7,* 239–243.

U.S. Department of Commerce. (2003). *STAT-USA market research report on telemedicine/ telehealth.* Retrieved October 14, 2004, from http://strategis.ic.gc.ca/epic/internet/ inimr-ri.nsf/en/gr-71552e.html

Vassallo, D. J., Hoque, F., Roberts, M. F., Patterson, V., Swinfen, P., & Swinfen, R. (2001). An evaluation of the first year's experience with a low-cost telemedicine link in Bangladesh. *Journal of Telemedicine and Telecare, 7,* 125–138.

Woods, K. F., Johnson, J. A., Kutlar, A., Daitch, L., & Stachura, M. E. (2000). Sickle cell disease telemedicine network for rural outreach. *Journal of Telemedicine and Telecare, 6,* 285–290.

Wootton, R. (2001). Telemedicine and developing countries—Successful implementation will require a shared approach. *Journal of Telemedicine and Telecare, 7*(1), 1–6.

Chapter 17

Internet in the War Against HIV/AIDS in Asia*

Indrajit Banerjee
*Nanyang Technological University and Asian Media
Information and Communication Centre*

Cecilia Hsi-Shi Leong
Nanyang Technological University

ICTS AND TREATMENT/PREVENTION OF HIV/AIDS

In a short span of less than 30 years, information and communication technologies (ICTs) have brought about many social changes in contemporary societies. The Internet, in particular, is said to have the potential to radically impact health care models and delivery systems. According to Gomez, Caceres, Lopez, and Del Pozo (2002), it is transforming relationships between health care administrations and companies, professionals, and patients. This process of transformation also extends to diseases such as Human Immunodeficiency Virus/Acquired Immune Deficiency Syndrome (HIV/AIDS) that have a poorer life expectancy forecast, making it vital for prevention efforts in the form of information.

As advances in antiretroviral therapy have made it possible to reduce AIDS-related deaths, health care professionals dealing with AIDS are beginning to view HIV infection as a long-term illness rather than a fatal disease (Reiter, 2000). Therefore, like all other serious illnesses, people living with HIV/AIDS (PLWHA) should be able to access information and resources, learn how to manage their disease, and have some form of self-monitoring system where PLWHAs look out for symptoms of the

---

*Most of the best practices and country statistics discussed in this chapter are part of a Regional Development Report, Promoting ICT for Human Development in Asia 2004 United Nations: Realising the Millennium Development Goals. Indrajit Banerjee was the Research Coordinator for this project.

disease and are the first line of defense in keeping watch over their own state of health. This is where disease management professionals are increasingly looking towards the Internet as a tool for this purpose. With the rise of technoliteracy and self-reliance, the Internet has the potential to empower HIV/AIDS patients and health care professionals in managing this disease.

On the other side of the coin is the preventive aspect in battling the HIV/AIDS epidemic. Mitchell, Nakamanya, Kamali, and Whitmore (2001) have shown that behavioral change interventions are still one of the best ways to counter HIV in developing countries. Stover, Walker, Garnett, Salomon, Stanecki, et al. (2002) estimated that almost two thirds of projected HIV/AIDS infections between 2002–2010 would have been preventable if existing HIV/AIDS prevention strategies had been significantly enlarged.

Thus, parallel to efforts in research to finding a cure or vaccine, equal effort has been put into AIDS education and prevention, leading to the use of the ICTs such as the Internet as major potential tools in global mobilization and response to the disease (Driscoll, 2001). Although some researchers such as Kalichman, Weinhardt, Benotsch, DiFonza, Luke, and Austin (2002), contended that the Internet provides *universal* access to information about HIV disease processes, AIDS clinical trials, medical treatments, alternative therapies, advocacy, legal advice, social support, and other aspects of living and coping with HIV/AIDS, in most developing countries studied in this chapter, universal access is not a certainty due to factors such as the digital divide, economic considerations, or literacy levels. Nevertheless, it is important to note that although the Internet does not provide universal access, it does provide an alternative avenue (and in that sense, increases the options) for access to information. More specifically, there are also AIDS-related Web sites that are targeted at specific audiences, such as women, adolescents, families affected by AIDS, and ethnic minorities.

This chapter discusses how ICTs, in particular the Internet, have been used in Asia in the battle against HIV/AIDS across nine Asian countries. They are countries from South Asia (India, Pakistan, Sri Lanka), South East Asia (Indonesia, Malaysia, Thailand, and Vietnam) and East Asia (China and Mongolia). We look at the prevalence of HIV/AIDS in these Asian countries, how widespread it has become and also how the Internet is being used by various HIV/AIDS interest groups for support. We also discuss the use of the Internet for HIV/AIDS monitoring, research and education, as well as how networking effects of the Internet has generated synergies between health care providers, researcher, policymakers and PLWHAs. Lastly, we review what all these mean in terms of implications and challenges for Asia.

THE PREVALENCE OF HIV/AIDS IN ASIA

It is estimated that 34 to 46 million people are living with AIDS in 2004. Out of that, 5 million were newly infected in 2003, 700,000 of them children. To date, the disease has killed more than 20 million people—3 million died in 2003. Asia is predicted to be the next continent after sub-Saharan Africa to see a rapid growth in the AIDS epidemic. One fifth of the People Living with HIV/AIDS (PLWHA) are currently from Asia. Not surprisingly, the two most populous countries in the world, China and India, are also housing the highest number of PLWHAs in Asia (World Health Report, 2004). High HIV infection rates are being discovered among specific groups—intravenous drug users, sex workers, and homosexuals—in countries across Asia and the Pacific (UNAIDS & WHO, 2002). Another worrying trend is that HIV/AIDS infections are increasingly being seen in heterosexuals. This, in turn, wreaks havoc on social structures as children become orphans and, in other cases, parents infect their children (Ireland & Webb, 2001). The time lag of 9 to 11 years between the start of infection to the manifestation of the disease means that for Asia, these numbers probably represent just the tip of the iceberg. The worst is yet to come.

In the case of China, although national scientifically valid data on current estimates and future trends remain incomplete, many national and international experts estimate that there were more than 1 million HIV infections in 2001 (UNAIDS, 2003). More than 70% of these infections were caused by intravenous drug use or faulty plasma-collection procedures. More than 80% of those infected are currently men (World Health Report, 2004). China's UNDP Representative Khalid (2004) cautioned that if efforts are not stepped up, HIV/AIDS infections could reach 10 million people by 2010.

After China, India has the second largest number of PLWHA (UNDP, 2002). The World Health Report 2004 estimates the number of HIV infections in India at 3.8 to 4.6 million people in 2003. Thus, the percentage of new infections at 0.11% is considered high, even for a populous country like India.

Among Asian countries, Thailand has been one of the worst hit by the AIDS epidemic. It has the highest prevalence rate of AIDS, with 1.5% of its adult population living with HIV (see Table 17.1). Although the Thai AIDS control campaign has attained international recognition as being the first in the developing world to halt the growing incidence of HIV new cases, the battle against the disease is far from over. HIV/AIDS is also a potentially explosive challenge to Vietnam's future as 0.40% of its adult population are living with HIV and 65,000 of its women are infected. In Malaysia, 0.4% of its adult population are infected although the

TABLE 17.1
Estimated People Living With HIV/AIDS
in Selected Asian Countries (2003)

Country	% Adults (age 15–49)	People Living With HIV/AIDS		
		Adults & Children	Women (age 15–49)	Children (age 0–14)
China	0.1	840,000	190,000	10,000
India	0.8	5,100,000	1,900,000	120,000
Indonesia	0.1	110,000	15,000	—
Malaysia	0.4	52,000	8,500	1,000
Mongolia	< 0.1	< 500	—	< 200
Pakistan	0.1	74,000	8,900	1,000
Sri Lanka	< 0.1	3,500	600	—
Thailand	1.5	570,000	200,000	12,000
Vietnam	0.4	220,000	65,000	—

Note. Source: Epidemiological Fact Sheet, 2004, World Health Organization 2004 (http://www.who.int/GlobalAtlas/PDFFactory/HIV/index.asp?strSelectedCountry=CN)

prevalence is more rampant in the male population. Both Mongolia and Sri Lanka have relatively low HIV/AIDS prevalence rates and their status is that of "low-risk" HIV/AIDS countries. The 2003 HIV prevalence rate is less than 0.10% for both countries. However, Indonesia is experiencing new, rapidly developing subepidemics of HIV/AIDS in several provinces and communities (Table 17.1). As of end 2003, the number of PLWHA was estimated to be 110,000 adults aged between 15 and 49. In Pakistan, there were an estimated 74,000 PLWHA, out of which most of the cases were men (World Health Report, 2004).

HIV/AIDS AND THE INTERNET

Internet as a Source of Information and Support in the War Against HIV/AIDS

For health care workers and PLWHA in developing countries, the increasing connectivity of the Internet and e-readiness of nations are indeed a much-needed help and support. As this section illustrates, Internet users can access HIV/AIDS related mailing lists, interactive Web sites, chat sessions, and online resources from around the world to improve their knowledge of the disease.

One of the main advantages of new ICTs is their ability to provide easy, relatively low-cost access to information that results in information sharing for different interest groups and global networking for health groups. This helps in providing informational support for health care providers as well as policy makers.

For example HIF-net (hif-net@dgroups.org), which was launched in July 2000 by the International Network for the Availability of Scientific Publication and the World Health Organization, is an e-mail discussion list targeted mainly for providers and users of health information in resource-poor settings. It currently has 1,400 subscribers spread over 130 countries. Another global networking health group is the Program for Monitoring Emerging Diseases (http://www.promedmail.org). This is an Internet-based reporting system that provides information on outbreaks of infectious diseases and acute exposures to toxins. In fact, the global health community was first alerted to Severe Acute Respiratory Syndrome (SARS) through ProMEDmail.

Thus, health researchers have come to see that the impact of HIV/AIDS can be reduced by generating and disseminating knowledge as different groups need different kinds of knowledge such as information specific to the disease, and its epidemiological patterns, prevention, treatment and care (Driscoll, 2001). So, rather than the lack of information, one of the problems now is the over abundance of information and misinformation (Gomez et al., 2002).

On another level, the Internet helps to support the PLWHAs by disseminating relevant information via the Internet and providing a form of social support network. One area where support for PLWHAs has been crucial is "treatment literacy" where people with HIV/AIDS are informed and educated on the availability and advantages of antiretroviral treatment. It is being acknowledged as an important aspect of health management for the disease (World Health Report, 2004). A study of Internet usage by PLWHA in the United States found that 31% of the study's participants used the information found on the Internet on HIV/AIDS for discussions with their health care provider (Kalichman et al., 2002; see also Rice & Katz, chap. 8, this volume). This supports the notion that the Internet can serve to foster patient-centered medicine, motivate patients to participate in their own care, and build effective coping strategies (Eysenbach, Ryoung, & Diepgen, 1999; Krumholz, Rathore, Chen, Wang, & Radford, 2002; Widman & Tong, 1997). For Berland, Elliot, Morales, Algazy, Kravitz, et al. (2001), the Internet can also be a powerful avenue by which patients with chronic health conditions can obtain information about their illness and treatment options. It is a communication tool for self-help group initiatives such as peer counselling and consultation leading to the process of building communities for those affected by HIV/AIDS and serving as an online source of mutual support.

PLWHAs are also actively using the Internet to organize informal support groups. Yahoo!® Groups has started an experimental occasional electronic newsletter called Welcome to AIDS_ASIA with an e-forum committed to the development of an Asian perspective on AIDS prevention and care issues. More than 4,000 subscribers are currently using this FORUM. When there are private initiatives such as those on public domain groups such as Yahoo!®, it is a sign that individuals are actively using the Internet as a means to connect and communicate about HIV/AIDS and it is not merely the civil groups that are pushing their efforts.

Web sites such as the AIDS Treatment Data Network (http://www .atdn.org), http://www.aidsinfonyc.org, www.unaidsapict.inet.co.th, and the AIDS Education Global Information System (http://www.aegis .com) may not cater specifically to developing Asian countries but, as they can be freely accessed, they serve as an information warehouse on policies and programs, on monitoring and surveillance results, guidelines and best practices relating to the war against HIV/AIDS.

However, there are now various specialized Web sites for Asian countries that cater to HIV/AIDS providing the latest updates of treatment and happenings on the disease. For example, www.youandaids.org was initiated by the UNDP and UNAIDS. It is an HIV/AIDS Internet portal for Asia Pacific that seeks to promote networking, strengthen advocacy, and catalyze civil society response by giving detailed information about HIV/AIDS as well as specific country management of the disease in Asia Pacific.

Thailand's *Kaew Diary* is one example of a civic movement that offers community support for HIV-infected and AIDS patients. When it first started in early 2001, it was posted as a personal diary on one of Thailand's most popular portal sites, www.pantip.com, by a HIV-infected woman, Ms. Kaew, who was in her early 20s. In it, Ms. Kaew wrote about her experiences after being diagnosed with the disease. "The only friend I had then was the Internet," wrote Ms. Kaew, who does not reveal her full name. "I could talk to anybody without feeling discrimination. I was sure HIV/AIDS cannot be spread through the computer" (Poonyarat, 2002). Feedback was encouraging as people volunteered to help with her "cybercommunity" by developing a Web site (http://www .kaewdiary.com), which enriched its content and design. About 3,000 people have applied to become members so that they can search and exchange information and experiences or seek consultation. Despite remaining anonymous, Ms. Kaew has put a young and personal face on HIV/AIDS, enabling her to reach out across a spectrum of people, from those infected with HIV to educating the young modern Thai.

Another use of the Internet is in the area of prevention and education of a population against HIV/AIDS. Some governments have launched initiatives with nongovernmental bodies to battle HIV/AIDS. Malaysia's Department of Public Health launched its PROSTAR program where youths aged between 16 and 25 are trained as peer educators who, in turn, plan and implement suitable activities to influence other youths to practice healthy lifestyles. There are 850 PROSTAR clubs throughout Malaysia, mostly in secondary schools, with a total membership of 20,000. There is also an e-forum on its Web site for discussions. China too has its own sexual health advice Web site for youths. The Web site (http://www.youandme.net.cn) is sponsored by the United Nations and Marie Stopes International, a nonprofit organization. Most Chinese people have little access to reliable and accurate information on sex due to traditional sensitivities (First Chinese, 2003). The interactive Web site encourages youths to discuss their love lives and matters on sex openly. Its ability to allow for interactive use while remaining anonymous is especially useful for HIV/AIDS education that can be spread through unsafe sex.

INTERNET FOR HIV/AIDS MONITORING

The Internet has also been used in HIV prevention and containment efforts. As the diversity of HIV epidemics around the world become more apparent, existing HIV surveillance systems are being improved on to capture this or explain changes over time in mature epidemics. According to the World Health Organization, countries affected by the HIV epidemic need efficient HIV-surveillance systems that provides data that reports on trends in the spread of HIV, such as risk behaviors, or which sector of the population that are most or least affected. In Asia, efforts are now being made to build on existing systems, strengthening their explanatory power and making better use of the information they generate. Strengthened systems, dubbed as "second generation surveillance systems," are being developed to yield information that is useful to reduce the spread of HIV and provide care for those affected by tailoring the surveillance system to the country's epidemic pattern. This also includes concentrating data collection in populations most at risk of becoming newly infected with HIV— populations with high levels of risk behavior or young people at the start of their sexual lives. In countries such as China and India where data is collated from such a vast area, the Internet has come in useful in helping to increase the efficiency of data collection. Distance has become less of a hindrance in coordinating data collection efforts. This inadvertently encourages transparency and makes it easier to carry out monitoring and evaluation of HIV/AIDS programs (Driscoll, 2001).

Since 1995, Thailand's Ministry of Public Health has been using ICTs in its Annual Surveillance of HIV Infection. ICTs have played a significant role in data collection, analysis, and dissemination of the results, and this has enabled the Ministry to have up-to-date surveillance data for better management and control of the AIDS epidemic. In China, a national sentinel surveillance system alerted authorities to the high needle-sharing rates among Intravenous Drug Users (IDUs) in Jiangxi province, reaching 74% in 1998 and 93% in 1999. Had this warning system been in place earlier, intensive intervention measures aimed at decreasing needle sharing among IDUs could have reduced China's 2000 epidemic. Clearly, these monitoring systems can be effective tools for controlling the spread of HIV/AIDS if used as an early prevention system.

USE OF THE INTERNET IN HIV/AIDS RESEARCH

ICTs, especially the Internet, can support HIV/AIDS research in many ways such as allowing better response to a disease pandemic through sharing lessons learned, treatment practices and guidelines with other health care professionals, researchers and policymakers during the outbreak (see also Murero, chap. 3, this volume). These prevention and educational uses of the Internet, which increases the quality and quantity of discussions between health care workers and researchers, have taken on a more significant meaning with the detection of multi-drug resistant tuberculosis and HIV/AIDS in some parts of Asia (World Health Report, 2004). There is also increasing enlightenment among research groups to make HIV/AIDS information freely available through the Internet. In 1997, HIV InSite Knowledge Base, a free online textbook with references and related links organized by textbook, was launched by the Center for HIV Information, a health sciences institution at the University of California, San Francisco. Most online journals are affordable, even by a developing country's standard. For example, The Journal of AIDS/HIV charges a yearly subscription of US$9.95 and this would entitle the subscriber to online diagnosis tools, online treatment, electronic textbooks, and articles.

Others have gone a step further by providing free access to countries that need it most. HINARI, a joint initiative between The World Health Organization and the world's six biggest medical journal publishers, was launched in 2002. Its Web site contains online versions of the information available in these journals and is freely accessible to almost 100 developing countries, enabling health care professionals and researchers to gain access to vital scientific information that they otherwise could not afford. HIV Medicine is an online medical textbook that provides a comprehensive and up-to-date overview of the treatment of HIV Infection and can be accessed freely. There is also a hard copy version available.

In Sri Lanka, ICTs are used for health care research in most medical research institutions. The Medical Research Institute (MRI) uses ICTs for research by maintaining various research databases; digitally transmitting medical information such as CT and MRI scans via e-mail; using specialized software packages as well as using common word processing and spreadsheet applications to conduct and report research. The Ceylon Medical Journal has also made itself available on the web. Meanwhile, Pakistan has PakMediNet, an online portal that facilitates research and provides access to Pakistani medical journals. So far, it has managed to archive and store 39 medical journals, a phenomenal achievement in the absence of financial support.

THE NETWORKING EFFECTS OF INTERNET IN HIV/AIDS INTEREST GROUPS

The effects of the Internet on health care is unique as ICT innovations and processes do not necessarily need to reach the final beneficiaries (i.e., the patients) as long as the participants in the delivery process of health care are reached. Cost reductions, faster turnaround time in terms of processing of information, and coordination ultimately serve to the benefit of the patient (Chandrasekhar & Ghosh, 2001). One such effect is how the Internet empowers stakeholders and encourages consultations on policy formulation through knowledge and networking. This allows health care providers, researchers, policymakers and even PLWHAs to communicate via local or global discussion groups and/or bulletin boards, which serve as a venue for sharing and consultations on health issues. This enables HIV health care providers and PLWHA to benefit from a global or regional joint efforts to manage and contain the disease. On an international level, the Asia Pacific PLWHA Resource Centre not only provides a regional hub of information and knowledge on HIV/AIDS, it also provides an avenue for networking among its members through online discussion forums and chat rooms.

SEA-AIDS is another good example demonstrating the use of electronic mail discussion and information service to promote people building and shaping the response to HIV and AIDS in the South East Asia region. Currently, SEA-AIDS provides three basic services:

- SEA-AIDS Link where participants can share experiences and information through an electronic mail network. Sent messages will be distributed to all colleagues throughout the region who have also joined the group.
- SEA-AIDS Files where participants can use e-mail commands to provide information and materials on HIV/AIDS in South East Asia.

- SEA–AIDS Flash is a biweekly online regional news digest on HIV and AIDS sent automatically through the Internet. It also covers information about new documents, news items, forthcoming training, and training in the South East Asian region.

In 1998, the forum moved to HIVNET that is hosted by the Foundation du Present (FdP). It is currently moderated and managed by Health and Development Network (HDN) with support from FdP. SEA–AIDS has proven to be more than just a mechanism for discussions, updates and articles. It has changed the way people involved in HIV/AIDS programs communicate and work on a daily basis. By facilitating fast, easy and open communication across geographic and sectoral borders, SEA–AIDS has shown that networking and information sharing are crucial to strengthening and uniting the response towards the epidemic. Porter (2004) quoted Deany who reported that half of SEA–AIDS members said that they had continued forum discussions one-on-one offline; thus Porter reasoned that networking benefits from the Internet extended beyond the forum.

India's Saathii (Solidarity and Action Against the HIV Infection in India) is an organization that seeks to disseminate research, training, and funding-related information on a real-time basis to those with limited access to libraries and the Internet. It publishes a weekly or daily e-newsletter, providing information on current research advances in behavioral, basic science and clinical aspects of HIV/AIDS that are relevant to resource-limited settings. There are updates on HIV-related national and international conferences, national and international training, funding announcements relevant to India, as well as news items and letters that merit political action. Saathii also collaborates with AIDS-India e-forum to disseminate India-relevant information daily and seeks to facilitate active discussions on current Indian HIV events, as well as the sharing of information on various programs, individuals and experiences. The AIDS-India e-forum is a virtual organization set up as a Yahoo!® e-group forum in response to India's AIDS crisis. It facilitates networking, communication and collaboration among those involved or interested in India's AIDS-related issues. It has more than 1,700 registered members, and is extremely active with four or more messages or responses circulated daily.

IMPLICATIONS AND CHALLENGES
FOR ASIAN COUNTRIES

Although the Internet has proven to be a boon in HIV/AIDS prevention and disease management efforts, there are numerous challenges involved. The UNAIDS and WHO (2001) estimates show that low- and middle-income countries account for about 81% of the global population (Population Reference Bureau, 2003), and 95% of those infected with HIV (UNAIDS & WHO, 2001), but just 5% of the world's Internet users (DOI, 2001). The problems of low Internet diffusion and the digital divide are obstacles that developing countries in Asia face in using the Internet for development purposes. Critics have also highlighted that the present paradigm is too technology driven, with profits as the overriding motive, and that saturated demands for ICT products in the North may just see these ICT products and technologies being dumped on the South (Driscoll, 2001).

DeGuzman and Ross (1999) noted that although there is an abundance of HIV/AIDS information on the Internet, applications beyond information retrieval are largely absent. Advanced use of the Internet such as interactive behavior change technology (IBCT) that delivers health behavior change counselling is yet to be realized for HIV/AIDS patients in Asia. As with other ICT innovations, there are also other challenges such as the issues of affordability by those in developing countries or marginalized groups in society who already have trouble paying for medical treatment. Results of a recent U.S. study showed that persons living with HIV/AIDS with 12 or fewer years of education were significantly less likely to have used the Internet, and were less likely to have been instructed in Internet use. In the study, participants with greater education were four times more likely to have current access to the Internet than their less educated counterparts (Kalichman et al., 2002). In Mumbai and Goa, India which has a larger population than Botswana and Zambia combined, more than 50% of its commercial sex workers are HIV-positive (World Health Report 2004). In Henan, China, impoverished farmers who sell their blood plasma are transfused back with pooled blood products to enable them to sell again in over a week are said to have contributed to the 1 million HIV infected in Henan (Russell, 2002). These are populations which may face the same Internet access barriers as those in the Kalichman et al. (2002) study.

The rural–urban divide where ICT diffusion is usually much higher in urban centers is problematic when implementing ICT programs in villages. One example is a program by Sri Lanka's Companions of Journey to build an island-wide database of HIV-infected individuals, which failed due to lack of financial resources and poor assistance from the community. Low Internet-penetration level was identified as a key issue in its failure.

Kalichman et al. (2002) also found evidence of a digital divide in PLWHA in the United States with a history of Internet use more common among Whites (77%) than African Americans (42%; but see Katz & Rice, 2002, for comparisons in the general population of users). In Asia, there are already major fault lines within the digital divide between minority groups and income groups. Racial, language, and cultural divides threaten any efforts to provide ICT support for PLWHA. In Asia where the population most at risk are the already socially disadvantaged sex workers, getting the message across through the use of the Internet alone is not enough. What most countries are doing is to use all avenues of ICTs, be it old ICTs such as the television and radio, as well as other forms of media such as print, billboards and theatre to bring the message home (see also Curioso, chap. 18, this volume). In Thailand, effective communication strategies involving the use of ICTs have been used to bolster public health campaigns since the 1990s. The results have been promising: 90% of sex workers now use condoms and the number of men visiting sex workers has dropped by 50% (World Health Report, 2004). The number of new HIV-infection cases in Thailand dropped from 143,000 in 1991 to 29,000 in 2000, which can be attributed partly to a US$48 million education and public health campaign. Led by a well-respected politician, Mr. Meechai Viravaidhya, 488 radio stations and 15 TV stations aired HIV/AIDS preventive messages for 30 seconds every hour such as advocating a "100% condom use" program aimed at commercial sex workers. These strategies helped Thailand to become the first developing country to successfully control AIDS (Singhal, 2002).

The audio and visual stimulation that the television provides have also proven to be an effective medium for creating health awareness in Sri Lanka, where almost all television channels have their own health programs. Some popular health shows include *Suva Hamuva* and *Lama Suvasetha* on Rupavahini, *Vaidya Hamuva* on TNL and *Suva Hamuva* on Swarnavahini. These weekly 30- to 45-minute programs usually involve interviews or discussions with medical specialists. On a daily basis, television news bulletins often carry health items, including advice about preventive measures, treatment, and national campaigns.

On the other hand, it cannot be denied that the Internet is also useful in reaching out to educate and inform the increasing online population as Internet penetration increases exponentially in Asian countries, especially those of India and China. In 2002, a penetration of 46 Internet users per 1,000 people in China translated into 59.1 million Internet users, whereas in India there were a total of 16.6 million Internet users (see Table 17.2). Such numbers of users cannot be ignored in any program concerned with information dissemination.

As the Internet becomes more accessible and more PLWHAs become online information consumers, increasing interventions will be needed to target behavioral skills for optimal Internet use (Kalichman, Benotsch, & Weinhardt, 2003).

Another implication to note is that there is a hype and reality to using the Internet for HIV/AIDS intervention and prevention purposes. The is-

TABLE 17.2
Internet Penetration in Selected Asian Countries (2002)

Country	Internet Users Per 1000 People	Internet Users
China	46	59.1 million
India	16	16.6 million
Indonesia	38	8 million
Malaysia	320	7.8 million
Mongolia	21	50,000
Pakistan	10	1.5 million
Sri Lanka	11	200,000
Thailand	78	4.8 million
Vietnam	18	1.5 million

Note. Source: Extracted from Development Data Group, World Bank (http://www.worldbank.org/data/countrydata/countrydata.html) and 2004 World Development Indicators (http://www.worldbank.org/data/wdi2004/pdfs/Table5_11.pdf).

sue of sustainability of many ICT projects is commonly ignored. Many countries in the developing world are conducting pilot projects or actual projects in health care that are funded through various sources from international donor and aid agencies to local nongovernmental organizations. In 2003, The Bill & Melinda Gates Foundation (2003) committed $200 million to Avahan, the foundation's India AIDS initiative, which has disbursed $126.9 million in grants to HIV-prevention programs across various Indian states. Various pharmaceutical companies are also working with local organizations to start HIV programs. There is also the REACH initiative started by the United Nations Development Program that brings together 13 countries in Asia to share their own experiences and get exposure to global expertise to combat the HIV/AIDS epidemic (UNDP, 2005).

Investments in ICTs for fighting HIV/AIDS are often scarce and low. The recipients of these projects are often poor and those who work among them have limited or no access to appropriate communication media. Therefore, the high costs of ICT applications and communications often make ICT-related services unaffordable for those who are most in need. This negates the "low costs of access" advantage enjoyed by ICTs, as users in this category will already face difficulties in getting the hardware and connecting to the Internet. This is especially true in countries such as Sri Lanka, Mongolia, China, India, Vietnam, and Thailand.

For countries experimenting with ICTs for health care, information transmission via Web sites is still mostly one-way, from experts to the public. Even when there is interactivity, these portals are accessible mainly to other experts, urban users and those literate in English. There

is still a lack of content in native languages for HIV/AIDS online resources presented in a simple and easily understood format without the
use of complicated medical jargon to cater to the local population.

Another challenge is the limited documentation of experiences in using
ICT to address the HIV/AIDS issue in poor countries. There is also a lack
of standard criteria for evaluating online HIV/AIDS information (Jadad,
Haynes, Hunt, & Browman, 2000). Currently, the criteria for evaluating
Internet health information usually takes on a developed country focus.
A study carried out by Kim, Eng, Deering, and Maxfield (1999) found
that most frequently cited criteria were content, design and aesthetics of
site, disclosure of authors, sponsors, or developers, currency of information (including frequency of update, freshness, maintenance of site), authority of source, ease of use, and accessibility and availability. Some researchers are beginning to examine how health Web sites are being used
in developing countries. Gummerson (2003) suggested that development
health sites should take into practical considerations such as supporting
lower version web browsers, offering simpler versions of the Web site
and catering to multiple language environment.

CONCLUSION

Although many HIV/AIDS programs and projects with ICT components,
especially computers and the Internet, were only recently implemented,
there are emerging signs that suggest that many working in HIV/AIDS
programs in poor countries are already benefiting from the Internet and
e-networking. Prior experiences in some developing countries like India
suggest that ICT use in enhancing delivery and providing better information to health care professionals have proven to be viable and important
as a means to improve public health conditions (Chandrasekhar & Ghosh,
2001). The two Asian countries (India and Thailand) discussed here
which have been most affected by HIV/AIDS, are the two most actively
using ICTs to battle this disease.

ICTs, especially the Internet, are facilitating knowledge sharing, increasing the number of people involved in HIV/AIDS policy dialogue,
promoting partnerships and networking, improving access to and quality of information, and increasing accountability and transparency in decision making. This not only shows how Internet can play a role in dealing with HIV/AIDS, but also points to the need to build content and
infrastructure in the overall battle against the epidemic.

Public health is a community concern. If health portals can partner local community portals and projects to elicit feedback and participation,
there will be multiplier effects. With advances in multimedia streaming,

chat and Internet phone capabilities, the application of the Internet beyond just merely information delivery is promising (DeGuzman & Ross, 1999). These ICT solutions have been implemented commercially but are sorely lacking in public health intervention initiatives.

However, most Asian governments have wisely used ICTs in health care for surveillance of diseases by maintaining patient database records. ICTs have made a great impact in improving the effectiveness of disease surveillance, early detection, treatment and control of communicable diseases such as HIV/AIDS. Thus, developing countries in Asia have realized that the potential benefits of ICTs are endless but as technological advances are not stand alone innovations, in order to reap the rewards there must be government resolve, civic participation and corresponding progress must also be made in other socio-economic areas such as literacy, ICT diffusion. The bottom line is that Internet initiatives in the War against HIV/AIDS have to be adapted to suit local conditions and must serve the real needs of the community.

REFERENCES

Berland, G. K., Elliot, M. N., Morales, L. S., Algazy, J. I., Kravitz, R. L., Broder, M. S., et al. (2001). Health information on the Internet: Accessibility, quality, and readability in English and Spanish. *Journal of the American Medical Association, 285*(20), 2612–2621.

Bill & Melinda Gates Foundation. (2003). Avahan: Indian AIDS initiative. Retrieved December 2, 2005, from http://www.gatesfoundation.org/GlobalHealth/Pri_Diseases/HIVAIDS/HIVProgramsPartnerships/Avahan.htm

Chandrasekhar, C. P., & Ghosh, J. (2001). Information and communication technologies and health in low income countries: The potential and the constraints. *Bulletin of the World Health Organisation, 79*(9), 850–855.

DeGuzman, M. A., & Ross, M. W. (1999). Assessing the application of HIV and AIDS related education and counselling on the Internet. *Patient Education and Counseling, 36*, 209–228.

DOI (Digital Opportunity Initiative). (2001, July). *Creating a development dynamic.* Retrieved August 8, 2003, from http://www.markle.org/news/onepage/onepage.html

Driscoll, L. (2001). *HIV/AIDS and Information and communication technologies: final report.* Ottawa: IDRC. Retrieved May 6, 2004, from http://www.lib.uct.ac.za/Training/driscoll%20report.pdf

Eysenbach, G., Ryoung, S., & Diepgen, T. (1999). Shopping around the Internet today and tomorrow: Towards the millennium of cybermedicine. *British Medical Journal, 319*, 1–5.

First Chinese. (2003). First Chinese website to give sex advice. *The Strait Times.* 12 July, 2003. Retrieved July 17, 2003, from http://straitstimes.asia1.com.sg/asia/story/0,4386,199310-1058047140,00.html

Gomez, E. J., Caceres, C., Lopez, D., & Del Pozo, F. (2002). A Web-based self monitoring system for people living with HIV/AIDS. *Computer Methods and Programs in Biomedicine, 69*, 75–86.

Gummerson, E. (2001). Is anybody out there? Accessing the global audience for healthcare web sites. Presentation at the workshop *"e-Health in Developing Countries: The Future of Healthcare,"* Center for International Development. Harvard University. June 18, 2001.

Retrieved May 29, 2003, from http://www.cid.harvard.edu/ciditg/Health/eHealth%20Workshop%20Presentations/ElizabethGummerson.ppt

Ireland, E., & Webb, D. (2001). *No quick fix: A sustained response to HIV/AIDS and children.* Save the Children UK. Retrieved August 25, 2003, from http://www.savethechildren.org.uk/hiv/pdfs/Quickfix.pdf

Jadad, A. R., Haynes, R. B., Hunt, D., & Browman, G. P. (2000). The Internet and evidence-based decision-making: A needed synergy for efficient knowledge management in health care. *Canadian Medical Association Journal, 162*(3), 362–365.

Kalichman, S. C., Benotsch, E. G., & Weinhardt, L. (2003). Health-related Internet use, coping, social support, and health indicators in people living with HIV/AIDS: Preliminary results from a community survey. *Health Psychology, 22*(1), 111–116.

Kalichman, S. C., Weinhardt, L., Benotsch, E., DiFonza, K., Luke, W., & Austin, J. (2002). Internet access and Internet use for health information among people living with HIV-AIDS. *Patient Education and Counselling, 46,* 109–116.

Katz, J. E., & Rice, R. E. (2002). *Social consequences of Internet use: Access, involvement and interaction.* Cambridge, MA: The MIT Press.

Khalid, M. (2004). *China's strides against HIV/AIDS.* Retrieved August 23, 2004, from http://www.youandaids.org/Guest%20Column/Khalid%20Malik/index.asp

Kim, P., Eng, T., Deering, M. J., & Maxfield, A. (1999). Published criteria for evaluating health related web sites: Review. *British Medical Journal, 318*(March 6), 647–649.

Krumholz, H., Rathore, S., Chen, J., Wang, Y., & Radford, M. (2002). Evaluation of a consumer-oriented Internet health care report card: The risk of quality ratings based on mortality data. *Journal of the American Medical Association, 287,* 1277–1287.

Mitchell, K., Nakamanya, S., Kamali, A., & Whitmore, J. (2001). *Community-based HIV/AIDS education in rural Uganda: Which channel is most effective? Health Education Research, 16.* Retrieved May 29, 2003, from http://www.id21.org/zinter/id21zinter.exe?a=30&i=h5jw3g6&u=3eecb600

Poonyarat, C. (2002). *Health—Thailand: Life continues even with HIV/AIDS.* InterPress Service. Feb 15, 2002. Retrieved December 5, 2004, from http://www.aegis.com/news/ips/2002/IP020211.html

Population Reference Bureau. (2001). *World population data Sheet 2001.* Retrieved May 29, 2003, from http://www.prb.org/Content/NavigationMenu/Other_reports/2000-2002/sheet1.html

Porter, C. (2004). Networking for health: Health professionals using email discussion forums for development. *Information Development, 20*(2), 117–121.

Reiter, G. (2000). *Comprehensive clinical care: Managing HIV as a chronic illness, AIDS Clinical Care.* Boston, MA: Massachusetts Medical Society.

Singhal, A. (2002). *How Communications Can Combat HIV/AIDS,* Office of Research Communications, Ohio University. Retrieved May 29, 2003, from http://www.ohiou.edu/researchnews/research/singhal_book.html

Stover, J., Walker, N., Garnett, G., Salomon, J., Stanecki, K., Ghys, P., Grassly, N., Anderson, R., & Schwartlander, B. (2002). Can we reverse the HIV/AIDS pandemic with an expanded response? *The Lancet, 360*(9326), 73–77.

UNAIDS. (2003). *A global overview of the epidemic.* UNAIDS. Retrieved August 25, 2003, from http://www.unAids.org/barcelona/presskit/barcelona%20report/chapter2.pdf

UNAIDS/WHO. (2002). *AIDS epidemic update December 2002.* Joint United Nations Programme on HIV/AIDS (UNAIDS) & World Health Organisation (WHO). Retrieved May 30, 2003, from http://www.who.int/hiv/facts/epiupdate2002_en.doc

UNAIDS/WHO. (2001). *AIDS epidemic update—December 2001.* Geneva. Retrieved August 19, 2003, from http://www.unAids.org/epidemic_update/report_dec01/index.html

UNAIDS/WHO. (2000). *Epidemological factsheet on HIV/AIDS and other sexually transmitted infections.* Retrieved March 18, 2003, from http://www.hivaidssearch.com/hiv-aids-links.asp?id=1246

UNDP. (United Nations Development Programme). (2002). *HIV/AIDS and poverty reduction strategies*. August 2002. Retrieved September 5, 2003, from http://www.undp.org/hiv/docs/hivprsEng25oct02.pdf

WHO. (World Health Organisation). (2002). *Follow up on the United Nations General Assembly special session on HIV/AIDS: Work of WHO (Progress Report)*. (2002). World Health Organisation. July 2002.

Widman, L. E., & Tong, D. A. (1997). Requests for medical advice from patients and families to health care providers who publish on the world wide web. *Archives of Internal Medicine, 157*, 209–212.

World Health Report 2004. (2004). *Changing history*. Geneva: World Health Organisation.

Chapter 18

New Technologies and Public Health in Developing Countries: The Cell PREVEN Project

Walter H. Curioso

Universidad Peruana Cayetano Heredia, Peru
University of Washington, Seattle

TELEHEALTH AND PUBLIC HEALTH

This chapter describes an application of telehealth using cell phones and the Internet to collect, transmit and monitor data in real-time from female sex workers (FSW) who are part of a large project in Peru to reduce sexually transmitted diseases (STD). According to a national survey conducted in Peru of 4479 FSW in 2002, the prevalence of STDs and bacterial vaginosis was 26% and 34% respectively (PREVEN, 2003). Early detection and treatment of STDs represents one major strategy for preventing transmission of STD, including infection with HIV (Sanchez, Campos, Courtois, Gutierrez, Carrillo, et al., 2003). New technologies and information systems can help public health in terms of prevention, surveillance, and management of public health data. Consider the following case.

> At 6 p.m. on a Friday night in a rural community in Piura, north of Peru, nurse Raquel Butron takes a taxi for the hour ride to the brothel. Raquel is part of a mobile team that screens female sex workers every 2 months as a sentinel surveillance. She provides medication for bacterial vaginosis, namely metronidazole. As part of her job, she carries three or more folders full of papers to track codes, medications, and adverse events such as nausea and vomiting that the participants might experience from the metronidazole they are receiving. This night, she is hoping that she won't be robbed like the week before. Although she recovered the folders and medications 3 days later, she is guarded about being robbed again.

Raquel and a peer-educator arrive early in order not to interrupt the women while they are working. They are well-received. Raquel starts screening "Paola," but Paola gets a call on her cell phone, so Raquel has to wait. Even among female sex workers who earn just 5 dollars a night, cell phones are a mainstay of life.

A year later, as Raquel heads to the brothel, she is going more discreetly. She is not carrying folders full of papers, just a cell phone. Helped with a hands-free device, she performs the interviews. Following a voice menu prompt on her cell phone, Raquel goes through a list of questions, pressing one and two on the phone's key pad for yes and no answers. She can also leave a voice message for a doctor in Lima at the end of the interview.

"A cell phone makes my job easier," she said. She doesn't worry as much about getting robbed because rather than sticking out, she appears like anyone else making a phone call. She also doesn't have to carry folders full of papers, or have to ship her reports every weekend to Lima. "I send the reports in real-time," she said.

Doctors in Lima, meanwhile, monitor in real-time the reactions female sex workers are having to medication and respond immediately if there is a strong reaction such as vomiting. Each time the system detects a serious adverse event, the system sends an alert to the cell phones of doctors in Lima. Using the Internet, the doctors can also monitor the activities of the health workers. After logging in, doctors can see the entire list of participants registered by the mobile team, day-by-day, or on a weekly basis. If Raquel leaves a voice message, the message is registered in the database as an audio file. Doctors in Lima can hear her message by accessing the database from the web. Doctors also have the capability to perform searches, and they can download the database for further analysis.

By using the cell phone, Rachel can enter the code for a female sex worker to get her past results from the lab. Because female sex workers do not stay in one place all the time, being able to tap into a database makes accessing records a world easier. "I don't have to wait weeks or months to share results with patients who may have traveled to another city".

CELL PREVEN: A MOBILE TELEHEALTH PROJECT

PREVEN (Prevencion comunitaria de enfermedades de transmision sexual; in English: Urban community randomized trial of STD prevention) is a collaborative effort between the Universidad Peruana Cayetano Heredia (Peru), Imperial College (London) and the University of Washington (Seattle). This project is a national urban community randomized trial in 20 Peruvian cities with populations more than or equal to 50,000 inhabitants. The cities were randomized into two groups: (1) 10 control sites with no intervention and (2) 10 intervention cities, with syndromic management of sexually transmitted diseases (STD), delivered primarily through pharmacies linked to referral networks of private physicians and health centers, and outreach to marginalized female sex workers (FSW). One of the primary scientific aims of the study is to determine the impact of the interventions on prevalence of gonococcal, chlamydial, trichomonal infection, syphilis and HIV seroreactivity in the general population of young adults through a population-based survey and in high-risk populations through sentinel surveillance of FSW and clients of FSW (PREVEN, 2003).

Workers in rural health care, who serve most of the population, are usually isolated from specialist support and up-to-date information because of poor roads and scarce access to information technologies. Many developing countries have a shortage of health care workers and most of the doctors, specialists and services are concentrated in the main cities (Fraser & McGrath, 2000).

Early detection and treatment of STDs represents one major strategy for preventing transmission of STD, including infection with HIV (Sanchez et al., 2003). Female sex workers (FSW), as other core groups, play a crucial role in STD transmission (Campos, Chiappe, Carcamo, Garcia, Buendia, et al., 2003). In a national survey conducted in 2002, the prevalence of STD and bacterial vaginosis in FSW in Peru was 26% and 34% respectively (PREVEN, 2003). Early detection of STD in FSWs, as well as promoting and providing condoms for commercial sex workers are needed to prevent HIV/STD in Peru, as in much of the developing world (Sanchez et al., 2003). New technologies and information systems can help programs and trials not only in STD/HIV, but in other fields of public health involving prevention, surveillance, and management of data.

Before the diffusion of new technologies among FSW in Peru, reports were collected on paper. Weeks or months could pass before public health workers, physicians, and team leaders learned of trends and patterns and were able to respond.

Using cell phone and the Internet technology, the aim of this project was to develop an interactive computer system for real-time collection and transmission of adverse events (e.g., vomiting, diarrhea) related with metronidazole administration as presumptive treatment for bacterial vaginosis in female sex workers. We developed a system that combines the phone and the Internet (Cell PREVEN). The idea was to design and implement a real-time surveillance system of adverse events as a component of the PREVEN Project. It also was a mean to optimize the data report efficiently, and improve time in sending the reports in order to have real-time decision-making.

We piloted the system in three cities of Peru: Chincha, Huanuco, and Piura. Data collection and transmission of AE information in the field began in early September, 2004. The system was incorporated in the mobile team activity of the PREVEN Project. The mobile team is composed mainly of nurses or obstetricians and a peer educator. They periodically screen female sex workers for STDs (gonococcal, chlamydial, trichomonal infection, and syphilis) and provide presumptive treatment of bacterial vaginosis. One week after they provide treatment, they return to the participants and ask for any adverse events. Six public health workers were trained to use the mobile phones and keep track of study participants. The report in the cell phone contained the same questions as on the paper form.

We developed an interactive voice response application for cell phones in Spanish, based on the infrastructure of Voxiva, a telecommunications company based in Peru (Voxiva, 2005). The architecture of the system has five elements: a central database and web server; remote access to the database from any Internet-connected computer; telephone audio computer-assisted personal interviewing; voice messages and short-message service (SMS)-based communications to and from the server via cell phones (Fig. 18.1).

Public health workers received an account number, personal identification number (PIN) and a plastic card with simple instructions and codes for all the symptoms they need to report (Fig. 18.2). By calling into a number in Lima using cell phones they could access the system and report adverse events from FSW systematically and in real time in urban and rural areas. Authorized users logged on and followed instructions on a wallet-sized card or a simple prompted menu and entered digital information about participants with adverse events. They could attach additional information in voice files.

Information was stored in an online database and could be immediately accessed worldwide and exported over a secure Internet connection. Safeguarding the privacy, confidentiality, and security of any public health informatics or e-health project is an important undertaking (O'Carroll, Yasnoff, Ward, Ripp, & Martin, 2002; see also Wallis & Rice, chap. 14, this volume). Our project does not collect the names on the database. The project works only with numbers. Each time that the health worker wants to make a report they have to enter a login, a password and the code number of the participant. If someone steals the cell phone, it could be easy to get access to the number that gets access to the system, but it is difficult to guess the login and the password and even more difficult to guess the code of the participants.

Team leaders (doctors) could receive the information immediately via the Internet, analyze the data, and use the system's communication and

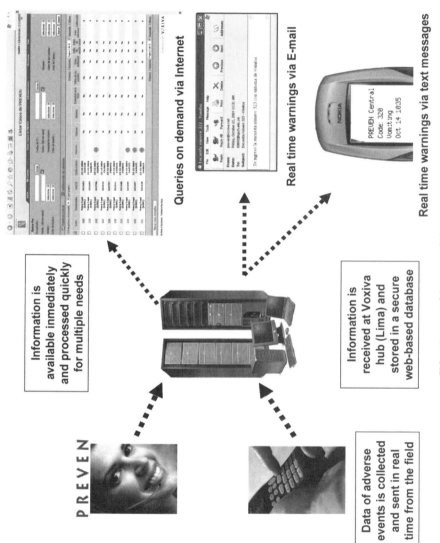

Queries on demand via Internet

Information is available inmediately and processed quickly for multiple needs

Real time warnings via E-mail

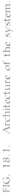

Real time warnings via text messages

Information is received at Voxiva hub (Lima) and stored in a secure web-based database

Data of adverse events is collected and sent in real time from the field

FIG. 18.1. Architecture of the system.

379

PREVEN	**Reporte de Eventos Adversos al Metronidazol**	Numero Telefónico: 01 317-5941 Nombre: Walter Curioso Código: 123456

PREVENCIÓN COMUNITARIA DE ENFERMEDADES DE TRANSMISIÓN SEXUAL

1. Acceso al Sistema	4. Detalle de Síntomas

Ingrese código de usuario, seguido marque #
Ingrese su clave secreta, seguido marque #
	Para cada síntoma marque 1 para SI ó 2 para NO:
	  Náuseas Cambio sabor comidas
	  Vómitos Dolor abdominal
	  Sequedad en Falto de apetito
	  la boca Dolor de cabeza

2. Registro de la Participante	**4.1 Si marcó SI responda:**
Ingrese código de la participante, seguido marque #	Cuando empezó? Ingrese el número de días, seguido marque # Cuando terminó? Ingrese el número de días, seguido marque # Tomó medicinas? Marque 1 (SI) ó 2 (NO) Afectó su rutina? Marque 1 (SI) ó 2 (NO) Volvería a tomar el medicamento? 1 (definitivamente si), 2 (no está segura), 3 (probablemente no), 4 (definitivamente no)
3. Alguna Molestia?	
Marque 1 para SI or 2 para NO SI marcó 1, después de la señal grabe el síntoma y los días de ocurrencia, seguido marque #	

FIG. 18.2. Example of the instruction card.

messaging tools to respond. Team leaders could monitor incoming reports through a Web interface (Fig. 18.3). Individual adverse event reports arrived in real time with full-case details. Authorized users could also listen to voice files recorded by the remote health workers. Data were available immediately and team leaders could export it to various programs for analysis and presentation.

Designated users received automatic notification of selected symptoms via e-mail and SMS messages. Health officials could communicate with remote health professionals using voice mails as well as e-mails. For example, Dr. Pablo Campos, one of the team leaders in Peru received e-mail messages and text messages on his cell phone. He accessed the database for the project at his work at University Cayetano Heredia. I was consulting on the project through e-mail, chat and telephone from Seattle before heading to Peru. In Seattle, I could access the database from my computer. The system was operational 24 hours a day, 7 days a week. Because data was entered directly, data errors were reduced.

During September through December 2004, the system collected 800 reports of adverse events. A formal evaluation is currently under development. For updates please refer to the Web site of the cell phone project: http://www.prevenperu.org

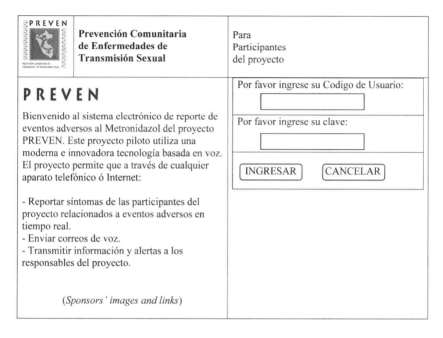

FIG. 18.3.   Basic text and elements of the Web page (https://www.preven .alertaperu.net/).

CONTEXTUAL BARRIERS AND OPPORTUNITIES IN DEVELOPING COUNTRIES

Socioeconomic and Technology Infrastructure Factors

There are many factors that limit the dissemination of e-health applications in developing countries. Technology distribution and access deficiencies are two factors (Rodrigues & Risk, 2003). For example, there is a huge variation in terms of access to computer-based information technologies, usually measured in terms of teleaccessibility, personal computer ownership, and Internet connectivity available to people (Rodrigues, 2003).

Other factors that contribute to the digital divide include insufficient telecommunications infrastructure, limited markets for information technologies (IT), high telecommunication tariffs, inappropriate or weak policies, organizational inefficiency and lack of locally created content. Inequalities in the utilization of information technologies by the general population are also found in developed countries determined by income and level of education. In the health sector, the divide between developed and developing countries in technology access is wider than the gap observed in social and commercial sectors (Rodrigues & Risk, 2003).

Poor telecommunications infrastructure, limited number of Internet service providers, lack of access to international bandwidth, limited wireless networks and affordable Internet access costs continue to be major impediments to the diffusion of Internet applications to the point-of-care in developing countries.

Good connectivity is needed for reliable transactions. In developing countries, fast connectivity is still limited and usually only dial-up access is available. As an example, a study by Harte Hanks in 2001 across different industries showed that only about one-third of the connected organizations in selected lower and upper middle income Latin American countries had access to connection speeds higher than 56 Kilobits per second (Table 18.1).

However, the reform of telecommunications in many sectors of developing countries has been bringing considerable improvements in services. As a result of greater competition, expanding markets, and rapid trade liberalization, telecommunications prices are dropping and the infrastructure has been improving worldwide. One-fourth or 22 of the 89 major public telephone operators that were privatized throughout the world by the end of 1999 were in Latin America and the Caribbean (Rodrigues & Risk, 2003).

New Technologies in Developing Countries

By 2002, telephones had reached more than 6,000 communities in Peru, with Internet access reaching 900 (Prahalad, 2005). A high demand for cell phones is occurring in many developing countries, a demand that was lag-

TABLE 18.1
Connectivity Speed in Selected Countries of Latin America

Countries	Organizations with Access > 56 kbps* (%)
Mexico	42
Peru	39
Chile	37
Regional average	35
Brazil	33
Argentina	31
Colombia	31
Venezuela	27
Ecuador	22

Note. *Kilobits per second. Source: Harte-Hanks CI Technology Database (Harte-Hanks Market Intelligence, 2001), cited by Rodrigues and Risk (2003).

ging behind with the installation of conventional land-based communications equipment. Approximately 50% of refurbished cell phones are sold in Latin America, Africa, Russia, India, China and Pakistan (Bhuie, Ogunseitan, Saphores, & Shapiro, 2004). In Peru, the market for cell phones has been increasing since 1993, with major growth from about 200,000 in 1996 to 2.5 million cell phones by mid-2003 (ONGEI, 2003).

In some countries, one user may access the Internet in numerous ways including wireless, Internet cafes, kiosks, home, work and/or school accounts. Other single accounts may be shared by many users. Some users are heavy and others light; some started long ago while others started recently. Internet cafes are popular access points in many developing countries, such as Peru. By the year 2003 more than 3,600 *"cabinas publicas"* or Internet cafes were operating in Peru, up from 417 in 1999 (Yachay, 2003). Recent estimates reported that, by February 2005, there were 10,000 *"cabinas publicas"* in Peru and at least 6,000 were in Lima (Villalobos, 2005).

In Peru, doctors have limited access to the Internet in their workplace. They access mainly from home and Internet cafes. Meanwhile, 54 countries and territories in Africa have Internet access—at least in the capital cities (Jensen, 2002)—and many acquired the connection in recent years, indicating the rapid pace of change. The dramatic falling costs of computers suitable for Internet use should go some way to closing the gap between rich and poor. This price drop and accessibility to computers brings a unique opportunity for health care research.

Lack of Proficiency in Using Computers, and the Internet

Several other factors have been identified as contributing to the digital divide in developing countries, chief among them a lack of proficiency in using computers (Chandrasekhar & Ghosh, 2001). Other factors that have contributed to the digital divide include a gap in the actual use, measured as the amount of time spent utilizing information technologies; and a gap in the impact of use, measured by financial, economic and clinical returns. In other words, equipment alone is useless unless people are able to use it effectively and informed of the potential benefits of its use (Samuel et al., 2004).

Inadequate education in informatics skills is a constraint among medical students, doctors, nurses and many other health care professionals who have different levels of computer competence. In our study (1999), 40% of the sample composed by medical students in Peru' reported lack of proficiency on the use of Internet. We also found that the proficiency on the use of the Internet was not related with the year of medical school nor with age (Horna, Curioso, Guillen, Torres, & Kawano, 2002).

Similarly, in 2003, Samuel et al. reported that only 52% of medical students in Tanzania felt that they understood the basic terminology and concepts of computing. Only 23% of their sample had ever consulted an electronic journal, and 70% did not use any electronic resource. The authors concluded that the sample had a low level of ability (very basic) to use information technology facilities (Samuel et al., 2004). In Nigeria, Ajuwon reported that only 42.6% of the sample studied could use a computer. Another study conducted in Nigeria reported that 79% of students had little or no computer skills (Ajuwon, 2003), and a study conducted in Nigeria reported that 79% of students had little or no computer skills (Odusanya & Bamgbala, 2002).

Absent or Costly Committed Human Resources

People are central for the success of any application of e-health products and services. Employees' skills are the most expensive and least elastic resource, and an obstacle to technological development in developing countries. Systems professionals, technology products, services providers, and project team must have superior skill levels and experience in the particularities of the area being automated (Curioso, Saldias, & Zambrano, 2002).

Managing IT personnel and projects in both developing and developed countries is a challenging undertaking (O'Carroll et al., 2002). Successful IT projects depend greatly on a project head's ability to identify and select the right people to work on the project, to communicate with technical people, to hire consultants appropriately, and to organize technical teams. Selecting the most appropriate technology is important when developing an e-health project, but also important are good managing skills. It is important to recognize that the latest technology does not necessarily solve all the problems (O'Carroll et al., 2002).

Lack of Vision of Public Health Authorities Regarding IT

In developing countries, most public health organizations have a very limited use of IT applications in day-to-day practice. Some public health authorities believe that using IT is limited to creating a chart of the epidemiological weekly report or to produce statistical reports. Collecting and presenting data in a chart is not necessarily of interest to health care professionals and managers when it comes to surveillance systems.

Most of the information systems in developing countries are inadequate to the current models of health care, and many public health authorities are not aware of the potential of IT to support public health. Moreover, the public health sector is behind business, banks and other sectors in terms of effectively using information technologies. There can be many reasons for resistance to chance in developing countries. These can be classified as resistance to a particular change or resistance to the changer, for example, the individual initiating the change. There are several strategies that can be used to address these factors. One strategy, the five-stage model, includes assessment, feedback and options, strategy development, implementation and reassessment (O'Carroll et al., 2002).

On the other hand, private providers and managed care groups have been recognizing that a different type of information system and data elements are required to run their organizations and to survive in a competitive environment driven by increasing consumer demands and expectations for the delivery of personalized evidence-based services (Curioso, Montori, & Curioso, 2004).

CAN INEXPENSIVE TECHNOLOGIES BE USED EFFECTIVELY IN PUBLIC HEALTH IN DEVELOPING COUNTRIES?

New technology offers much better ways to collect data; for example, it can be collected more easily over much shorter periods of time (McCoy, 2002). Although the use of computers or PDAs are limited in developing countries because of their expense and requirement for additional equipment such relatively complex network connections, cell phones are proving a simple solution. Cell phones are ubiquitous and cheaper than most computers and PDAs. Cell phones are showing how easy it is to collect data electronically in developing countries even in remote settings.

Currently, one of the simplest solutions to collect data is to call a telephone number that links to the investigator's computer via the Internet. In our project, subjects accessed the system, and provided data using the push buttons on the telephone. Data was automatically inserted into the subjects' data files. The Internet provided the team leaders the possibility to access to all reports made by the field workers so doctors can monitor what is going in the field on a daily or weekly basis. The team leaders could perform searches of participants, and hear the voice files that the health workers recorded. Use of such technology depends on various factors—cost and availability, the socioeconomic status and education level of the subjects, and/or the amount of money available for the research. However, the cost of new technology tends to decrease over time, and it offers much improved methods for collecting more accurate data while involving less time and inconvenience for subjects and researchers alike (McCoy, 2002).

APPLICATIONS OF THE SYSTEM
IN OTHER CONTEXTS

There are other applications of the system in both developing and developed countries. Alerta is a system that involves phone and the Internet for communications and disease surveillance in real-time in Peru. Health professionals, using available telephones and the Internet (whichever was available), submitted real-time, electronic reports of mandated diseases and disasters. Alerta required a substantially lower allocation of resources, lower operating costs, and resulted in a threefold increase in reporting coverage (Prahalad, 2005). Overall, the system required 40% lower costs of operations than the traditional paper system. The application was incorporated in health clinics and health centers of the Ministry of Health (Prahalad, 2005). The study also concluded that the use of voice mail for communication was 7.8 times less expensive than written communication.

Lescano et al. (2003) reported that the introduction of the application has led to early outbreak identification/response, timely case management, and increased review of clinical procedures within reporting units. The investment required by the system was small compared to alternative approaches to building disease surveillance capabilities, particularly in terms of infrastructure and maintenance expenses. The combination of scalable technology, accurate and close monitoring of performance, controlled growth, and effective mechanisms for information sharing, feedback and data-driven decision making has turned the application into a highly innovative, cost-effective, and replicable surveillance model (Lescano et al., 2003).

Applications Outside Peru

The U.S. Food and Drug Administration developed a Web-based system using Voxiva's platform for monitoring blood shortages in the United States. After discovering that 40 % of the nation's blood centers did not have ready access to the Internet, they used a system based on the use of the phone as well as the Internet to track blood shortages. The U.S. Department of Defense developed a disease surveillance system for Washington D.C., and San Diego County regarding a smallpox vaccination monitoring system (Voxiva, 2004).

In the developing world, similar systems have deployed health solutions in Latin America, Africa, Iraq, and India. For example, in Africa, they created a national HIV/AIDS information system for eight countries that among other things, monitors current data for national and global reporting requirement and manages the use of antiretrovirals to reduce the spread of viral resistance. In India, a surveillance system for Japanese encephalitis was created in a month (Prahalad, 2005).

OTHER TELEMEDICINE APPLICATIONS IN PERU

There is a great potential to improve health through the use of telecommunications and information technologies in developing countries. Installing more computers or connecting a computer to the Internet is not necessarily the answer to public health problems. One answer could be using cell phones, public phones or *"cabinas publicas"*.

Other telemedicine projects have been developed in Peru. One of the most relevant is The Enlace Hispano Americano de Salud (EHAS; Hispanic American Health Link) (Martinez, Villarroel, Seoane, & del Pozo, 2004). EHAS has developed a system that facilitates the exchange of information between health centers and health workers in a rural area. The EHAS system uses radio (VHF, HF and WiFi) for voice and data communication. Information exchange is by e-mail, and is focused on distance training, the exchange of epidemiological reports and patient transfer. The system was installed in the province of Alto Amazonas in Peru. EHAS demonstrated that: (1) voice and e-mail communication via VHF radio is technically and economically sustainable for rural telemedicine; (2) rural health workers, in many cases nursing technicians with no university education, are capable of learning to use computers for basic office tasks and e-mail, by attending training sessions of no more than 10 days' duration; (3) only through a scheme involving the active participation of all users can a sustainable service be achieved. Currently, EHAS is working in four Latin American countries as well as Spain (EHAS, 2002).

TeleMedMail (Fraser, Jazayeri, Bannach, Szolovits, & McGrath, 2001) is a software application to facilitate store-and-forward telemedicine by secure e-mail of images from digital cameras. TeleMedMail is written in Java and allows structured text entry, image processing, image and data compression, and data encryption. This web-based telemedicine system is currently under evaluation in South Africa and Peru and is available for free at http://www.sourceforge.net/projects/telemedmail/

Lastly, but not least, training in telemedicine is a key aspect. In Peru, for example, a collaboration between the University of Washington (UW) and the Universidad Peruana Cayetano Heredia, allows better training. The training includes a combination of short-term training for resource personnel in Peru, and bringing many of the information integration and organizational tools from ongoing information technology projects at the UW (Karras et al., 2001).

LESSONS LEARNED WITH CELL PREVEN
IN A DEVELOPING COUNTRY

1. Even in a challenging social setting with limited infrastructure it is possible to develop an effective surveillance system. It is not necessary to have the latest Palm Pilot or Tablet PC to create a sophisticated public health surveillance system (Chin, 2005). It is possible to deploy a health information system much more quickly and cost-effectively than systems that require a lot of logistics and expensive network requirements and devices.

2. The system described in this chapter is applicable to a range of health problems—from reporting and monitoring adverse events during clinical trials or vaccination campaigns to reporting disease outbreaks. We can even apply the system to nonhealth settings like reporting crime or potentially tracking commercial orders and distribution.

3. Systems implementers need a clear idea of the problem. Many technologies failed because of lack of careful planning and evaluation of the necessities. Factors to consider include: scan assessment of barriers, technology, training, cost and sustainability. Even in 20 years this example could be still used by health professionals for different purposes. This system addresses three key ingredients of an effective surveillance system: (a) Real-time data collection, from health workers reporting an adverse event or a doctor reporting a disease outbreak, for example; (b) Rapid analyses of data to make opportune decisions and allocation of resources; and (c) Communications back to the field to coordinate response.

4. Two-way information systems are more than just collecting data. They provide feedback and support to health care workers in the field. Many times, only managers have information that allows them to monitor and evaluate data but these systems do not prove any aggregate value to health care workers in the field. A well-designed information system has to support and enhance the performance of all user levels in a secure environment.

5. Information systems should be carefully planned and integrated across different programs. Prahalad (2005) has reported that health workers in some developing countries spend as much as 40% of their time filling out forms, compiling and copying data from different pro-

grams (e.g., tuberculosis, malaria, HIV/AIDS, etc.). By choosing the most appropriate information technology, we can avoid duplication and deploy different devices—i.e., cell phones, Internet—to report from each public health program.

6. Partnership is key to overcome technology barriers. We can attract top-tier industry partners if we have a comprehensive public health initiative. Public private partnerships can increase developing country access to improved health technologies.

7. Installing programs and PCs in public health organizations does not mean that we are creating an integrated system. It is necessary to have a robust, scalable, integrated information system that connects health care professionals from the local to the national level and provide them with the most appropriate information and support they each need. To accomplish this, it may be necessary to have a different technology architecture and different approach for each demand.

8. Any new technology will fail if there is not support for management change by leaders or chief information officers. Many public health authorities in developing countries are not accustomed to real-time information. They have to understand that helping decision-making and response with information technologies is critical to the success of their mission. This change requires considerable teamwork, leadership with solid strategic planning, training, and capacity-building efforts that go together with the deployment of a robust information system.

9. We need to understand the culture and to select the most appropriate technology for a determined necessity.

FUTURE DEVELOPMENTS

Telecommunications and information technology breakthroughs hold great potential if properly harnessed. We must understand the rich array of information-based technologies that support public health goals, and which communications technologies are the most appropriate for a specific cause (intervention, prevention, etc.). We must also understand who needs to know about these new public health solutions and how to educate and training them.

Telemedicine holds the promise of improving access to health care, especially in areas where there are geographical barriers, and of reducing costs (Wootton, 2001). Telehealth in developing countries is a reality and offers tremendous opportunities that need to be explored more in the future. One of the problems with telehealth is that telecommunications companies often try to force a technical "solution" in public health services without understanding the problems in the field. Some new technologies may become more important in the future, as wireless access improves (for example, Wireless Application Protocol -WAP- phones) (Hung & Zhang, 2001, 2003). Karras et al. reported that a Java-enabled wireless phone could be potentially used in disaster response and public health informatics. They emphasized that the technology was inherently deployable, portable and that minimal orientation to new hardware was needed since everyone was comfortable with entering numbers on a phone keypad and pushing the send button (Karras, Huq, Bliss, & Lober, 2002). Any application that can run on a PC can potentially run on a portable phone using Java applets.

In teleconsultation, cell phones has been proven that is feasible to capture and transmit images using e-mail for care of chronic wounds (Braun et al., 2005). However, the main problem in telemedicine is not the lack of technology; rather, it is the organizational problem of knowing how to take advantage of the technology. For example, how communities may benefit from the right information technology application. In some countries, cell phones may be a better application than using Tablets PCs, smart cards, or satellite communications (Wootton, 2001).

A Web-based electronic medical record system has shown that effective information management is also possible in a poor community with no modern infrastructure. In Peru, Fraser et al. (2004) described a web-based medical record system to support the management of multidrug resistant tuberculosis. Web-based analyses have been developed to track drug sensitivity test results, patterns of sputum smear and culture results and time to conversion from positive to negative cultures (Fraser, Jazayeri, Mitnick, Mukherjee, & Bayona, 2002). Jazayeri et al. (2003) described a prototype Electronic Medical Record system the "HIV-EMR" to support treatment of HIV and tuberculosis in remote and impoverished areas in Haiti. The EMR allows physicians to order medicines and laboratory tests, and provides alerts based on clinical status and test results (see also Wallis & Rice, chap. 14, this volume).

Recently, we developed a web-based electronic report system for STD for the PREVEN project. Interviewers entered their data directly into a single database as they progress through the reports, thereby saving time and costs over having the data entry done after data is collected. The system collects new participants and generates alert reports defined by the number of missed treatment that must be provided by the health care interviewers. The system has the capability of searching so the interviewers can check past laboratory results and medications. The system allows real-time access of the database (only available for the team leaders) via the web. We believed that web-based data collection may provide better access to difficult-to-reach populations and cities considering the great popularity and cheap cost of Internet cafes or *"cabinas publicas"* in Peru (Curioso, Campos, Buendia, Butron, & Kimball, 2005). The unique popularity and low-cost of Internet cafes in some countries open new possibilities to developing future web-based systems to show that effective information management can be possible in poor communities with no modern infrastructure but widespread use of *"cabinas publicas."*

REFERENCES

Ajuwon, G. A. (2003). Computer and internet use by first year clinical and nursing students in a Nigerian teaching hospital. *BioMed Central Informatics and Decision Making*, *3*(1), 10.

Bhuie, A. K., Ogunseitan, O. A., Saphores, J.-D. M., & Shapiro, A. A. (2004). Environmental and economic trade-offs in consumer electronic products recycling: A case study of cell phones and computers. *Electronics and the Environment, 2004. Conference Record* (pp. 74–79). Scottsdale, AZ, 10–13 May. Retrieved January 30, 2006, from http://ieeexplore.ieee.org/xpls/abs_all.jsp?isnumber=28876&arnumber=1299691&count=61&index=13

Braun, R. P., Vecchietti, J. L., Thomas, L., Prins, C., French, L. E., Gewirtzman, A. J., et al. (2005). Telemedical Wound Care Using a New Generation of Mobile Telephones: A Feasibility Study. *Archives of Dermatology*, *141*, 254–258.

Campos, P. E., Chiappe, M., Carcamo, C., Garcia, P., Buendia, C., Segura, P., et al. (2003, December 2–5). *STI Prevalence among Female Sex Workers from 24 Peruvian Cities*. Paper presented at the 8th World STI/AIDS Congress/40th IUSTI World General Assembly/XIV Panamerican STI/AIDS Congress, Punta del Este, Uruguay.

Chandrasekhar, C. P., & Ghosh, J. (2001). Information and communication technologies and health in low income countries: The potential and the constraints. *Bull World Health Organ*, *79*(9), 850–855.

Chin, T. (2005). *Cell phones help doctors collect data in new ways*. Retrieved January 30, 2006, from http://www.ama-assn.org/amednews/2005/02/21/bise0221.htm

Curioso, W. H., Campos, P. E., Buendia, C., Butron, R., & Kimball, A. M. (2005). *Design and implementation of a Web-based system to transmit STD reports in communities of Peru*. Retrieved January 30, 2006, from http://www.prevenperu.org/preven/std.htm

Curioso, W. H., Montori, V. M., & Curioso, W. I. (2004). Evidence based medicine for the gastroenterologist. *Revista de Gastroenterologia de Peru*, *24*(1), 75–91. Retrieved January 30, 2006, from http://www.waltercurioso.com/uw/ebm.pdf (In Spanish)

Curioso, W. H., Saldias, J. A., & Zambrano, R. (2002). Electronic medical records: A Peruvian experience in a National Hospital. Health care staff and patient's satisfaction. *Revista de la Sociedad Peruana de Medicina Interna.*, *15*(1), 22–29. Retrieved January 30, 2006, from http://www.waltercurioso.com/uw/emr.pdf

EHAS. (2002). *Information technology in rural areas of Latin America*. Retrieved January 30, 2006, from http://www.isf.uva.es/cursotsd/tsd4/Tecnologias_de_la_Informacion_y_Comunicacion_I.pdf

Fraser, H. S., Jazayeri, D., Bannach, L., Szolovits, P., & McGrath, S. J. (2001). TeleMedMail: Free software to facilitate telemedicine in developing countries. *Medinfo*, *10*(Pt 1), 815–819.

Fraser, H. S., Jazayeri, D., Mitnick, C. D., Mukherjee, J. S., & Bayona, J. (2002). Informatics tools to monitor progress and outcomes of patients with drug resistant tuberculosis in Peru. *Proceedings American Medical Informatics Symposium, 270–274.*

Fraser, H. S., Jazayeri, D., Nevil, P., Karacaoglu, Y., Farmer, P. E., Lyon, E., et al. (2004). An information system and medical record to support HIV treatment in rural Haiti. *British Medical Journal, 329*(7475), 1142–1146.

Fraser, H. S., & McGrath, S. J. (2000). Information technology and telemedicine in sub-saharan Africa. *BMJ, 321*(7259), 465–466.

Horna, P., Curioso, W., Guillen, C., Torres, C., & Kawano, J. (2002). Knowledge, abilities and characteristics of the Internet access in medical students of a Peruvian university. *Anuales de la Facultad de Medicina, 63*(1), 32–39. Retrieved January 30, 2006, from http://www.waltercurioso.com/uw/internet.pdf

Hung, K., & Zhang, Y. T. (2001). WAP-based telemedicine applications. *Australas Phys Eng Sci Med, 24*(4), 196–200.

Hung, K., & Zhang, Y. T. (2003). Implementation of a WAP-based telemedicine system for patient monitoring. *IEEE Trans Inf Technol Biomed, 7*(2), 101–107.

Jensen, M. (2002). *African Internet Connectivity.* Retrieved January 30, 2006, from http://www3.sn.apc.org/africa/

Karras, B. T., Huq, S. H., Bliss, D., & Lober, W. B. (2002). National Pharmaceutical Stockpile drill analysis using XML data collection on wireless Java phones. *Proceedings American Medical Informatics Symposium, 365–391.*

Karras, B. T., Kimball, A. M., Gonzales, V., Pautler, N. A., Alarcon, J., Garcia, P., & Fuller, S. (2001). Informatics for Peru in the new millennium. *Medinfo, 10*(Pt 2), 1033–1037.

Lescano, A., Ortiz, M., Elgegren, R., Gozzer, E., Saldarriaga, E., Soriano, I., Martos, I., Negrete, M., & Batsel, T. (2003, December). *Alerta DISAMAR: Innovative disease surveillance in Peru.* Paper presented at the American Society of Tropical Medicine and Hygiene, Philadelphia.

Martinez, A., Villarroel, V., Seoane, J., & del Pozo, F. (2004). A study of a rural telemedicine system in the Amazon region of Peru. *J Telemed Telecare, 10*(4), 219–225.

McCoy, N. L. (2002). Longitudinal study of menopause and sexuality. *Acta Obstet Gynecol Scand, 81*(7), 617–622.

O'Carroll, P. W., Yasnoff, W. A., Ward, E., Ripp, L., & Martin, E. (2002). *Public health informatics and information systems.* New York: Springer-Verlag.

Odusanya, O. O., & Bamgbala, O. A. (2002). Computing and information technology skills of final year medical and dental students at the College of Medicine University of Lagos. *Nigerian Postgraduate Medical Journal, 9*(4), 189–193.

ONGEI. (2003). *Peru: The use of information and communication technologies.* Retrieved January 30, 2006, from http://www.pcm.gob.pe/portal_ongei/publica/indicadores/Lib0365/Libro.pdf

Prahalad, C. (2005). The Voxiva Story. In *The Fortune at the Bottom of the Pyramid: Eradicating Poverty Through Profits* (pp. 361–379). New Jersey: Wharton School Publishing.

PREVEN. (2003). *Urban Community Randomized Trial of STD Prevention.* Retrieved January 30, 2006, from http://www.upch.edu.pe/faspa/preven/

Rodrigues, R. J. (2003, October 12–18). *Deploying e-Health Solutions in Latin America and the Caribbean: Development and Policy Issues.* Paper presented at the Proceedings of the International Telecommunications Union Telecom World, Forum PL11: Workshop on Telemedicine, Geneva, Switzerland.

Rodrigues, R. J., & Risk, A. (2003). eHealth in Latin America and the Caribbean. Development and policy issues. *Journal of Medical Internet Research, 5*(1), e4.

Samuel, M., Coombes, J. C., Miranda, J. J., Melvin, R., Young, E. J., & Azarmina, P. (2004). Assessing computer skills in Tanzanian medical students: An elective experience. *BioMed Central Public Health, 4*(1), 37.

Sanchez, J., Campos, P. E., Courtois, B., Gutierrez, L., Carrillo, C., Alarcon, J., et al. (2003). Prevention of sexually transmitted diseases (STDs) in female sex workers: Prospective evaluation of condom promotion and strengthened STD services. *Sexually Transmitted Diseases, 30*(4), 273–279.

Villalobos, H. (2005). Solo 22 distritos regulan el uso de filtros. *El Comercio Peru*. Retrieved January 30, 2006, from http://www.elcomercioperu.com.pe/EdicionImpresa/Html/2005-02-21/ImpTemaDia0263138.html

Voxiva. (2005). United States SAFEVAX. Adverse event reporting solution. Retrieved January 30, 2006, from http://www.voxiva.net/safevax.asp

Voxiva. (2005). *Voxiva News*. Retrieved February 24, 2005, from http://www.voxiva.net/news.asp

Wootton, R. (2001). Recent advances: Telemedicine. *British Medical Journal, 323*(7312), 557–560.

Yachay. (2003). *Internet cabinas ("Internet cafes")*. Retrieved January 30, 2006, from http://www.yachay.com.pe/especiales/cabinas/

Author Index

Subject Index

399

diabetes information on the web, 204
future research directions, 209–210
policy implications, 206–209
reliability, 203–204
sampling strategy, 202–203
structural and performance criteria,
197, 204–206
Web site quality, 204–206

R

Reimbursement issues, 77–78
Reinvention, 15, 282, 299, 303–308
Rise in use of Internet for health care,
reasons for, 83
Role model, 321, 325–327, 330

S

Salience, 85, 88, 95
Scalable health community system,
265–266, 386, 389
Scale economies, 69, 80
Security, 31, 33, 36–37, 44, 49, 76,
79–80, 197, 265, 283–287, 296,
298, 302, 348–349, 378
Search modes, 131, 138, 140, 143–144
Selective processing theories, 84, 86–87
Self-efficacy, 93, 94, 107–108, 111,
120–121, 297, 299, 306, 317–328
Self-help groups
eating disorders, 219–224
suicidal, 224–228
Self-monitoring, 15, 92, 357
Sensation seeking, 92
Singapore Internet users' health informa-
tion search, 107
Social influence, 317–323, 327
Social support, 142–143
Source credibility, 119–120
Stepwise model, 130, 304
Subjective norms, 15, 317
Supply chain management, 15, 75
Surveillant, 113

T

Technology acceptance model, 282
Tele-Homecare, 36–37
Telemedicine, 35–36
Theories and constructs, 15–16, *see also*
Users and gratifications approach
and motivations
Theory of channel complementarity,
89–90
Third-party Web site accreditation, 15,
197
Transaction cost theory, 39, 75–76, 273
Transtheoretical model, 95–96
Trends, 24, 25

U

Use of information sources, 113
Users and gratifications approach and
motivations, 109–111, *see also* Theories and constructs
Uses and gratifications perspective, 84–86

V

Verifier, 113
Virtual communities
Community Platform Engineering
Process (COPEP), 261–271
field studies, 256–259
mobile services, 273–275
online communities, 216
requirements and the development
process, 259–264
Virtual environments, 58

W

Weak ties, 15, 235
Web fluency, 298, 301, 306